Sexual Deviance

Sexual Deviance

Understanding and Managing Deviant Sexual Interests and Paraphilic Disorders

Edited by

Leam A. Craig
Forensic Psychology Practice Ltd, The Willows Clinic, Birmingham, UK
Centre for Applied Psychology, University of Birmingham, UK
School of Social Sciences, Birmingham City University, UK
School of Psychology, University of Lincoln, UK

Ross M. Bartels
School of Psychology, University of Lincoln, UK

WILEY Blackwell

This edition first published 2021
© 2021 John Wiley & Sons Ltd.

All rights reserved. No part of this publication may be reproduced, stored in a retrieval system, or transmitted, in any form or by any means, electronic, mechanical, photocopying, recording or otherwise, except as permitted by law. Advice on how to obtain permission to reuse material from this title is available at http://www.wiley.com/go/permissions.

The right of Leam A. Craig and Ross M. Bartels to be identified as the author(s) of the editorial material in this work has been asserted in accordance with law.

Registered Office(s)
John Wiley & Sons, Inc., 111 River Street, Hoboken, NJ 07030, USA
John Wiley & Sons Ltd, The Atrium, Southern Gate, Chichester, West Sussex, PO19 8SQ, UK

Editorial Office
The Atrium, Southern Gate, Chichester, West Sussex, PO19 8SQ, UK
For details of our global editorial offices, customer services, and more information about Wiley products visit us at www.wiley.com.

Wiley also publishes its books in a variety of electronic formats and by print-on-demand. Some content that appears in standard print versions of this book may not be available in other formats.

Limit of Liability/Disclaimer of Warranty
The contents of this work are intended to further general scientific research, understanding, and discussion only and are not intended and should not be relied upon as recommending or promoting scientific method, diagnosis, or treatment by physicians for any particular patient. In view of ongoing research, equipment modifications, changes in governmental regulations, and the constant flow of information relating to the use of medicines, equipment, and devices, the reader is urged to review and evaluate the information provided in the package insert or instructions for each medicine, equipment, or device for, among other things, any changes in the instructions or indication of usage and for added warnings and precautions. While the publisher and authors have used their best efforts in preparing this work, they make no representations or warranties with respect to the accuracy or completeness of the contents of this work and specifically disclaim all warranties, including without limitation any implied warranties of merchantability or fitness for a particular purpose. No warranty may be created or extended by sales representatives, written sales materials or promotional statements for this work. The fact that an organization, website, or product is referred to in this work as a citation and/or potential source of further information does not mean that the publisher and authors endorse the information or services the organization, website, or product may provide or recommendations it may make. This work is sold with the understanding that the publisher is not engaged in rendering professional services. The advice and strategies contained herein may not be suitable for your situation. You should consult with a specialist where appropriate. Further, readers should be aware that websites listed in this work may have changed or disappeared between when this work was written and when it is read. Neither the publisher nor authors shall be liable for any loss of profit or any other commercial damages, including but not limited to special, incidental, consequential, or other damages.

Library of Congress Cataloging-in-Publication Data
Names: Craig, Leam, editor. | Bartels, Ross M., editor. | John Wiley & Sons, Inc., publisher.
Title: Sexual deviance : understanding and managing deviant sexual interests and paraphilic disorders / edited by Leam A Craig, Ross M Bartels.
Description: Hoboken, NJ : Wiley-Blackwell, [2021] | Includes bibliographical references and index.
Identifiers: LCCN 2020047914 (print) | LCCN 2020047915 (ebook) | ISBN 9781119705833 (paperback) | ISBN 9781119706007 (pdf) | ISBN 9781119705987 (epub) | ISBN 9781119771401 (ebook)
Subjects: LCSH: Paraphilias. | Deviant behavior. | Psychosexual disorders.
Classification: LCC HQ71 .S3983 2021 (print) | LCC HQ71 (ebook) | DDC 616.85/83--dc23
LC record available at https://lccn.loc.gov/2020047914
LC ebook record available at https://lccn.loc.gov/2020047915

Cover image: © hauged/iStock/Getty Images
Cover design by Wiley

Set in 10/12, WarnockPro by Integra Software Service, Pondicherry, India.
Printed and bound by CPI Group (UK) Ltd, Croydon, CR0 4YY

C108437_050421

Contents

About the Editors

Leam A. Craig, PhD, C.Psychol, CSci, MAE, FBPsS, FAcSS, EuroPsy, is a Consultant Forensic and Clinical Psychologist and Partner at Forensic Psychology Practice Ltd. He is Professor, Visiting Chair of Forensic Psychology, University of Lincoln, UK, a Visiting Professor of Forensic Clinical Psychology at Birmingham City University, UK, and an Hon. Professor of Forensic Psychology at the Centre for Applied Psychology at the University of Birmingham, UK. He is a Chartered and dual Registered [Forensic and Clinical] Psychologist, a Chartered Scientist, holder of the European Certificate in Psychology and a Full Member of the Academy of Experts. He was awarded Fellowship of the British Psychological Society and the Academy of Social Sciences for distinguished contributions to psychology and the social sciences. He has previously worked in forensic psychiatric secure services, learning disability hospitals and consultancy to prison and probation services throughout England, Wales, and Northern Ireland, specializing in high-risk, complex cases. He was previously Consultant Lead to three community forensic psychiatric hospitals for people with personality disorders, learning disabilities and challenging behavior. He is currently a Clinical Lead to the National Probation Service on working with offenders with personality disorders. He acts as an expert witness to civil and criminal courts in the assessment of sexual and violent offenders and in matters of child protection. He has previously received instruction from the Salvation Army, Catholic and Church of England Dioceses, South African Police Service, the UK Government Legal Department (GLD) and currently receives instruction from the Criminal Case Review Commission (CCRC) and the United States Air Force European Area Defence Counsel. He has over 120 publications including 12 books. In 2013 he received the Senior Academic Award by the Division of Forensic Psychology for distinguished contributions to academic knowledge in forensic psychology and in 2018 received the Emerald Literati Award for a Highly Commended paper. In 2015 he co-authored a Ministry of Justice research funded report into the use of expert witnesses in family law and in 2016 he was appointed as Chair of the British Psychological Society, Expert Witness Advisory Group. His research interests include sexual and violent offenders, personality disordered offenders, forensic risk assessment and the use of psychologists as expert witnesses.

Ross M. Bartels, PhD, is Senior Lecturer in Forensic Psychology at the University of Lincoln in the UK. He also leads the "Forensic and Clinical Research Group" (FCRG) within the School of Psychology at the same university. Dr Bartels's research interests focus on understanding and investigating typical and atypical sexual interests, as well as the psychology of sexual thoughts and sexual fantasizing, within forensic and community populations. His research also includes examining offense-supportive cognition using self-report and indirect measures and exploring the public's perception/attitudes towards people who have offended or have an atypical sexual interest. Dr Bartels recently set up the Forensic Cognition Lab (FCL) whose aim is the study of the above topics. The FCL consists of current PhD students, research assistants, and collaborators. He also sits on the editorial board for the *Sexual Abuse* journal and conducts peer reviews for a number of forensic and sex-related journals. He has, himself, published numerous peer-reviewed journals and book chapters on his specialist areas, and regularly presents his work at national and international conferences.

About the Contributors

Ross M. Bartels, PhD, is Senior Lecturer in Forensic Psychology and the current group leader of the "Forensic and Clinical Research Group" (FCRG) in the School of Psychology at the University of Lincoln (UK). His research is primarily focused on understanding the psychological underpinnings, facilitators, and effects of sexual thoughts and sexual fantasizing. He also actively researches atypical sexual interests and offense-supportive cognition, within both forensic and community populations. Dr. Bartels has published numerous peer-reviewed papers and book chapters on these particular topics, and regularly presents his work at national and international conferences.

Anthony R. Beech, DPhil, CSci, FBPsS, CPsychol, has authored over 200 peer-reviewed articles, 50+ book chapters and 10 books in the area of forensic science/criminal justice. His particular areas of research interests are: risk assessment; the neurobiological bases of offending; reducing online exploitation of children; and increasing psychotherapeutic effectiveness of the treatment given to offenders. In 2009 he received the Significant Achievement Award from the Association for the Treatment of Sexual Abusers in Dallas, Texas, and the Senior Award from the Division of Forensic Psychology, British Psychological Society, for recognition of his work in this area.

Klaus M. Beier, MD, PhD, is Director at the Institute of Sexology and Sexual Medicine at the Charité–Universitätsmedizin Berlin and in charge of the undergraduate and postgraduate training in his field as well as the outpatient clinic dealing with the full range of sexual disorders and gender dysphoria. His main focus in research is the prevention of child sexual abuse (CSA). The goal is to encourage self-identified undetected pedophiles to seek professional help in order to avoid committing CSA or consuming child sexual abuse material (CSAM). In 2005 he initiated the "Prevention Project Dunkelfeld," which has now extended to 10 additional locations all over Germany (www.dont-offend.org), as well as a prevention approach to recruit juveniles with sexual interests towards children (www.just-dreaming-of-them.org), financed by the German insurance system for the next three years. In 2017 he started the internet-based self-management tool "Troubled Desire" for assessment and treatment of pedophilia to prevent CSA and the use of CSAM, currently available in English, French, German, Hindi, Marathi, Portuguese and Spanish (www.troubled-desire.com).

Peer Briken, MD, FECSM, is a full Professor for Sex Research, Sexual Medicine, and Forensic Psychiatry and Director of the institute of the same name at the University Medical Center Hamburg-Eppendorf. From 2010 to September 2016 he was the president of the German Society for Sexual Research (DGfS) and from 2012 to September 2016 vice-president of the International Association for the Treatment of Sexual Offenders (IATSO). He is editor of the

Zeitschrift für Sexualforschung and authored or co-authored more than 300 scientific papers. Since January 2016, Briken has been a member of the Independent Inquiry into Child Sexual Abuse in Germany.

Leam A. Craig, PhD, FBPsS, FAcSS, is a Consultant Forensic and Clinical Psychologist and Partner at Forensic Psychology Practice Ltd. He is a Professor, Visiting Chair of the School of Psychology at the University of Lincoln, UK, a Visiting Professor of Forensic Clinical Psychology at Birmingham City University, UK, and a Hon. Professor of Forensic Psychology at the Centre for Applied Psychology at the University of Birmingham, UK. He is a Fellow of the British Psychological Society and of the Academy of Social Sciences and a Full Member of the Academy of Experts. He has experience working in various forensic settings including prisons, probation and secure forensic psychiatric services throughout England and Wales and Northern Ireland. He is currently a Clinical Lead to the National Probation Service working on the Offenders with Personality Disorder Pathway. He has over 120 publications including 12 books. He is a series editor for the *What Works in Offender Rehabilitation* book series for Wiley-Blackwell. His research interests include sexual and violent offenders, personality disorder, forensic risk assessment and the use of psychologists as expert witnesses (see "About the Editors" section for more detail).

Elizabeth Deehan, MS, is currently a PhD student at the University of Lincoln (UK), having previously completed a BSc (Hons) in Psychology with Forensic Psychology, and an MSc in Forensic Psychology at the same institute. Her primary research interest is on paraphilias and sexual deviance, particularly somnophillia (a sexual interest in sleeping partners), which formed the focus of her MSc research and her current PhD research. Through conducting research on somnophilia, a complementary paraphilia was identified (a sexual interest in being asleep during sexual activity), which was designated "dormaphilia." Elizabeth's research on sleep-related paraphilias has been published in a leading journal and presented at major conferences, such as the Division of Forensic Psychology (DFP) and the International Association for the Treatment of Sexual Offenders (IATSO). Elizabeth also works as an Offending Behaviour Programme Facilitator for Her Majesty's Prison Service. Currently, she delivers RESOLVE and the Thinking Skills Programme in a Category B male prison.

Deirdre D'Orazio, PhD, is the CEO of Central Coast Clinical and Forensic Psychological Services. She provides psychotherapy services, forensic expert services, professional training, outcome evaluation, and program development. She also works as a psychologist consultant to the California Department of State Hospitals, to programs for forensically committed individuals with sexual offenses. She is a member of the California Sex Offender Management Board, the leadership board for the Association for the Treatment of Sexual Abusers, and the Sexual Offender Civil Commitment Network. Dr D'Orazio is a recipient of the Fay Honey Knopp award by the California Coalition on Sexual Offending for positive and sustained contributions to the field of sexual offending. Dr. D'Orazio has publications, professional training, and research projects in forensic risk assessment, paraphilic disorders, best practices in sexual offense specific treatment, program development and evaluation, and professional ethics and supervision. Dr. D'Orazio has provided evaluations, expert witness testimony, and direct treatment services for more than 1,000 individuals identified as perpetrators or victims of violent or sexual crimes over the past 25 years. She holds psychologist licenses in California, Minnesota, and North Dakota. She is a certified trainer for the Static99R, the Structured Risk Assessment—Forensic Version, the Violence Risk Scale Sexual Offense Version, and the Stable and Acute 2007.

Yolanda Fernandez, PhD, is a registered clinical psychologist and currently holds the position of Special Advisor to the Sexual Misconduct Response Centre at the Department of National Defence in Canada. Her previous position was Regional Manager Institutional Mental Health for the Ontario region of Correctional Services of Canada. She has extensive experience supervising multi-disciplinary teams of mental health professionals providing services to minimum, medium, and maximum-security federally incarcerated offenders in Canada. Earlier in her career Dr. Fernandez worked as the Clinical Director at Rockwood Psychological Services, providing a sex offender treatment program at a medium security federal penitentiary and supervising all intake assessments of sex offenders entering the Ontario region of CSC. Dr. Fernandez is a certified Master Trainer and member of the development team for the Dynamic Supervision Project providing training in Static-99/R, STABLE-2007 and ACUTE-2007. She was the lead author on the extensive revisions to the STABLE-2007 manual and the ACUTE-2007 manual and is the second author for the revised 2016 Static-99R manual. Dr. Fernandez has multiple presentations at international conferences and publications in peer-reviewed journals as well as a number of co-authored and co-edited books.

Charles A. Flinton, PhD, has been engaged in research, assessment, and treatment of child abuse since 1986. Since 1992, his work has focused on assessing and treating sexual offenders. His work includes consulting on the management of sexual offenders with various local and national organizations, including the Center on Sex Offender Management (CSOM), Generation 5, the National Organization of Women (NOW), and the California Sexual Offender Management Board (CASOMB). In 2004, he was appointed Co-Chair of the San Francisco Sex Offender Management Alliance (SFSOMA) by the San Francisco's Mayor's Office. In 2006, Dr. Flinton co-authored *Engaging Resistance*, a book that explores the manner in which sexual offenders resist change and how this resistance both mirrors and is facilitated by treatment providers, the criminal justice/child welfare systems, and society. In 2008, he founded the San Francisco Forensic Institute, a state of the art forensic psychological assessment center. In 2010, as chair of the Adult Standards Committee of the California Coalition on Sexual Offending, he was the primary author for the *Guidelines and Best Practices: Adult Male Sex Offender Treatment.* Most recently, he co-founded the Blue Rock Institute, an organization aimed to prevent sexual abuse through early intervention and education.

Alexandre Gauthier is a master's candidate in criminology at the University of Montreal, and a research assistant at the National Institute of Forensic Psychiatry Philippe-Pinel. He is currently conducting a study on sexual sadism, more specifically on its manifestations and origins.

Etienne Garant is a doctoral candidate in criminology at the University of Montreal and a research assistant at the National Institute of Forensic Psychiatry Philippe-Pinel. He is currently conducting research on child sex offenders and the maintenance of abstinence trajectories of adults who recognize sexual interest for children.

Leigh Harkins, PhD, is an Associate Professor at the University of Ontario Institute of Technology in Canada. Her current research interests focus on understanding sexual aggression and aggression in groups including factors influencing perceptions of the acceptability of sexually coercive behavior, technology and sexual violence, and multiple perpetrator sexual offending. Dr. Harkins's work has focused on understanding and improving assessment and treatment of sexual offenders. This combined work has highlighted the importance of accurate and evidence-based approaches to assessment and treatment. She also has practice experience working in treatment groups for sexual offenders, and completing psychological assessments in prisons and community criminal justice settings in Canada and the UK. Leigh has published numerous manuscripts in peer-reviewed journals and book chapters, and has co-edited a book in the area of forensic psychology and has presented her research at international conferences. Leigh has supervised Honour's thesis, MA, MSc, ForenPsyD and PhD students in forensic psychology.

Craig Harper, PhD, is a Senior Lecturer in Psychology at Nottingham Trent University. His research interests lie in the psychological processes that underpin decision making in relation to controversial social and political topics, with most of his research focused on how people form and express attitudes towards people with sexual convictions. He is a member of the Heterodox Academy, which seeks to promote viewpoint diversity and reduce political polarization in higher education.

Tamsin Higgs, DForenPsy, is an Assistant Professor in the Department of Psychology, University of Montreal, Canada, and is affiliated with the International Centre for Comparative Criminology and the research center of the National Institute of Forensic Psychiatry Philippe-Pinel. She is a Registered Forensic Practitioner Psychologist with the Health Professions Council, UK, and a member of the Québec Order of Psychologists, Canada. Her main research interests are in the trajectories that lead to violent and sexual offending, and risk evaluation and interventions for the perpetrators of this type of offense. She has published 12 peer reviewed articles and 5 book chapters on these subjects.

Roland Imhoff, PhD, is a Professor of Social and Legal Psychology at the University of Mainz in Germany. He considers himself to be a cognitively oriented social psychologist with an interest in the underpinnings and measurement of sexual interest.

Jonathan James, PhD, is an Assistant Professor at the Department of psychology at the Université du Québec à Trois-Rivières, Canada, and a researcher affiliated at the Behavioral Science Unit (French Gendarmerie). He is currently conducting research on the developmental and psychological processes involved in the commission of a sexual homicide.

Elizabeth L. Jeglic, PhD, is a Professor of Psychology at John Jay College of Criminal Justice in New York and co-director of the Sex Offender Research lab (SORL). Her research interests include sexual violence prevention and evidence-based public policy.

Christian Joyal, PhD, is a full Professor at the Psychology Department of the University of Quebec at Trois-Rivières (Canada) and co-director of the International Research Center of Comparative Criminology (University of Montreal). His research interests encompass forensic neuropsychology and forensic neuro-imaging, as well as paraphilic interests and sexual fantasies of sexual offenders and the general population.

Leah Kaylor, PhD, graduated from John Jay College of Criminal Justice with a master's degree in Forensic Mental Health Counseling. She earned her PhD in clinical psychology from Saint Louis University. She is currently completing a post-doctoral fellowship at the Forensic Evaluation Services in the South Carolina Department of Mental Health.

Raymond Knight, PhD, is Professor Emeritus of Human Relations at Brandeis University. He has been doing research on sexual aggression for more than four decades. He has developed and validated taxonomic models for rapists and child molesters and has completed a 25-year follow-up of sex offenders released from the Massachusetts Treatment Center. He is currently validating the Multidimensional Inventory of Development, Sex, and Aggression (the MIDSA), which is a computerized contingency-based inventory that provides a comprehensive assessment of multiple critical areas of adaptation for juvenile and adult sexual offenders. He has served as president of both the Society for Research in Psychopathology and the Association for the Treatment of Sexual Abusers. Recently, his work has been recognized with the Joseph Zubin Lifetime Achievement Award for Research in Psychopathology and the Theoharis Seghorn Award for Professional Achievement in Preventing Sexual Abuse.

Tillmann H. C. Kruger, MD, is a medical doctor and Associate Professor at the Department of Psychiatry, Social Psychiatry and Psychotherapy at the Hannover Medical School (MHH), where he received his MD degree in 1999. He works as a consultant and is Head of the Section Clinical Psychology and Sexual Medicine as well as Deputy Head of the Department of Psychiatry. He is a board-certified psychiatrist and psychotherapist as well as neurologist. Training locations include the Hannover Medical School and the University Clinics of Essen, both in Germany, and the University Hospital and Swiss Federal Institute of Technology in Zurich, Switzerland. He has published numerous of papers on the neurobiology of human and deviant sexual behavior and related neurobehavioral topics and has continuously been supported by national and international grants. Tillmann Kruger coordinates a research consortium dedicated to basic and clinical understanding of child sexual abuse and pedophilia (NeMUP) which is funded by the Federal Ministry of Research and Education (BMBF). In 2018 he was elected as an ordinary member of the Center for Systems Neuroscience, Hannover. At MHH he is medical head of two clinical prevention programs against child sexual offending ("Don't offend") and sexual violence towards women ("I CAN CHANGE"). Apart from this his clinical and scientific expertise includes clinical neuroscience of affective and personality disorders. Main topics are the modulation and treatment of mood states and affective/personality disorders by novel neuropsychiatric interventions such as treatment with botulinum toxin. Tillmann Kruger has been a Fellow of the European Committee of Sexual Medicine (FECSM) since 2012 and a EFS-ESSM certified Psycho-Sexologist (ECPS) (European Federation of Sexology, European Society of Sexual Medicine) since 2018. He has had a special authorization for consultation hours in sexual medicine and sex therapy from the Association of Statutory Health Insurance Physicians in Lower Saxony, Germany since 2012. In his consultation hours he meets people with all kind of sexual disorders and problems with a special emphasis on the interface of psychiatry, neurology and sexual medicine.

Rebecca Lievesley, PhD, is a Senior Lecturer in Psychology at Nottingham Trent University. She has conducted research within the criminal justice system since 2008, with projects including an investigation of reoffending and desistance in those serving short sentences, the evaluation of anti-libidinal medication for individuals convicted of a sexual offense, and help seeking prior to committing a sexual offense. She is also co-founder of the Safer Living Foundation charity.

Nicholas Longpré, PhD, is a Lecturer in the Department of Psychology at the University of Roehampton. He acts as Modules Convenor for the third year BSc in forensic psychology and for the MSc in forensic psychology. His research interests principally revolve around sexual and nonsexual violent offending. More specifically, his work focuses on the study of the latent structure and etiology of sexual sadism and sexually coercive behaviors, the Agonistic Continuum, the measurement of offense-supportive cognitions among sexual offenders, as well as the exchange and consumption of child pornography. He is currently studying the latent structure of sexual harassment and sexually coercive behaviors among college students and their correlates with personality disorders, hypersexuality, and emotion processing.

Patrick Lussier, PhD, is a Full Professor of Criminology at the School of Social Work and Criminology at Université Laval, in Quebec city, Canada. After completing a PhD in criminology at the University of Montreal, he completed postdoctoral studies at the Institute of Criminology at the University of Cambridge under the supervision of Prof. David P. Farrington. He was Professor at the School of Criminology at Simon Fraser University for eight years. Professor Lussier is currently a regular researcher at the International Center for Comparative Criminology (CICC). His field of expertise is at the intersection of criminology and criminal justice and includes, among other things, the etiology of antisocial and criminal behavior, sexual offending, risk assessment and management as well as quantitative research methods. He has published five books and about 150 publications, including scientific articles published in journals such as *Criminology, Criminal Justice and Behavior, Justice Quarterly, Journal of Interpersonal Violence, Psychology, Public Policy & Law, Sexual Abuse: A Journal of Research and Treatment.* Professor Lussier is the Editor-in-chief of the *Canadian Journal of Criminology and Criminal Justice* and a member of the editorial board of the *Journal of Criminal Justice.* He has also been a member of the American Society of Criminology for more than 15 years. In 2005, Professor Lussier received the Academic Gold Medal from the Governor General of Canada for the excellence of his doctoral dissertation on the origins and the development of sexual aggression.

Evan McCuish, PhD, received his PhD in Criminology in 2016. He is currently an Assistant Professor at Simon Fraser University, in Burnaby, Canada. He is the Principal Investigator of the Incarcerated Serious and Violent Young Offender Study, which is a longitudinal study on young offenders in Canada followed through adulthood. His research interests include criminal careers, desistance, developmental criminology, foster care, gang involvement, psychopathy, sexual offending, and violence. His work is published in *Psychological Assessment, Crime and Delinquency, Sexual Abuse, Justice Quarterly,* and *Journal of Quantitative Criminology.* He is on the editorial boards of the *Journal of Criminal Justice* and *Youth Violence and Juvenile Justice.* He is the recipient of the Simon Fraser University Dean's Convocation Medal for Academic Excellence, the American Psychology-Law Society Outstanding Dissertation Award, and the American Society of Criminology Division of Developmental and Life Course Criminology Early Career Award.

Lauren McIvor holds a bachelor's degree in behavioral psychology. She currently works as a behavioral technologist in Correctional Service Canada's Ontario region. She also provides risk assessments and treatment for sexual offenders, in the community. Some of her research interests include applications of behavioral and mindfulness techniques in sexual offender treatment as well as psychopathy in sexual offenders.

Michael H. Miner, PhD, LP, is Professor of Family Medicine and Community Health and Research Director for the Program in Human Sexuality at the University of Minnesota Medical School. He began his research in sexual aggression as the experimental psychologist for the Sex Offender Treatment and Evaluation Project at the California Department of Mental Health and has continued exploring causes of sexual perpetration in adolescent males since joining the faculty of the Program in Human Sexuality. Dr. Miner is past president of Association for the Treatment of Sexual Abusers and a founding vice-president of the International Association for the Treatment of Sexual Offenders.

Rosemary Munns, PsyD, is an Assistant Professor at the University of Minnesota Program in Human Sexuality. She has extensive clinical experience in compulsive sexual behavior, relationship and sex therapy, gender diverse clients, and sex offender treatment. Dr Munns's therapeutic work extends to partners and families of people who have compulsive sexual behavior issues or offenses. She is an AASECT (American Association of Sex Educators, Counselors, and Therapists) certified sex therapist as well as an AASECT certified sex therapist supervisor and serves on the AASECT committee for reviewing sex therapy certification applications. Dr. Munns is a member of ATSA (Association for the Treatment of Sex Abusers), MnATSA (Minnesota Chapter: Association for the Treatment of Sexual Abusers), as well as serving on the board of MnATSA. She is a member of the American Psychological Association and the Minnesota Psychological Association. Dr. Munns earned her PsyD at Minnesota School of Professional Psychology.

Mark Pettigrew, PhD, is an award winning researcher and criminologist. After completing his doctoral research on death row incarceration in the United States, Mark has published extensively on whole life imprisonment in England and Wales and the crimes, specifically aggravated forms of homicide, that give rise to the sentence. His current research interests include sexual paraphilias and adult homicide, homicide dynamics, and crime scene behaviors of sexually motivated killers.

Jean Proulx, PhD, is Professor and the Director of the School of Criminology at the University of Montreal, and a researcher at the International Centre for Comparative Criminology. Since 1987, he has also been active, both as a researcher and forensic psychologist, in treatment programs for sex offenders at the Philippe-Pinel Institute of Montreal, a maximum security psychiatric institution. His main research interests are the pathways in the offending process, personality profiles, and sexual preferences and recidivism risk factors in sexual murderers, rapists, paedophiles, and incest offenders. Over the last 35 years, he has published 10 books, and more than 150 book chapters and peer-reviewed articles in French and in English.

Ethel Quayle, PhD, is Professor of Forensic Clinical Psychology in the School of Health in Social Science at the University of Edinburgh and Director of COPINE. A clinical psychologist who has worked with both sex offenders and their victims for over 20 years, she has researched technology mediated crimes against children, collaborating internationally with government and non-government agencies in the context of research, policy and practice. Recent EU-funded research examined the function of coercive and non-coercive self-produced sexual images by adolescents and NSPCC-funded research on deterrence of possession of images. She plays an active role in a number of government and non-government organizations.

Alexander F. Schmidt, PhD, is a Senior Lecturer in Social and Legal Psychology at the University of Mainz in Germany. He is a licensed cognitive-behavioral therapist and does forensic expert assessments in court. His research interests focus on the indirect assessment of sexual interests as well as atypical/paraphilic interests and their link to sexual offending.

David Thornton, PhD, is a psychologist in private practice based in Wisconsin and holds a part time position as a professor in the Department of Clinical Psychology at the University of Bergen in Norway. He is licensed to practice as a psychologist in Wisconsin and Minnesota in the United States, and also in the United Kingdom. He was research director for Wisconsin's program for sexually violent persons for three years and previously was the treatment director for that program for over a decade. He has published on evidence-based standards for effective correctional programs and on the importance of therapist style. He has been involved in the development of static actuarial instruments to assess sexual recidivism risk, contributing to the development of such scales as Static-99, Static-2002, Static-99R, Static-2002R, and Risk Matrix 2000. He has been involved in the development of psychological risk assessment, creating the Structured Risk Assessment (SRA) framework. His research is currently focused on clinically useful ways of assessing protective factors. He has published three books, over 15 chapters in edited books, and over 80 papers in peer-reviewed scientific journals.

Daniel Turner, PhD, first achieved his master's degree in psychology at the University of Frankfurt, Germany. Afterwards he completed his medical studies at the University of Hamburg, where he also achieved his PhD degrees in psychology and medical studies. He has worked as a PhD student at the Institute for Sex Research, Sexual Medicine, and Forensic Psychiatry, at the University Medical Center Hamburg, Eppendorf and is now working as a post-doc researcher and medical resident at the Department of Psychiatry and Psychotherapy at the University Medical Center Mainz, Germany. His research interests are pharmacological offender treatment, neuropsychological assessment of sexual offenders, sexuality education within medical studies and sexual behavior in patients with psychiatric disorders.

Jayson Ware, PDD, is currently the Group Director, Offender Services & Programs, Corrective Services New South Wales, Australia. He has researched or worked with sexual offenders for the past 20 years and has authored over 40 journal articles or book chapters primarily relating to the treatment of sexual or violent offenders. He has particular research interests in offender denial, group work, enhancing treatment effectiveness, and therapeutic communities.

Jamie Walton, PhD, is a practitioner psychologist (forensic) registered with the Health and Care Professions Council (HCPC). Jamie is an Associate Fellow of the British Psychological Society (AFBPS). Jamie has worked in the Her Majesty's Prison Service (HMPPS) and the National Health Service in England for over 12 years. Jamie is current National Specialist Lead within the High Intensity programs team in HMPPS. He has co-authored a number of rehabilitative programs in HMPPS for people convicted of sexual offenses. His research interests include compassion interventions, the causes of pedophilia and child sexual offending, and the evaluation of rehabilitative programs for individuals convicted of sexual offenses.

Pamela M. Yates, PhD, R Psych, is a forensic psychologist, researcher, and Adjunct Professor at Saint Mary's University, and is a Fellow of the Association for the Treatment of Sexual Abusers (ATSA). Formerly with the Correctional Service of Canada, Dr. Yates has worked extensively and internationally in forensic settings as a clinician, researcher, program developer, trainer, and consultant. She has authored numerous books and publications related to risk assessment, correctional intervention, and evidence-based practice in rehabilitation with individuals in conflict with the law. She has written extensively on offender rehabilitation, risk assessment, treatment, treatment effectiveness, psychopathy, and sexual sadism, as well as the Self-Regulation and Good Lives Models of sexual offender intervention. Dr. Yates is the primary author of *Applying the Good Lives and Self-Regulation Models to Sex Offender Treatment: A Practical Guide for Clinicians*, and, *Building a Better Life: A Good Lives and Self-Regulation Workbook.*

Acknowledgments

We are grateful to the contributors of this volume for sharing their experience and expertise and who have worked tirelessly on this project alongside their hectic schedules.

We would like to thank all those at Wiley-Blackwell for their patience and guidance in bringing this project together.

Part I

Sexual Deviance and Paraphilic Disorders

1

An Overview of Sexual Deviance and Paraphilic Disorders

Leam A. Craig[1] *and Ross M. Bartels*[2]

[1] *Forensic Psychology Practice Ltd, The Willows Clinic, Sutton Coldfield, UK, Centre for Applied Psychology, University of Birmingham, UK School of Social Sciences, Birmingham City University, UK School of Psychology, University of Lincoln, UK*
[2] *School of Psychology, University of Lincoln, UK*

Introduction

Paraphilias (parəˈfɪlɪə from Greek *philos*, loving) are difficult to define, contentious as a basis for legal processes, and their classification is prone to criticism. In the purist sense of the word, *para*—going beside or beyond, amiss; *philia*—attachment, is typically defined as a condition characterized by abnormal sexual desires, typically involving extreme or dangerous activities (Collins English Dictionary, 2018). According to the *Diagnostic and Statistical Manual of Mental Disorders*, 5th ed. (DSM-5: APA, 2013), a sexual fantasy (SF) is paraphilic if it concerns activities outside the realm of "genital stimulation or preparatory fondling with phenotypically normal, physically mature, consenting human partners" (normophilic). Intensity of the paraphilic SF is also "greater than or equal to normophilic interests."

In the DSM-5, paraphilias are distinct from paraphilic disorders. A paraphilic disorder denotes a paraphilia that is accompanied by distress or impairment in functioning. This indicates that paraphilias are necessary but not sufficient for determining the presence of a paraphilic disorder. According to the DSM-5, a sexual interest is anomalous if its intensity is equal or superior to that of a "normophilic" sexual interest. Eight paraphilias are specifically listed in the DSM-5: pedophilia (prepubescent children), exhibitionism (exposing the genitals to an unsuspecting stranger), voyeurism (spying on unsuspecting strangers in normally private activities), sexual sadism (inflicting humiliation, bondage, or suffering), sexual masochism (experiencing humiliation, bondage, or suffering real or not, physical or not), frotteurism (touching/rubbing against an non-consenting person), fetishism (non-sexual object), and transvestism (cross- dressing). While each paraphilic disorder in this list has its own specific diagnostic criteria, there is an acknowledgment by the American Psychiatric Association (2013) that the list is not exhaustive.

Prevalence rates for paraphilias are difficult to obtain due to changes in criterion over time (Joyal, 2021, chap. 6 in this book) and between cultures (Bhugra et al., 2010). In a sample of 1,915 German men aged between 40 and 79, Ahlers et al. (2011) reported that 62.4% reported at least one paraphilia-associated sexual arousal pattern, and that this caused distress in only 1.7% of cases (Ahlers et al., 2011).

A general interest in paraphilia is not uncommon within non-offending populations. For example, Joyal and Carpenter (2017) found that nearly 50% of non-offending adults expressed an interest in at least one paraphilic category, with approximately one-third having experience with such a practice at least once. Makanjuola et al. (2008) found that between 22% and 44% of men and women admitted to at least one paraphilic interest, while Bártová et al. (2020) found that 31.3% of men and 13.6% of women reported at least one paraphilic interest. Paraphilic sexual fantasies are also common among college students (Leitenberg & Henning, 1995). For

Sexual Deviance: Understanding and Managing Deviant Sexual Interests and Paraphilic Disorders,
First Edition. Edited by Leam A. Craig and Ross M. Bartels.
© 2021 John Wiley & Sons, Ltd. Published 2021 by John Wiley & Sons, Ltd.

example, Williams et al. (2009) found that 95% of their male college sample reported at least one paraphilic or offense-related sexual fantasy. Within non-offending samples, an interest in voyeurism, fetishism, frotteurism, sadism and masochism are most common (Ahlers et al., 2011; Bártová et al., 2020; Joyal & Carpenter, 2017; Leitenberg & Henning, 1995; Williams et al., 2009).

Survey results from Långström and Seto (2006) sample of Swedish adults ($N = 2433$) revealed a lifetime prevalence of 3.1% for exhibitionistic behavior (4.1% for males and 2.1% for females), broadly consistent with the DSM-5's prevalence estimate of exhibitionistic disorder, which range between 2 and 4% in the general population (APA, 2013). Also, 8% of their Swedish sample admitted to being sexually aroused by spying on others having sex (Långström & Seto, 2006). While exhibitionistic and voyeuristic acts have been identified as sexually deviant behaviors for centuries, the research on these disorders is scarce. Kaylor and Jeglic (2021, chap. 11 in this book) note that exhibitionistic and voyeuristic behaviors frequently occur together, as well as with other mental health issues, such as depression, substance use, anxiety, hypersexuality, bipolar disorder, attention-deficit/hyperactivity disorder, and antisocial personality disorder. A number of theories have been posited to explain paraphilic interests, including Courtship Disorder Hypothesis, Psychoanalytic Theory, Evolutionary Theory, Behavioral and Social Learning Theory, as well as increased availability with developments in technology. Of these various theories, Kaylor and Jeglic note that the Courtship Disorder model is favored in the field as it explains the high comorbidity rates amongst sexual paraphilias, as well as the escalation toward more serious sexual offending behavior. This hypothesis posits that deviant sexual behavior follows the template of normal dating behaviors, such as visually selecting a partner (voyeuristic behavior), nonphysical interactions (exhibitionistic behavior), physical touching (toucherism/frottuerism), and intercourse (rape).

Fantasies involving masochistic or sadistic content are more atypical, in that they are reported to be experienced by fewer people, although not so infrequently that they may be called rare (16–19% and 9–22% respectively). In fact, the prevalence rates of men who self-identify as BDSM practitioners vary between 2.2% and 7.6% (De Neef et al., 2019). Most people with atypical sexual interests do not have a mental disorder, and thus a paraphilic disorder, where a mental disorder is defined by DSM-5 as:

> A mental disorder is a syndrome characterized by clinically significant disturbance in an individual's cognition, emotional regulation, or behaviour that reflects a dysfunction in the psychological, biological or developmental processes underlying mental functioning. Mental disorders are usually associated with significant distress or disability in social, occupational or other important activities. An expectable or culturally approved response to a common stressor or loss, such as the death of a loved one, is not a mental disorder, socially deviant behaviour (e.g., political, religious, or sexual) and conflicts that are primarily between the individual and society are not mental disorders unless the deviance or conflict results from a dysfunction in the individual as described above. (p. 20)

To be diagnosed with a paraphilic disorder, DSM-5 requires that people with these interests: feel personal distress about their interest, not merely distress resulting from society's disapproval; or have a sexual desire or behavior that involves another person's psychological distress, injury, or death, or a desire for sexual behaviors involving unwilling persons or persons unable to give legal consent. However, critics have argued that the current criteria for paraphilia are too inclusive, with the crucial difference being the intensity of a sexual fantasy, which must be greater or equal than that of "normophilia."

Miner and Munn (2021, chap. 17 in this book) highlight that compulsive sexual behavior (CSB) presents even more definitional problems. Indeed, it has been described as "sexual addiction" (Carnes, 1983), "compulsive sexual behavior" (Coleman, 1991), "paraphilia related disorder" (Kafka & Hennen, 1999), "hypersexual disorder" (Kafka, 2010), and "out of control sexual behavior" (Braun-Harvey & Vigorito, 2015). Common across these various descriptors is hypersexual behavior, which has been linked to sexual recidivism (Thornton, 2021, chap. 16 in this book).

If a person denies distress in the form of guilt, shame, or anxiety about their paraphilic impulses; are not impaired in important areas of their functioning due to this interest; and their urges are not acted upon, then they would not meet criteria for a paraphilic disorder (APA, 2013). Diagnostic systems in determining the presence of a paraphilic disorder are not without controversy and the DSM-5, in particular, has been criticized for lacking specificity. This includes an unclear definitional strategy for each paraphilia, whether paraphilias should be construed as categorical or dimensional, whether each paraphilia is properly subtyped, and whether the paraphilias are natural kinds or social constructions. These are but four of the 25 critical points regarding the DSM-5 diagnostic criteria (O'Donohue, 2016). This is demonstrated in a study by Joyal (2015). Using a general community sample ($N = 1{,}501$), Joyal (2015) found that the most intense "normophilic" sexual fantasy (receiving oral sex) is statistically more intense, on average, than the most intense "paraphilic" sexual fantasy. However, in four participant subgroups (combined $n = 851$), the most intense paraphilic sexual fantasy was statistically as intense as the most intense "normophilic" sexual fantasy. In other words, 57% of the study sample had met the DSM-5 definition of paraphilia (*not* paraphilic disorder). Joyal (2021, chap. 6 in this book) discusses the problems with psychiatric diagnoses of paraphilia in more depth, offering a number of possible solutions, including a more global diagnostic term (e.g., "sexual interest disorder" or a harmful dysfunction definition) and the need to consider different dimensions when diagnosing paraphilias.

Like Joyal (2020), D'Orazio and Flinton (2021, chap. 7 in this book) also highlight the diagnostic limitations of a categorical system when considering the diagnosis of paraphilic disorder and argue that salient aspects of sexual preferences are more accurately understood as occurring on continuums rather than as discrete categorical entities. This means there is a progression in values from one end to the other, and that adjacent points on the continuum are very similar whereas distant points are distinct. They argue that an agonistic continuum model acknowledges that what is commonly referred to as sexual sadism occurs along a continuum much like any other disorder. Sexual scripts and other diagnostic indicators, such as information from self-reports, collateral interviews, information from psychological tests or tools, police reports, crime scene reports/photographs, prison and community supervision records, victim statements, medical reports, previous psychological evaluations, and school records will be useful in the assessment of sexual sadism. D'Orazio and Flinton provide a detailed explanation as to how paraphilic disorder diagnoses can be improved based on a continuum approach. They suggest it is important that differential diagnosis is considered when assessing for agonistic disorders and that diagnoses can be tendered for any preference point on the agonistic continuum but must meet the general criteria for paraphilic disorder, i.e., intense, persistent, atypical sexual interest plus clinically significant negative consequences.

Theory of Sexual Deviance and Paraphilias

To fully understand the development of sexual deviance, and the role of deviant sexual interest, it is crucial to examine how sexual offending behavior unfolds over time, in terms of its onset, frequency, persistence, and desistance. By charting a fascinating overview of the history of sex offending research from the end of the 19th century to the early part of the 21st century, Lussier et al. (2021, chap. 2 in this book) highlight the developmental insights that have been gained along the way, as well as the methodological issues that have prevented the formation of reliable causal conclusions. To address these limitations, Lussier et al. (2021, chap. 2 in this book) discuss the benefits of adopting a developmentalist approach to studying sexual deviance, demonstrating how it can provide a clearer insight into how sexual offending behavior develops and fluctuates over one's life course. As Lussier et al. (2021) argue, the understanding, assessment, and management of sexual deviance can be greatly advanced by examining developmental pathways using a life course or developmentalist perspective.

Numerous multifactorial theories of sexual offending behavior have been put forward over the decades (e.g., Finkelhor, 1984; Marshall & Barbaree, 1990; Seto, 2019; Ward & Beech, 2006). Each of these theories regards deviant sexual interest as a core explanatory factor. In spite of this, however, there are comparatively fewer theories aimed at explaining deviant sexual interest, the most well-known being the learning-based theories of McGuire et al. (1964) and Laws and Marshall (1990). Although these theories were seminal and informed the development of several reconditioning treatment strategies, much more has been learned about human sexuality through empirical study since these earlier theories were proposed (see Lehmiller, 2017; Toates, 2014). In spite of this, no recent theories of deviant sexual interest have been developed. In fact, as Schmidt and Imhoff (2021, chap. 3 in this book) note, a general theory of how sexual interest develops is lacking within the literature. Schmidt and Imhoff (2021) argue that filling this theoretical gap should be a priority as it provides a more scientifically parsimonious approach to explaining deviant interests, as well as sexual offending behavior. As such, Schmidt and Imhoff (2021) offer a theoretical approach for understanding chronophilic interests in heterosexual males, one that provides testable hypotheses, which they demonstrate by presenting some preliminary data.

One variable that has remained key to understanding deviant sexual interest is "sexual fantasy." However, the theoretical landscape on sexual fantasy is sparse, primarily based on a behaviorist perspective, and confined to the development of fantasy content (McGuire et al., 1964; Stockwell & Moran, 2014). Thus, the cognitive processes that underpin the *cognitive act* of sexual fantasizing have been largely ignored. To address this, Bartels et al. (2014) developed the Dual-Process Theory of Sexual Thinking (DPM-ST), aimed at explaining the psychological processes that underpin fleeting sexual thoughts and the act of prolonged sexual fantasizing operate. Thus, the DPM-ST offers new perspectives on sexual fantasy that contribute greatly to our understanding of deviant sexual interest and behavior. In chapter 4 of this book Bartels et al. (2021) provide an in-depth overview of the DPM-ST, along with suggestions for practice and research.

Another route to understanding deviant sexual interest and behavior is to examine the neurobiological factors and processes at play. While still in its infancy, there has been a notable increase in neurobiological research. In chapter 5 of this book, Kruger and Kneer provide a discussion of this literature. Specifically, they bring together and review research on the differences in brain structure, brain activation, endocrinology, and epigenetics, particularly in relation to pedophilia and sadism (and their respective offense-related manifestations). This research is beginning to reveal the neural structures involved in the processing of sexual preferences, and why some people might be directed toward paraphilic stimuli. Also, recent studies suggest that the differences in brain structure and function may be more related to the sexual act (e.g., child sexual abuse) than the sexual preference. Thus, the neurobiological research is beginning to provide crucial insights that contribute to our understanding of sexual deviance.

Sexual Deviance and Paraphilic Disorder

While some paraphilias are commonplace within the general population, they become pathological (a paraphilic disorder) when they are illegal if acted upon or associated with clinically significant distress or impairment in social, occupational, or other areas of functioning (APA, 2013). Within structured risk assessment frameworks, sexual deviance is defined as a stable pattern of deviant sexual arousal. Related terms and concepts include psychosexual disorder, deviant sexual preference, paraphilia, and perversion. Specifically, "a sexual interest, preference arousal or behavior that involves a focus on inappropriate persons or objects (i.e., those falling outside of the realm of what is considered legal or conventional in consenting adult sexual relationships) ... manifest by fantasies, urges, or repeated acts of a sexually deviant nature" (Hart et al., 2003, p. 63).

While many consenting paraphilias do not appear to be associated with mental disorders, one exception is child sexual abuse, with or without pedophilia. For the diagnosis of a pedophilic disorder, it is required that (a) the patient exhibits recurrent, intense, sexually arousing fantasies or *behaviors* involving sex with prepubescent children, and (b) he has *acted* on these urges or is at least markedly distressed and/or experiences interpersonal difficulties as a consequence of these urges or fantasies. DSM-5 further discriminates between an "exclusive type" and a "non-exclusive type" of pedophilia, and whether the individual is attracted to males, females, or both, as well as whether the behavior or the fantasies/urges are limited to incest or not. According to Seto's chronophilia (2016), a sexual orientation is something that has an early age of onset, is resistant to attempts to change it, and contributes to a congruence between the targets of sexual and romantic attractions, with pedophilia in particular meeting these criteria.

Sexual interest in children (usually defined as aged 12 years or less), or sometimes referred to as "minor attraction" (Lievesley & Harper, 2021, chap. 8 in this book), is rare among adults recruited in non-forensic/non-clinical populations, with an estimated prevalence rate within the general (male) population being less than 10% (Ahlers et al., 2011; Dawson et al., 2016; Dombert et al., 2016; Joyal & Carpenter, 2017; Santtila et al., 2015) or between <.1–5% (Dombert et al., 2016; Seto, 2008). Indeed, in a non-offending sample, sexual fantasies of having sex with a child under the age of 12 (0.8% of women and 1.8 of men, not significantly different) were found to be statistically rare (Joyal, 2014). As Lievesley and Harper (2021, chap. 8 in this book) note, there are substantial issues with some of the criteria used to diagnose pedophilic disorder (Schmidt et al., 2013). Having not acted on pedophilic impulses or urges, or having no feelings of guilt, shame, or anxiety or not being limited by such impulses of fantasies, however, would not justify a diagnosis of pedophilic disorder but rather a pedophilic sexual orientation. Lievesley and Harper argue, in line with the DSM-5 criteria, that being attracted to minors is not problematic in and of itself, but rather becomes so when there is harm or distress being caused to oneself or others. They suggest a humanistic approach when presenting information about pedophilia to persons attracted to children and advocate a health- and wellbeing-based approach to the management of minor attraction, with sexual abuse prevention being a secondary aim within this paradigm.

Generally, paedophilia is diagnosed at a prevalence of 30–70% in samples of men who have sexually abused children (Eher, 2017), although there is some evidence that DSM-diagnosed pedophiles and non-pedophiles differ on fewer variables than expected (Kingston et al., 2007), with the most relevant differences being observed when groups were divided by phallometric results. Blanchard et al. (2001) investigated the prevalence rate of pedophilia using phallometric procedures and found a lower base rate of DSM-diagnosed pedophiles of about

50% (n = 85 pedophiles versus n = 79 non-pedophiles) in their sample. A positive pedophile assault index would not necessarily indicate the existence of an absolute pedophilic preference, since it measures the relative arousal to assault in children and, therefore, might be more specific to a sexual preference for violence than to a sexual preference specific for children (Eher, 2017).

Although phallometry can be seen as an established and well-validated indirect measure of deviant interests, it is expensive, generally unavailable, and "labour intensive as a method in everyday routine practice" (Schmidt et al., 2013, p. 110). Yates (2021, chap. 10 in this book) explores several methods of assessing deviant sexual interests in men, including self-report measures, indirect measures, viewing time measures, and phallometric measures. Yates highlights that low reliability has been, and remains, an ongoing concern with phallometric assessment with marked variations in sensitivity of phallometric assessment in relation to PPG assessments with men who have offended against children and assessments of men who have sexually assaulted adults. As Yates highlights, measurement of sexual interests is complicated by a number of factors, not the least of which being that there are different approaches to sexual offending and hypotheses about how information is processed. For example, diagnostic measures rely on self-report with arbitrarily defined criteria that focus on an individual's behavior, while indirect measures rely on attentional factors and response times, thereby highlighting the role of sexual interest. Further, phallometric assessment and viewing time measures rely on physiological sexual arousal. Sexual interests, preferences, and arousal are complex processes involving emotions, cognition, personal history, context, and a multitude of other factors. As such, it is not surprising that, within research, there is variability across different measures.

Perhaps more unusual as a paraphilic interest is the sexual attraction to corpses (necrophilia) and the sexual attraction to those who are sleeping or unconscious (somnophilia), both of which have long been under-researched sexual paraphilias. DSM-5 lists necrophilia as a Paraphilia Not Otherwise Specified (PNOS), and as Pettigrew and Deehan (2021, chap. 9 in this book) observe, although those with true/genuine necrophilia have a primary and persistent attraction to corpses, it is probable that the majority will never actually sexually abuse a corpse but instead confine their necrophilic interest to private sexual fantasies and perhaps, for some, the use of "pornographic" material. True prevalence rates are largely unknown and there is currently no prevailing aetiological theory of necrophilia. However, as Pettigrew and Deehan note, common across the few theoretical accounts is that the person with necrophilia has complete dominion over the corpse, the corpse cannot resist or reject them, the corpse cannot argue, retaliate, or defend themselves, and the corpse cannot demand anything of the person with necrophilia. Pettigrew and Deehan suggest there is a unifying attraction to passivity and the control/dominion over the body of another person, not dissimilar to that of another under-researched paraphilia: somnophilia. Sometimes referred to as Sleeping Beauty Syndrome, this paraphilia is an interest in fondling or having sex with a sleeping or unconscious person and has been linked to the act of rape (Deehan & Bartels, 2019; Pettigrew, 2019). However, there is some definitional confusion as to the awareness or participation of the target person. Fantasies of sexually abusing a person who is drunk, asleep, or unconscious are statistically rare in women and more common in men (Joyal et al., 2015). Pettigrew and Deehan note that somnophilia and necrophilia may fall along a spectrum of passivity paraphilias both being confined to the permanence of the passive state with overlapping motivations including: dominion and passivity; power and defencelessness; and the elimination, in degrees, of the possibility of rejection.

There is much work still to do in understanding the aetiology of such paraphilias, which can be particularly difficult with regards to individuals convicted of sexual offenses, as disclosing specific paraphilic interests may increase their risk and prevent progression through their sentence. This is particularly concerning as men with these interests will require paraphilia-specific work in order to reduce the risk that they pose to the public, as well as future partners.

Sexual Deviance and Offending Behavior

It is not uncommon for persons with convictions for sexual offense (PCSOs) to have multiple paraphilias (Abel et al., 1988), with 43% of PCSOs having diagnosed paraphilic disorders (Eher et al., 2019). However, as Kaylor and Jeglic (2021, chap. 11 in this book) note, studies on recidivism and escalation from paraphilic "nuisance" behaviors (exhibitionistic and voyeuristic) to more serious sexual offending is scarce. While there is some evidence that points to increased likelihood for escalation (e.g., exhibitionistic behavior toward children, rape fantasies that accompany voyeuristic behavior), the determining factor in escalating to contact offenses is unclear. Exhibitionism, as an example of an atypical sexual outlet, has previously been related to rape offenses (Paitich et al., 1977). Gebhard et al. (1965) suggested that one in 10 exhibitionists have seriously thought about or attempted rape.

Arguably, many adult PCSOs begin their offending as adolescents (Zolondek et al., 1996). The self-report of juvenile PCSOs suggests the sexual abuse of children is the highest frequency offense (Davis & Leitenberg, 1987). Compared with adult males, juveniles had greater frequencies of fetishism, obscene phone calls, child sexual abuse, and phone sex. They report the age of first offense to be around 13 to 14 years, with the modal age of offending at 14 to 15 years. Victims are more likely to be younger female siblings or acquaintances. Most are verbally coercive (bribes or threat of force), not aggressive or violent. As with other groups of PCSOs, there is great variation in victim characteristics, degree of force, chronicity, variety of sexual outlets (paraphilias), arousal, motivation and intent (Weinrott, 1996). Although this suggests the processes contributing to sexual offending may remain constant during the stages of the life-span, the relationship between factors, and their strengths of influence, may be susceptible to change.

It appears that young men may be generally more inclined to perform sexually aggressive behaviors (e.g., rape), while older men may generally be more inclined to perform sexually seductive behaviors (e.g., child sexual abuse offenses). Younger (<24 years old) PCSOs are significantly more likely to attack stranger victims, be single, and use non-sexual violence during the index offense compared with older PCSOs (Craig, 2011). As Prentky and Lee (2007) argued, rape is fundamentally predatory anti-social behavior that is more likely to occur within five years of release. However, those who offend against children display persistent patterns of sexual deviance over longer time frames over the passage of time. Dickey et al. (2002) found that age over 40 may mitigate incidence of recidivism in rapists but not in pedophiles or sexual sadists. These differences may indicate that male sexuality, activities, and targets (interests and fantasies) may vary across the life-span from early adolescent exploration, discovery, and experimentation, through consolidation and practice within the partnership of relationships. It may be reasonable to assume that satiation and habit dull the sexual experience (perhaps sexual fantasy has a positive function in prolonging sexual interest by exploring variations either within fantasy or in activity). Indeed, the idea of change in sexual behaviors is consistent with sex offender treatment programs, which are predicated on the assumption that cognitive aspects of male sexual behavior are susceptible to change. Men who age past 60 after their last sex offense may pose different risk characteristics from those who last offended when aged 60+.

More extreme, atypical interests, such as sexual sadism and BDSM, have a long history dating back to the writings of Richard Von Krafft-Ebing (1886), who adopted the term from the name of the infamous Marquis de Sade (Donatien Alphonse François de Sade), who lived in France from 1740 to 1814. Prevalence rates of men who self-identify as BDSM practitioners varies between 2.2% and 7.6% (De Neef et al., 2019), with sexually sadistic activities including body torture (46.8%) and humiliation (34.6%). Key features of sexual sadism represented in DSM-5 involves the infliction of physical and psychological suffering, distinguishing sexual sadists from those who engage in more benign acts by requiring the victim of the sexual sadist to be non-consenting.

Sexual sadism has been described as "an elusive concept to define and measure" (Yates et al., 2008, p. 13) with different variations of assessment reported in different studies most likely due to an absence of agreed conceptual and methodological frameworks to guide the study of sadism (Healey et al., 2012), leading some to argue there are no valid and reliable measures of sexual sadism to assist researchers and clinicians (Proulx & Beauregard, 2009). Marshall et al. (2017) provided a detailed discussion on the various assessment methods, including phallometry, diagnostic criteria, crime scene data, and the use of rating scales. They concluded that the DSM diagnosis relies too heavily on insufficiently precise criteria and the accuracy (or otherwise) of clinical inference, especially since phallometric diagnostic tests have not yet proved to be satisfactory. This is primarily because the stimuli employed in almost all studies bear, at best, a tangential relationship with the purported features of sadists. Although not without limitations, clinician rated scales show the most promising results.

Higgs et al. (2021, chap. 12 in this book) discuss the psychopathology of BDSM practitioners who, for the most part, do not necessarily display psychopathology. When considering sadistic sexual aggressors, like Marshall et al. (2017), Higgs et al. comment on the difficulties associated with the reliable identification of sexual sadism and observe that not all perpetrators of sexualized murders meet DSM or ICD diagnostic criteria for sexual sadism, nor do they necessarily score highly on clinician-rated scales. For example, sexual sadism is typically found in one-third of all sexual murderers and even smaller numbers among sexual murderers of children. Higgs et al. consider the aetiology of sadistic sexual aggression and observe that psychological and sexual abuse—but not physical abuse—during childhood contributes to both juvenile externalizing behaviors (e.g., fighting, juvenile delinquency) and hypersexuality (e.g., sexual compulsion, sexual preoccupation, and sexual drive). Sadistic sexual aggressors more often present with schizoid and avoidant personality disorders, a range of paraphilias (i.e., exhibitionism, voyeurism and frotteurism; Longpré et al., 2018), and substance abuse issues, particularly alcohol consumption, which serves as a disinhibitor and favours aggressive behavior. Higgs et al. report that the psychosocial profile of sadistic sexual aggressors and male BDSM dominants differ in several ways, with BDSM dominants being generally well-adapted socially, report being sexually fulfilled, and present personality strengths and positive adaptative traits. Conversely, sadistic sexual aggressors are sexually and socially unfulfilled, and present with a diversity of personality disorders, notably schizoid, avoidant, antisocial, and narcissistic.

Continuing these observations, Knight and Longprè (2021, chap. 13 in this book) suggest that sadism comprises aspects of both control/coercion arousal and brutality, indicating two organizational models: one for arousal to coercion and one for arousal to pain. They suggest that the two should be parsed into two distinct paraphilias and propose a separate mental disorder diagnosis for paraphilic coercive disorder (PCD) that is distinct from sadism. Knight and Longprè (2021) further discuss how the two constructs are distributed along a single continuum called the Agonistic Continuum, which varies from no coercive fantasies, through fantasies of forcing sexual compliance, to fantasies and behaviors of hurting, humiliating, and torturing during sex. Based on data obtained from a validated sadism scale, a factor analysis revealed a three-factor solution—General Paraphilia, Pedophilia, and Agonistic Continuum—where paraphilic coercion loaded substantially and solely on the Agonistic Continuum factor, and Sexual Preoccupation loaded only on the General Paraphilia scale. This suggests that high sexual drive may be important in both their cohesion and aetiology.

Few studies have specifically examined the causal relations or the developmental factors that contribute to an aetiological model, and as such, aetiological models for sexual sadism have remained elusive. More recent explanatory models have revealed that sexual sadism appears to be a progressive disorder that begins with abusive experiences in childhood, has negative consequences for adaptation in adolescence, is mediated by cross-temporally stable traits, and eventually manifests as sadistic behaviors in adulthood (Knight & Longpré, 2020). Sadism arises from a series of aversive events during childhood where associative links between states of sexual arousal and feelings of aggression that arise from abuse are hypothesized to sow the seeds of subsequent sadistic fantasy. These states are mediated and emerge during adolescence in the form of externalizing behavioral problems, where early sexualization may antecede both involvement in violent sexual fantasies and a proclivity to view violent pornography, covarying in turn with sexual sadism. In adulthood, Knight and Longpre note that sadistic offenders are also marked with multiple adaptation difficulties, general antisocial lifestyles with criminal peers, a distorted sense of entitlement, and emotional dysregulation problems, which have also been associated with both psychopathy and sexually coercive behavior in general. Although the nomological network of the Agonistic Continuum is still in its early stages, the proposition of reconceptualizing sadism as a continuum from no coercive fantasies at the low end, moving through coercive/control fantasies and behaviors, to sadistic fantasies and torture at the higher end, is a developing area of research.

While deviant sexual interest and sexual arousal have consistently been reported as one of the strongest risk factors for sexual recidivism in men who have sexually abused children (Hanson & Bussiére, 1998; Hanson & Morton-Bourgon, 2005; Helmus et al., 2015; Mann et al., 2010; Seto, 2019), as noted above, accurate assessments of sexual interests are hard to come by. Schmidt et al. (2013) found that fewer than half of all individuals convicted of child abuse actually have a predominant sexual preference for children, raising questions as to the link between minor attraction and sexual offending. More complicated still is the advent of technology where it is often difficult to separate online sexual deviance and pedophilia from online sexual offending. The use of online pornography continues to grow with a reported 42 billion visits to Pornhub in 2019, which equates to an average of 115 million visits per day (Pornhub, 2019). Some of the most popular search terms in 2019 included Alien, Cosplay[1] and Autonomous Sensory Meridian Response (ASMR), which can be described as fetishistic interests. During the COVID-19 pandemic in 2020, Pornhub reported a 24.5% and 23.2% increase in online traffic during the European and United States lockdown periods, respectively.

Of particular concern in relation to sexual deviance and pedophilic interest is the availability and use of online child sexual exploitation materials (CSEMs). As Quayle (2021, chap. 14 in this book) observes, CSEM-offenders show greater sexual arousal to children than adults and differ from groups who have committed contact sexual offenses against children, sex offenses against adults, and general sexology patients, with CSEM offending being a stronger indicator of pedophilia than contact sex offending against a child (Seto et al., 2006). Indeed, there appear to be important demographic differences between CSEM users and contact sexual offenders, wherein some CSEM users may have more psychological barriers to contact offending, seen more typically in "fantasy driven/solicitation" offenders versus "contact driven/solicitation" offenders. Fantasy driven/solicitation offenders are those who restrict their online offending behavior to the internet (accessing indecent images) and who may connect to victims for cybersex/masturbation, whereas "contact driven/solicitation" offenders are those who attend meetings with minors to act out their deviant fantasies (Briggs et al., 2011; Merdian et al., 2013). As Quayle explains, online sexual offense-supportive cognitions may not be criminogenic, with the overall endorsement by CSEM offenders of cognitive distortions traditionally associated with contact sex offenders being low. This has led some to question the efficacy of existing sex offender instruments for use with CSEM offenders (Steel et al., 2020), leading to the development of the Child Pornography Offender Risk Tool (Seto & Eke, 2015).

The question most often asked is, to what extent will an individual who has viewed indecent images of children commit a contact sexual offense against a child? Research into internet solicitation, and online grooming of children for sexual purposes has attracted relatively less attention than the production and consumption of indecent images of children. The recidivism data would suggest that internet offenders with no known contact offense history are at relatively low risk of contact offending (Eke et al., 2011; Seto et al., 2011), and if anything, are more likely to commit a further "internet" offense than a new contact offense. Approximately 4.6% of online offenders committed a new sexual offense of some kind during a six-year follow-up: 2.0% committed a contact sexual offense and 3.4% committed a new child pornography offense (Seto et al., 2011). Initial research suggests the same kinds of risk factors, including criminal history, history of deviant sexual interest, and previous convictions for sexual offenses predict recidivism in this sexual offender population (Seto & Eke, 2005; Wakeling et al., 2011). Generalist (internet and non-internet) PCSOs have a significantly higher sexual reoffending rate at the two-year follow-up compared to internet-only sexual offenders (Elliott et al., 2019; Wakeling et al., 2011).

Managing Sexual Deviance and Paraphilic Disorder

As First (2014) noted, the determination of the presence (or absence) of a paraphilic disorder is likely to have a significant impact on sentencing recommendations and the categorization of persons convicted of sexual offenses into low, medium, or high risk under community-notification statutes. For example, some United States Federal sentencing guidelines require that the sentence take into account the need to "protect the public from further crimes of the defendant" (18 U.S.C. § 3553(a)(2)(C)). Actuarial risk assessment instruments (ARAIs) are widely used to provide baseline indications of a person's level of risk and have permeated the criminal justice system to such an extent that their use has been written into legislation when considering the sentencing or release of persons convicted of sexual offenses in Canada, the United States, and the United Kingdom (see Craig & Beech, 2010), with the STATIC family of risk scales (Hanson & Thornton, 2000, 2003; Phenix et al., 2008) being the most widely used globally, and the Risk Matrix-2000 scale (Thornton et al., 2003) used routinely in prison and probation services throughout England and Wales and Northern Ireland (Craig & Rettenberger, 2016). Indeed, risk scales such as the STATIC-99 and Risk Matrix-2000 make explicit the risk item, "non-contact offenses," suggesting paraphilic origins to be an aggravating risk item, the presence of which increases a person's overall actuarial level of risk.

The extent to which PCSOs are generally preoccupied with sex is also related to sexual reoffending (Craig et al., 2006), with sexual preoccupation being evidenced by a high frequency of impersonal sex, general sexual dissatisfaction, and repeat convictions for sexual offenses. Given that the presence of a paraphilic disorder is associated with an increased risk of recidivism (Mann et al., 2010), some have argued that a diagnosis of a paraphilic disorder is likely to result in the imposition of a longer sentence or the assignment of the individual to a higher risk category after being released into the community (First, 2014).

As Thornton (2021, chap. 15 in this book) argues, sexual deviance does not exist in a vacuum but rather, there will be internal and external triggers that activate the arousal pattern leading to urges and fantasies, and there will be both distal and proximate approach behaviors woven through a person's lifestyle that lead to opportunities to offend. Understanding how PCSOs respond to triggers pre-intervention and assessing change in responses post-intervention can provide a measure of change in terms of reductions in the intensity or the effects of sexual deviance. Using the Change score from the Violence Risk Scale – Sex Offense Version (Olver et al., 2007), Thornton illustrates the kinds of change that can occur, and which should be looked for in an institutional setting. Thornton highlights that breadth and duration of change is important. Where sexual deviance is a substantial part of the individual's need profile, changing non-sexual risk factors can help but will be insufficient to produce a substantial reduction in risk and that change will need to be demonstrated for at least two years to indicate reductions in risk.

In addition to actuarial style frameworks to assess behavioral change, there is an abundance of case studies and meta-analytical reports on the effectiveness of psychological and pharmacological interventions for sexual deviance and paraphilic disorders. Treatment of PCSOs has focused attention on both the sexual arousal (paraphilias) and the ability to control one's sexual behavior. As Miner and Munns (2021, chap. 16 in this book) note, the treatment of paraphilias has been conducted mainly with sexual offending samples, with the aim of affecting sexual arousal to children, sexual arousal to violent or sadistic themes, and sexual arousal to consensual sexual behavior. Ware et al. (2021, chap. 20 in this book) describe behavioral control procedures used by individuals to modify their deviant arousal, where the aim of treatment is to focus on the enhancement of appropriate arousal alongside the reduction or extinction of deviancy. In seeking to explain the development of sexual deviance, Laws and Marshall (1990) developed the conditioning theory of deviant sexual interests, which focuses on the involvement of both classical and operant conditioning processes. This led to the reintroduction of a range of behavioral interventions that were developed throughout the 1960s, 1970s, and 1980s (e.g., covert sensitization, olfactory aversion, orgasmic reconditioning, masturbatory satiation, verbal satiation) with varying degrees of success. These techniques employ two main principles of conditioning: classical and operant. Classical conditioning is often used as a technique to obtain a similar response (typically behavioral) by an individual to one which may be produced by some other stimulus (Pavlov, 1927). Operant conditioning follows an individual's response and may increase or decrease the probability of that response occurring through methods of punishment and reward (Skinner, 1953). Operant conditioning is based upon similar principles to that of a classically conditioned response. While initial results suggest a reduction in deviant fantasies when using behavioral techniques, over time, the frequency of non-deviant fantasies reduces. The initial increase in non-deviant fantasy is consistent with research noting the rapid and effective use of behavioral therapy procedures referred to as a "honeymoon effect" (Laws, 2001), which wanes with time, resulting in an "extinction effect" and the deviant arousal returns (Campbell-Fuller & Craig, 2009). Although some more recent studies have focused less on individuals with paraphilias and more on those identified as PCSOs and have demonstrated positive results in programs that have included behavioral techniques for addressing paraphilic arousal (Gannon et al., 2019), Ware et al. (2021) urge caution. They conclude that there is a lack of well-controlled studies and evidence-based practice to support such techniques, and that a number of practical issues remain regarding the use of behavioral interventions and the clinical utility of behavioral control procedures with individuals who have engaged in sexual offending.

As Miner and Munn (2021) observe, the underlying assumption is that paraphilias are unlikely to change and that individuals will continue to think about things they find sexually arousing. As such, any change in arousal patterns seen with masturbatory reconditioning is likely due to changes in cognition. Miner and Munn discuss interventions based on the addiction literature where sexual preoccupation and sexual behaviors have a medication effect for various emotions and family and life problems. Other intervention models, such as integrated biopsychosocial and sex positive models, define impulsive/compulsive sexual behavior as a clinical syndrome characterized by intense, distressing, and recurrent sexual urges and fantasies that significantly interfere with a person's daily functioning. Here, the assumption is that there are a multitude of underlying mechanisms that come together to create this problem and so treatment requires a thorough assessment of the individual to determine the biological, psychological, and sociocultural factors that have contributed to the development and maintenance of impulsive/compulsive sexual behavior. Combining both behavioral and cognitive techniques seeks to modify both the cognitive processes underlying the behavior and the habitual mechanisms associated with the behavior and underlies many cognitive behavioral techniques in this field (Marshall et al., 1999).

Much of the research into the treatment of sexual deviance and paraphilic disorders is based on incarcerated samples where, of people convicted of sexual offending, the prevalence of paedophilia is about 50% (see Seto, 2018). In working with men incarcerated for committing sexual offenses, Walton (2021, chap. 19 in this book) explains there are number of rehabilitation techniques that can be used to support people with paraphilic disorders to lead non-harmful lives. In addition to managing external factors, such as prison social climate, Walton describes how programs such as the Healthy Sex Programme (HSP) includes procedures such as behavior therapy, functional analysis, and the management of contingences surrounding sexual arousal, cognitive reappraisal, mindfulness, urge management, values clarification, compassion training, and intimacy and interpersonal competency, which can be used to achieve the functions of paraphilic arousal in alternative ways. Walton highlights that for some people convicted of sexual offenses, the stability of paraphilia along with the effects of Adverse Childhood Experiences (ACEs) and stigmatization, will make leading a continually non-harmful life challenging. Thus, practitioners will need to use multimodal, brain-friendly approaches to broadly appeal to neurodiversity. Methods for sensory learning (e.g., visual, auditory, and kinaesthetic) are used as much as possible beside reading and for people with high levels of shame linked to trauma and stigmatization, it is helpful to recognize that distress is experienced in the body.

Acknowledging the distinction between pedophilic sexual interest and child sexual abuse, Beier (2021, chap. 17 in this book) discusses the work that he and his colleagues have pioneered, namely, the management and treatment of pedophillically-inclined individuals within the community who have not offended. In 2005, in Berlin, the Prevention Project Dunkelfeld (PPD) was launched—a preventative approach to reducing sexual offending. It involved encouraging (via media advertisements) pedophilic and hebephilic persons to come forward and seek professional help with their interests in order to avoid committing a sexual offense in the future. Using CBT techniques and sexological strategies designed to address how one perceives and understands their sexual preference, as well as pharmacological strategies (as an option), the PPD aims to help minor-attracted individuals effectively control their sexual preference impulses and live offense-free lives. Beier discusses the empirical work and therapeutic perspective that guided the development and expansion of the PPD, as well as recent outcome data showcasing the efficacy of the program and how it has been applied to adolescent individuals. Beier urges for the prevention approach to be internationally extended and discusses the strategies required to achieve this.

In addition to psychotherapeutic interventions for the treatment of paraphilic urges and sexual fantasies, pharmacological agents have also shown to be effective in reducing deviant sexual arousal. Turner and Briken (2021, chap. 18 in this book) describe how the most commonly used testosterone-lowering medications (TLM) such as Cyproterone acetate (CPA),

Medroxyprogesterone acetate (MPA), and Gonadotropin-Releasing-Hormone (GnRH-) agonists are used in the treatment of paraphilic disorders and can lead to considerable decrease in the frequency and intensity of paraphilic sexual fantasies and behaviors in PCSOs. They note that it is generally recommended that pharmacological treatment should in all cases be used as an add-on to psychotherapeutic interventions and that the selection of the most appropriate medication should be based on the individual's risk to show sexually violent behaviors as well as on the intensity of the self-reported and observed paraphilic urges. The use of pharmacological agents should be monitored closely due to potential side effects including weight gain, pain at the site of injection, lethargy and depression, gynecomastia, thromboembolic events as well as liver and kidney dysfunctions, and loss of bone mineral density. Similarly, such treatments should never be terminated abruptly, and termination should be closely monitored, including frequent measurements of serum testosterone concentrations as well as assessments of paraphilic sexual fantasies and behaviors. The use of the Change or Stop Testosterone Lowering Medication (COSTLow)-Scale (Briken et al., 2019) appears to be particularly useful in this regard and can be used to structure the process of changing or discontinuing TLM.

Common across all intervention models is that sexual deviance and paraphilic disorder behaviors are considered maladaptive and are used as a way of soothing or coping with various emotions and life events and interventions focus on identifying behavior and thought patterns that reinforce the sexual behaviors, developing skills for intervening in these patterns, and developing a support system and stopping the problematic sexual behaviors.

Conclusions

There remains some controversy concerning paraphilias in terms of defining what is "normal" or typical versus what is "deviant" or atypical, as well as what is can be consider a disordered behavior. As such, this impacts on how best to understand, assess, and manage such interests and behaviors. As discussed in this chapter, and throughout this volume, paraphilias, paraphilic disorders, and sexual deviance exemplify the difficulty of integrating psychiatric concepts and concerns with those of the legal system and society in general.

This volume on *Sexual Deviance and Paraphilic Disorder* is designed to provide an introduction to a diversity of theories and diagnostic considerations of sexual fantasy, paraphilic interests, paraphilic disorders and sexual aggression, and approaches to the assessment, treatment, and management of potentially offense-related sexual interests. With changing diagnostic criteria and advances in research and treatment, it can be difficult for professionals new to the field to know where to start and, for those who are not new to the field, to know what the latest thinking and research tells us about sexual deviance and paraphilias. We believe this volume provides easily accessible answers to these questions. In addition, it provides specialized references for those interested in diagnostic, treatment, and management of paraphilic disorders and sexual deviance.

Note

1. Performance art in which participants called cosplayers wear costumes and fashion accessories to represent a specific character.

References

Abel, G. G., Becker, J. V., Cunningham-Rathner, J., Mittelman, M., & Rouleau, J.-L. (1988). Multiple paraphilic diagnoses among sex offenders. *Journal of the American Academy of Psychiatry and the Law Online, 16*(2), 153–168.

Ahlers, C. J., Schaefer, G. A., Mundt, I. A., Roll, S., Englert, H., & Willich, S. N. (2011). Beier KM: How unusual are the contents of paraphilias? Paraphilia-associated sexual arousal patterns in a community- based sample of men. *The Journal of Sexual Medicine, 8*, 1362–1370. https://doi.org/10.1111/j.1743-6109.2009.01597.x

American Psychiatric Association (APA). (2013). *Diagnostic and statistical manual of mental disorders* (5th ed.). American Psychiatric Association.

Bartels, R. M., Beech, A. R., & Harkins, L. (2014, September). *Reacting fast, imagining slow: The dual-process model of sexual thinking. Presented at the 13th Annual Conference of the International Association for the Treatment of Sexual Offenders*, Porto, Portugal.

Briken, P., Turner, D., Thibaut, F., Bradford, J., Cosyns, P., & Tozdan, S. (2018). Validation of the change or stop testosterone-lowering medication (costlow) scale using the delphi method among clinical experts. *Journal of Sex & Marital Therapy*. Advance online publication. https://doi.org/10.1080/0092623X.2018.1491910

Bartels, R.M., Beech, R. B., & Harkins, L. (2021). Understanding sexual thoughts and sexual fantasizing: The Dual-Process Model of sexual thinking. In L. A. Craig, & R. Bartels (Eds.), *Sexual deviance: Understanding and managing deviant sexual interests and paraphilic disorders* (pp. 53–66) Wiley-Blackwell.

Bártová, K., Androvičová, R., Krejčová, L., Weiss, P., & Klapilová, K. (2020). The prevalence of paraphilic interests in the Czech population: Preference, arousal, the use of pornography, fantasy, and behavior. *Journal of Sex Research*, Advance online version. https://doi.org/10.1080/00224499.2019.1707468

Beier, K. M. (2021). Managing paraphilic interests in the community: An international perspective. In L. A. Craig, & R. Bartels (Eds.), *Sexual deviance: Understanding and managing deviant sexual interests and paraphilic disorders*. (pp. 268–281). Wiley-Blackwell.

Bhugra, D., Popelyuk, D., & McMullen, I. (2010). Paraphilias across cultures: Contexts and controversies. *Journal of Sex Research, 47*, 242–256. https://doi.org/10.1080/00224491003699833

Blanchard, R., Klassen, P., Dickey, R., Kuban, M. E., & Blak, T. (2001). Sensitivity and specificity of the phallometric test for pedophilia in nonadmitting sex offenders. *Psychological Assessment, 13*(1), 118–126. https://doi.org/10.1037/1040-3590.13.1.118

Braun-Harvey, D., & Vigorito, M. (2015). *Treating out of control sexual behavior: Rethinking sex addiction*. Springer Publishing Company, LLC.

Briggs, P., Simon, W. T., & Simonson, S. (2011). An exploratory study of internet-initiated sexual offences and the chatroom sex offender: Has the internet enabled a new typology of sex offender? *Sexual Abuse: A Journal of Research and Treatment, 23*, 72–91. https://doi.org/10.1177/1079063210384275

Briken, P., Turner, D., Thibaut, F., Bradford, J., Cosyns, P., & Tozdan, S. (2019). Validation of the 'change or stop testosterone lowering medication (COSTLow)-scale' using delphi method among clinical experts. *Journal of Sex & Marital Therapy, 45*(2), 148–158. https://doi.org/10.1080/0092623X.2018.1491910

Campbell-Fuller, N., & Craig, L. A. (2009). A critical review of the use of olfactory aversion and directed masturbation in modifying deviant sexual interest. *Journal of Sexual Aggression, 15*(2), 179–192. https://doi.org/10.1080/13552600902759556

Carnes, P. (1983). *The sexual addiction*. CompCare.

Coleman, E. (1991). Compulsive sexual behavior: New concepts and treatments. *Journal of Psychology and Human Sexuality, 4*, 37–52. https://doi.org/10.1300/J056v04n02_04

Collins English Dictionary (15th ed.). (2018). HarperCollins.
Craig, L. A. (2011). The effect of age on sexual and violent reconviction. *International Journal of Offender Therapy and Comparative Criminology, 55*(1), 75–97. https://doi.org/10.1177%2F0306624X09353290
Craig, L. A., & Beech, A. R. (2010). Towards a guide to best practice in conducting actuarial risk assessments with sex offenders. *Aggression and Violent Behavior, 15*, 278–293. https://doi.org/10.1016/j.avb.2010.01.007
Craig, L. A., Browne, K. D., Beech, A., & Stringer, I. (2006). Psychosexual characteristics of sexual offenders and the relationship to reconviction. *Psychology, Crime and Law, 12*, 231–243. https://doi.org/10.1080/10683160500151084
Craig, L. A., & Rettenberger, M. (2016). A brief history of sexual offender risk assessment. In D. R. Laws, & W. O'Donohue (Eds.), *Treatment of sexual offenders: Strengths and weaknesses in assessment and intervention* (pp. 19–44). Springer.
Dawson, S. J., Bannerman, B. A., & Lalumière, M. L. (2016). Paraphilic interests: An examination of sex differences in a nonclinical sample. *Sexual Abuse, 28*, 20–45. https://doi.org/10.1177%2F1079063214525645
Davis, G., & Leitenberg, H. (1987). Adolescent sex offenders. *Psychological Bulletin, 101*, 417–427. https://doi.org/10.1037/0033-2909.101.3.417
De Neef, N., Coppens, V., Huys, W., & Morrens, M. (2019). Bondage-Discipline, Dominance-Submission and Sadomasochism (BDSM) From an Integrative Biopsychosocial Perspective: A Systematic Review. *Sexual Medicine, 7*(2): 129–144. https://doi.org/10.1016/j.esxm.2019.02.002
Deehan, E. T., & Bartels, R. M. (2019). Somnophilia: Examining its various forms and associated constructs. *Sexual Abuse*, Advance online version. https://doi.org/10.1177%2F1079063219889060
Dickey, R., Nussbaum, D., Chevolleau, K., & Davidson, H. (2002). Age as a differential characteristic of rapist, pedophiles and sexual sadists. *Journal of Sex and Marital Therapy, 28*, 211–218. https://doi.org/10.1080/009262302760328253
Dombert, B., Schmidt, A. F., Banse, R., Briken, P., Hoyer, J., Neutze, J., & Osterheider, M. (2016). How common is men's self-reported sexual interest in prepubescent children? *The Journal of Sex Research, 53*(2), 214–223. https://doi.org/10.1080/00224499.2015.1020108
D'Orazio, D. M., & Flinton, C. A. (2021). Diagnosing sexual sadism and other paraphilic disorders on the Agonistic Continuum. In L. A. Craig, & R. Bartels (Eds.), *Sexual deviance: Understanding and managing deviant sexual interests and paraphilic disorders* (pp. 117–131). Wiley-Blackwell.
Eher, R. (2017). The forensic relevance of paedophilia in the assessment of child molesters. In D. P. Boer, A. R. Beech, T. Ward, L. A. Craig, M. Rettenberger, L. E. Marshall, & W. L. Marshall (Eds.), *The Wiley handbook on the theories, assessment, and treatment of sexual offending* (pp. 863–875). Wiley Blackwell.
Eher, R., Rettenberger, M., & Turner, D. (2019). The prevalence of mental disorders in incarcerated contact sexual offenders. *Acta Psychiatrica Scandinavia, 139*(6), 572–581. https://doi.org/10.1111/acps.13024
Eke, A. W., Seto, M. C., & Williams, J. (2011). Examining the criminal history and future offending of child pornography offenders: An extended prospective follow-up study. *Law and Human Behaviour, 35*(6), 466–478. https://doi.org/10.1007/s10979-010-9252-2.
Elliott, I., Mandeville-Norden, R., Rakestrow-Dickens, J., & Beech, A. (2019). Reoffending rates in a U.K. community sample of individuals with convictions for indecent images of children. *Law and Human Behavior, 43*(4), 369–382. https://doi.org/10.1037/lhb0000328
Finkelhor, D. (1984). *Child sexual abuse: New theory and research*. Free Press.
First, M. B. (2014). DSM-5 and paraphilic disorders. *Journal of the American Academy of Psychiatry and the Law Online, 42*(2), 191–201. Print ISSN 1093-6793

Gannon, T. A., Olver, M. E., Mallion, J. S., & James, M. (2019). Does specialized psychological treatment for offending reduce recidivism? A meta-analysis examining staff and program variables as predictors of treatment effectiveness. *Clinical Psychology Review*, 101752. https://doi.org/10.1016/j.cpr.2019.101752

Gebhard, P. H., Gagnon, J., Pomeroy, W. B., & Christensen, C. (1965). *Sex offenders: An analysis of types*. Harper Row.

Hanson, R. K., & Bussière, M. T. (1998). Predicting relapse: A meta-analysis of sexual offender recidivism studies. *Journal of Consulting and Clinical Psychology, 66*(2), 348–362. https://doi.org/10.1037/0022-006X.66.2.348

Hanson, R. K., & Morton-Bourgon, K. E. (2005). The characteristics of persistent sexual offenders: A meta-analysis of recidivism studies. *Journal of Consulting and Clinical Psychology, 73*, 1154–1163. https://doi.org/10.1037/0022-006X.73.6.1154

Hanson, R. K., & Thornton, D. (2000). Improving risk assessment for sex offenders: A comparison of three actuarial scales. *Law and Human Behavior, 24*, 119–136. doi: 10.1023/a:1005482921333

Hanson, R. K., & Thornton, D. (2003). Notes on the development of a static-2002. Public Safety Canada. Retrieved January 2009, from http://ww2.psepc-sppcc.gc.ca/publications/corrections/200103_Static_2002_e.asp

Hart, S. D., Kropp, R. P., Laws, D. R., Klaver, J., Logan, C., & Watt, K. A. (2003). *The Risk for Sexual Violence Protocol (RSVP): Structured professional guidelines for assessing risk of sexual violence.* Mental Health, Law, and Policy Institute, Simon Fraser University.

Healey, J., Lussier, P., & Beauregard, E. (2012). Sexual sadism in the context of rape and sexual homicide: An examination of crime scene indicators. *International Journal of Offender Therapy and Comparative Criminology, 57*, 402–424. https://doi.org/10.1177/0306624x12437536PMID: 22436735.

Helmus, L., Hanson, R. K., Babchishin, K. M., & Thornton, D. (2015). Sex offender risk assessment with the Risk Matrix 2000: Validation and guidelines for combining with the STABLE-2007. *Journal of Sexual Aggression, 21*(2), 136–157. https://doi.org/10.1080/13552600.2013.870241

Higgs, T., Proulx, J., Gauthier, A., Garant, E., & James, J. (2021). Sexual sadism and offending. In L. A. Craig, & R. Bartels (Eds.), *Sexual deviance: Understanding and managing deviant sexual interests and paraphilic disorders* (pp. 189–206). Wiley-Blackwell.

Joyal, C. C. (2014). How anomalous are paraphilic interests? *Archives of Sexual Behavior, 43*, 1241–1243.

Joyal, C. C. (2015). Defining "normophilic" and "paraphilic" sexual fantasies in a population-based sample: On the importance of considering subgroups. *Sexual Medicine, 3*, 321–330. https://doi.org/10.1002/sm2.96

Joyal, C. (2021). Problems and controversies with psychiatric diagnoses of paraphilia. In L. A. Craig, & R. Bartels (Eds.), *Sexual deviance: Understanding and managing deviant sexual interests and paraphilic disorders* (pp. 91–116). Wiley-Blackwell.

Joyal, C. C., & Carpenter, J. (2017). The prevalence of paraphilic interests and behaviors in the general population: A provincial survey. *The Journal of Sex Research, 54*(2), 161–171. https://doi.org/10.1080/00224499.2016.1139034

Joyal, C.C., Cossette, A., & Lapierre, V. (2015). What exactly is an unusual sexual fantasy? *The Journal of Sexual Medicine, 12*, 328–340. https://doi.org/10.1111/jsm.12734

Kafka, M. P., & Hennen, J. (1999). The paraphilia-related disorders: An empirical investigation of nonparaphilic hypersexual disorders in 206 outpatient males. *Journal of Sex and Marital Therapy, 25*, 305–319. https://doi.org/10.1080/00926239908404008

Kaylor, L., & Jeglic, E. L. (2021). Non-contact paraphilic disorders and offending. In L. A. Craig, & R. Bartels (Eds.), *Sexual deviance: Understanding and managing deviant sexual interests and paraphilic disorders* (pp. 171–188). Wiley-Blackwell.

Kingston, D. A., Firestone, P., Moulden, H. M., & Bradford, J. M. W. (2007). The utility of the diagnosis of pedophilia: A comparison of various classification procedures. *Archives of Sexual Behavior, 36*(3), 423–436. https://doi.org/10.1007/s10508-006-9091-x

Knight, R., & Longpré, N. (2021). The structure and measurement of sadism: Implications for validation. In L. A. Craig, & R. Bartels (Eds.), *Sexual deviance: Understanding and managing deviant sexual interests and paraphilic disorders* (pp. 207–221). Wiley-Blackwell.

Kruger, T. H. C., & Kneer, J. (2021). Neurobiological basis of sexual deviance. In L. A. Craig, & R. Bartels (Eds.), *Sexual deviance: Understanding and managing deviant sexual interests and paraphilic disorders* (pp. 67–88). Wiley-Blackwell.

Långström, N., & Seto, M. C. (2006). Exhibitionistic and voyeuristic behavior in a Swedish national population survey. *Arch Sex Behav, 35*, 427–435. https://doi.org/10.1007/s10508-006-9042-6

Laws, D. R. (2001). Olfactory aversion: Notes on procedure, with speculations on its mechanism of effect. *Sexual Abuse: A Journal of Research and Treatment, 13*, 275–287. https://doi.org/10.1023/A:1017522515854

Laws, D. R., & Marshall, W. L. (1990). A conditioning theory of the etiology and maintenance of deviant sexual preferences and behaviour. In W. L. Marshall, D. R. Laws, & H. E. Barbaree (Eds.), *Handbook of sexual assault: Issues, theories, and treatment of the offender* (pp. 209–230). Plenum Press.

Lehmiller, J. J. (2017). *The psychology of human sexuality*. John Wiley & Sons.

Leitenberg, H., & Henning, K. (1995). Sexual fantasy. *Psychological Bulletin, 117*, 469–496. https://doi.org/10.1037/0033-2909.117.3.469

Lievesley, R., & Harper, C. (2021). Understanding minor attraction. In L. A. Craig, & R. Bartels (Eds.), *Sexual deviance: Understanding and managing deviant sexual interests and paraphilic disorders* (pp. 132–144). Wiley-Blackwell.

Longpré, N., Guay, J.-P., & Knight, R. A. (2018). The developmental antecedents of sexual sadism. In J. Proulx, A. Carter, E. Beauregard, A. Mokros, R. Darjee, & J. James (Eds.), *Routledge international handbook of sexual homicide* (pp. 283–302). Routledge.

Lussier, P., McCuish, E., & James, J. (2021). The developmental pathways of sexual deviance: More than 100 years of research in context. In L. A. Craig, & R. Bartels (Eds.), *Sexual deviance: Understanding and managing deviant sexual interests and paraphilic disorders* (pp. 25–40). Wiley-Blackwell.

Makanjuola, A. B., Adegunloye, O. A., & Adelekan, M. L. (2008). Disorders of sexual preference among secondary school teachers in Ilorin, Nigeria. *Nigerian Journal of Psychiatry, 6*, 26–30. https://doi.org/10.4314/njpsyc.v6i1.39907

Mann, R. M., Hanson, R. K., & Thornton, D. (2010). Assessing risk for sexual recidivism: Some proposals on the nature of psychologically meaningful risk factors. *Sex Abuse, 22*, 191–217. https://doi.org/10.1177%2F1079063210366039

Marshall, W. L., Anderson, D., & Fernandez, Y. M. (1999). *Cognitive behavioural treatment of sexual offenders*. John Wiley & Sons.

Marshall, W. L., & Barbaree, H. E. (1990). An integrated theory of the etiology of sexual offending. In W. L. Marshall, D. R. Laws, & H. E. Barbaree (Eds.), *Handbook of sexual assault: Issues, theories, and treatment of the offender* (pp. 257–275). Plenum.

Marshall, W. L., Hucker, S. J., Nitschke, J., & Mokros, A. (2017). Assessment of sexual sadism. In D. P. Boer, A. R. Beech, T. Ward, L. A. Craig, M. Rettenberger, L. E. Marshall, & W. L. Marshall (Eds.), *The Wiley handbook on the theories, assessment, and treatment of sexual offending* (pp. 849–862). Wiley Blackwell.

McGuire, R. J., Carlisle, J. U., & Young, B. G. (1964). Sexual deviations as conditioned behaviour: A hypothesis. *Behaviour Research and Therapy, 2*, 185–190. https://doi.org/10.1016/0005-7967(64)90014-2

Merdian, H. L., Curtis, C., Thakker, J., Wilson, N., & Boer, D. P. (2013). The three dimensions of online child pornography offending. *Journal of Sexual Aggression, 19*(1), 121–132. https://doi.org/10.1080/13552600.2011.611898

Miner, M. H, & Munns, R. (2021). Psychological treatments for paraphilia and sexually compulsive behaviour. In L. A. Craig & R. Bartels (Eds.), *Sexual deviance: Understanding and managing deviant sexual interests and paraphilic disorders* (pp. 253–267). Wiley-Blackwell.

O'Donohue, W. (2016). Problems in the classification and diagnosis of the paraphilias: What is the evidence that the DSM warrants use? In D.R. Laws, & W.T. O'Donohue (Eds.), *Treatment of sex offenders: Strengths and weaknesses in assessment and intervention* (pp. 1–17). Springer.

Olver, M. E., Wong, S. C. P., Nicholaichuk, T. P., & Gordon, A. (2007). The validity and reliability of the Violence Risk Scale – Sex Offender version: Assessing sex offender risk and evaluating therapeutic change. *Psychological Assessment, 19*, 318–329. https://doi.org/10.1037/1040-3590.19.3.318

Paitich, D., Langevin, R., Freeman, R., Mann, K., & Handy, L. (1977). The Clarke SHQ: A clinical sex history questionnaire for males. *Archives of Sexual Behavior, 6*, 421–435.

Pavlov, I. P. (1927). *Conditioned reflexes: An investigation of the physiological activity of the cerebral cortex*. Oxford University Press.

Pettigrew, M. (2019). Biastophilia, raptophilia, and somnophilia: The blurred distinctions and comorbidity of sexual paraphilias in a homicidal offender. *The Journal of Forensic Psychiatry & Psychology, 30*, 401–408. https://doi.org/10.1080/14789949.2018.1560490

Pettigrew, M., & Deehan, E. T. (2021). Passivity paraphilias: Understanding necrophilic and somnophilic interest. In L. A. Craig, & R. Bartels (Eds.), *Sexual deviance: Understanding and managing deviant sexual interests and paraphilic disorders*. (pp. 145–155) Wiley-Blackwell.

Phenix, A., Doren, D., Helmus, L., Hanson, R. K., & Thornton, D. (2008). *Coding rules for static-2002*. Retrieved electronically on March 21, 2012, from www.static99.org/pdfdocs/static2002codingrules.pdf

Pornhub (2019). The 2019 year in review. Retrieved May 12, 2020, from https://www.pornhub.com/insights/2019-year-in-review.

Prentky, R. A., & Lee, A. F. S. (2007). Effect of age-at-release on long-term sexual re-offense rates in civilly committed sexual offenders. *Sexual Abuse: A Journal of Research and Treatment, 119*, 43–59. https://doi.org/10.1177/107906320701900105

Proulx, J., & Beauregard, E. (2009). Decision making during the offending process: An assessment among subtypes of sexual aggressors of women. In A. R. Beech, L. A. Craig, & K. D. Browne (Eds.), *Assessment and treatment of sex offenders: A handbook* (pp. 181–197). John Wiley & Sons, Ltd.

Quayle, E. (2021). Online sexual deviance and pedophilia. In L. A. Craig, & R. Bartels (Eds.), *Sexual deviance: Understanding and managing deviant sexual interests and paraphilic disorders* (pp. 222–237). Wiley-Blackwell.

Santtila, P., Antfolk, J., Räfså, A., Hartwig, M., Sariola, H., Sandnabba, N. K., & Mokros, A. (2015). Men's sexual interest in children: One-year incidence and correlates in a population-based sample of Finnish male twins. *Journal of Child Sexual Abuse, 24*, 115–134. https://doi.org/10.1080/10538712.2015.997410

Seto, M. C. (2008). *Pedophilia and sexual offending against children: Theory, assessment, and intervention*. American Psychological Association. doi: 10.1037/11639-000

Seto, M. C. (2016). The puzzle of male chronophilias. *Archives of Sexual Behavior, 46*, 3–22. https://doi.org/10.1007/s10508-016-0799-y

Seto, M.C., Cantor, J.M., & Blanchard, R. (2006). Child pornography offenses are a valid diagnostic indicator of pedophilia. *Journal of Abnormal Psychology, 115*(3), pp. 610–615. https://doi.org/10.1037/0021-843X.115.3.610

Schmidt, A. F., Mokros, A., & Banse, R. (2013). Is pedophilic sexual preference continuous? A taxometric analysis based on direct and indirect measures. *Psychological Assessment, 25*, 1146–1153. https://doi.org/10.1037/a0033326

Seto, M. (2018). *Pedophilia and sexual offending against children: Theory, assessment, and intervention* (2nd ed.). American Psychological Association.

Seto, M. C. (2019). The motivation-facilitation model of sexual offending. *Sexual Abuse, 31*, 3–24.

Seto, M. C., & Eke, A. W. (2005). The future offending of child pornography offenders. *Sexual Abuse: A Journal of Research and Treatment, 17*, 201–210.

Seto, M., & Eke, A. (2015). Predicting recidivism among adult male child pornography offenders: Development of the Child Pornography Offender Risk Tool (CPORT). *Law and Human Behavior, 39*(4), 416–429.

Seto, M. C., Hanson, R. K., & Babchishin, K. M. (2011). Contact sexual offending by men arrested for child pornography offences. *Sexual Abuse: A Journal of Research and Treatment, 23*, 124–145. https://doi.org/10.1177%2F1079063217720919

Schmidt, A. F., & Imhoff, R. (2021). Towards a theory of chronophilic sexual orientation in heterosexual men. In L. A. Craig, & R. Bartels (Eds.), *Sexual deviance: Understanding and managing deviant sexual interests and paraphilic disorders*. (pp. 41–52) Wiley-Blackwell.

Skinner, B. F. (1953). *Science and human behaviour*. The Free Press.

Steel, C., Newman, E., O'Rourke, S., & Quayle, E. (2020). A systematic review of cognitive distortions in online child sexual exploitation material offenders. *Aggression & Violent Behaviour, 51*, 101375. https://doi.org/10.1016/j.avb.2020.101375

Stockwell, F. M., & Moran, D. J. (2014). A relational frame theory account of the emergence of sexual fantasy. *Journal of Sex & Marital Therapy, 40*, 92–104. https://doi.org/10.1080/0092623X.2012.736921

Thornton, D. (2021). A generalized model for identifying risk-related change in sexual deviance. In L. A. Craig, & R. Bartels (Eds.), *Sexual deviance: Understanding and managing deviant sexual interests and paraphilic disorders*. (pp. 241–252). Wiley-Blackwell.

Thornton, D., Mann, R., Webster, S., Blud, L., Travers, R., Friendship, C., & Erikson, M. (2003). Distinguishing and combining risks for sexual and violent recidivism. In R. A. Prentky, E. S. Janus, & M. C. Seto (Eds.), *Sexually coercive behavior: Understanding and management* (Vol. 989, pp. 225–235). New York Academy of Sciences.

Toates, F. (2014). *How sexual desire works: The enigmatic urge*. Cambridge University Press.

Turner, D., & Briken, P. (2021). Pharmacological treatments for sexual deviance. In L. A. Craig, & R. Bartels (Eds.), *Sexual deviance: Understanding and managing deviant sexual interests and paraphilic disorders* (pp. 282–294). Wiley-Blackwell.

von Krafft-Ebing, R. (1886). *Psychopathia sexualis*. F. A. Davis.

Wakeling, H. C., Howard, P., & Barnett, G. (2011). Comparing the validity of the RM2000 scales and OGRS3 for predicting recidivism by internet sexual offenders. *Sexual Abuse: A Journal of Research and Treatment, 23*, 146–168. https://doi.org/10.1177%2F1079063210375974

Walton, J. S. (2021). Rehabilitating paraphilic disorder in prisons: Interventions sensitive to shame and trauma and the importance of safe prisons. In L. A. Craig, & R. Bartels (Eds.), *Sexual deviance: Understanding and managing deviant sexual interests and paraphilic disorders* (pp. 295–310). Wiley-Blackwell.

Ward, T., & Beech, A. (2006). An integrated theory of sexual offending. *Aggression and Violent Behavior, 11*, 44–63. https://doi.org/10.1016/j.avb.2005.05.002

Ware, J., McIvor, L., & Fernandez, Y. (2021). Behavioural control models in managing sexual deviance. In L. A. Craig, & R. Bartels (Eds.), *Sexual deviance: Understanding and managing deviant sexual interests and paraphilic disorders* (pp. 311–323). Wiley-Blackwell.

Weinrott, M. R. (1996). Juvenile sexual aggression: A critical review. Boulder, CO: Center for the Study and Prevention of Violence.

Williams, K. M., Cooper, B. S., Howell, T. M., Yuille, J. C., & Paulhus, D. L. (2009). Inferring sexually deviant behavior from corresponding fantasies: The role of personality and pornography consumption. *Criminal Justice and Behavior, 36,* 198–222. https://doi.org/10.1177%2F0093854808327277

Yates, P. (2021). Measures of male sexual interest. In L. A. Craig, & R. Bartels (Eds.), *Sexual deviance: Understanding and managing deviant sexual interests and paraphilic disorders.* (pp. 156–167). Wiley-Blackwell.

Yates, P. M., Hucker, S. J., & Kingston, D. A. (2008). Sexual sadism: Psychopathy and theory. In D. R. Laws, & W. T. O'Donohue (Eds.), *Sexual deviance: Theory, assessment, and treatment* (pp. 213–230). Guilford Press.

Zolondek, S. C., Abel, G. G., Northey, W. F., & Jordan, A. D. (1996). The self reported behaviors of juvenile sex offenders. *Journal of Interpersonal Violence, 17,* 279–295. https://doi.org/10.1177%2F088626001016001005

Part II

Theory of Sexual Deviance and Paraphilias

2

The Developmental Pathways of Sexual Deviance

More than 100 Years of Research in Context

Patrick Lussier[1], Evan McCuish[2], and Jonathan James[3]

[1] *School of social work and criminology, Université Laval, Québec, Canada*
[2] *School of Criminology, Simon Fraser University, Burnaby, Canada*
[3] *Psychology Department, Université du Québec à Trois-Rivières, Québec, Canada*

Introduction

Since the pioneering work of Sheldon and Eleanor Glueck (1930), there has been a long tradition of developmental criminology research. Developmentalists have examined the origins of antisocial and criminal behavior, how it develops over time, and their associated risk and protective factors (e.g., Robins, 1978; West & Farrington, 1973). Developmentalists recognize the importance of human development and life stages (e.g., prenatal, perinatal, infancy, early childhood) to contextualize and understand antisocial and criminal behavior (Loeber & Farrington, 1998; Tonry et al., 1991). Historically, criminology focused on the period of adolescence because it corresponds to the stage during which the prevalence of official offending peaks (see Cullen, 2011). However, developmental and life course criminology have recognized the importance of looking prior to and after the period of adolescence to understand antisocial and criminal behavior more fully. On one hand, developmentalists recognized the importance of looking earlier in a person's development to examine the onset and persistence of antisocial and criminal behavior (Loeber & Farrington, 1998). On the other hand, life course researchers have also shown the importance of looking well beyond adolescence, especially in order to explain the process of desistance from crime (Maruna, 2001).

Developmental and life course research provides a more dynamic viewpoint that has contributed to the identification of various developmental patterns of antisocial and criminal behavior (Farrington, 2003). The search for developmental pathways is characterized by two interrelated streams of research: (a) the identification of the sequence of risk factors leading to antisocial and criminal behavior, and (b) the identification of sequences of development of antisocial and criminal behavior. The first stream is primarily concerned with variability in patterns of predictors (i.e., risk factors; Moffitt, 1993; Patterson & Yoerger, 1993), while the second stream is primarily concerned with variability in patterns of outcomes (i.e., antisocial and criminal behavior).

Regarding the first stream of research, explanatory developmental models have not been very popular because they have been perceived as too deterministic by some and too complex by others (Sampson & Laub, 2003). Deterministic criticisms were perhaps a mischaracterization by those that were unfamiliar with developmentalists' emphasis on change. Generally speaking, developmental models propose explanations of antisocial and criminal behavior that are framed around the role of person-level factors, environmental-level factors, and their interactions (Morizot & Kazemian, 2014). These models recognize the importance of genetic and biological factors in creating early predispositions that can shape a person's life course

Sexual Deviance: Understanding and Managing Deviant Sexual Interests and Paraphilic Disorders,
First Edition. Edited by Leam A. Craig and Ross M. Bartels.
© 2021 John Wiley & Sons, Ltd. Published 2021 by John Wiley & Sons, Ltd.

(Caspi, 2000). They also recognize that humans interact with multiple environments throughout their life course, starting in utero, moving to the familial, school, and then other social environments. After birth, each environment provides different biopsychosocial learning experiences that can impact a person's life course. Developmentalists have been working on the identification of these learning experiences and opportunities, as well as significant life events that can exacerbate, facilitate, or promote the development of antisocial and criminal behavior.[1] Despite this complexity in human development, researchers have shown that there are certain developmental patterns that routinely emerge. In fact, variability in initial conditions (e.g., socioeconomic status, familial environment, parental skills, childhood experiences) does not preclude two individuals from experiencing the same outcome (e.g., antisocial and criminal behavior), also known as equifinality. These findings stress the need to broaden the scope of risk factors (e.g., genes, exposure to teratogens) and to look well beyond the familial environment (e.g., social-peer environment) to describe risk pathways.

The second stream of research is mainly concerned with the measurement of antisocial and criminal behavior (Loeber & Le Blanc, 1990; Piquero et al., 2003), specifically the *longitudinal sequence of antisocial and criminal behavior over time*. This involves the measurement of a series of developmental parameters that capture this evolution (Le Blanc & Fréchette, 1989), including antisocial and criminal behavior age of onset, frequency, diversity, duration, escalation, and the process leading to termination. The latter is often referred to as desistance and includes parameters such as de-escalation and deceleration of antisocial and criminal behavior over time. Within this stream of research, some have been concerned with the measurement, identification, and explanation of developmental trajectories of antisocial and criminal behavior. These trajectories refer to quantitative longitudinal patterns: At what age does the behavior start? How frequent and how stable is it? And for how long does it persist until termination (Nagin et al., 1995)? Others have focused on qualitative developmental pathways: Do individuals confine themselves to a particular type/s of behavior? Do individuals move from less to more serious types of behavior? And is involvement in certain types of behavior informative of the nature of the most serious offense an individual will commit? (Loeber et al., 1993). Breaking down antisocial and criminal behavior into a set of quantitative and qualitative developmental parameters has shown that its development is much more dynamic than first thought and has helped debunk misconceptions such as "once a criminal always a criminal" and "he who steals an egg steals a cow."

Together, these two streams of research provide a more dynamic view of antisocial and criminal behavior during a person's life course. The developmental approach was formalized in the 1990s (e.g., Loeber & Le Blanc, 1990). Researchers recognized the presence of two meta-trajectories of risk (e.g., adolescence-limited; life course persistent) and up to four possible patterns of antisocial and criminal behavior (e.g., high-chronic, low-chronic, adolescence-limited/classic desistance, low rate). While knowledge about the development of antisocial and criminal behavior is certainly valuable for the understanding of sexual offending (Lussier, 2017), it has its limitations for the understanding of sexual deviance more generally (e.g., deviant sexual interests, paraphilia) and sex crimes driven by sexual deviance more specifically. Many researchers have stressed the need to study sexual deviance from a developmental perspective given that sexual deviance includes a broad spectrum of behavior at different age stages, such as childhood sexual problems (Chaffin, 2008; Elkovitch et al., 2009; Lussier et al., 2018), juvenile sexual offending (McCuish & Lussier, 2017) and adult sexual offending (Lussier, 2005). However, such studies are more the exception than the rule when it comes researching sexual deviance. Rather than focus on the behavior and its qualitative and quantitative patterns, research has primarily focused on risk factors for sexual deviance. While many risk factors are developmentally informed (e.g., early sexual victimization experiences), researchers have not approached sexual deviance from a developmental perspective, at least as it is known by those studying antisocial and criminal behavior more broadly. Below, we unravel the history of research on sexual deviance, the extent to which a developmental perspective informed this research, and the implications of this perspective for understanding developmental pathways to sexual offending.

Developmental Research on Sexual Deviance

"Sexual Perverts" in Asylums (1880s–1930s)

The study of the developmental antecedents of deviant sexual behavior emerged in Europe in the late 19th century in *asylums*. Until von Krafft-Ebing's (1886; 1895) well-known book *Psychopathia Sexualis*, there was little to no systematic classification of what constituted deviant sexual behavior. There were, however, several European physicians who provided detailed accounts of clinical cases (Magnan, 1885; Prince, 1898). At that time, sexual deviance loosely referred to behaviors that were unrelated to human reproduction or what was considered to be, at that time, humans' natural instinct (e.g., sexual masochism, homosexuality). Physicians emphasized the distinction between sexual instinct (e.g., sexual interest) and sexual behavior (Moreau, 1859), but this line of research was not extended to the understanding of sexual deviance. After all, physicians of the time believed that physical and mental health were critical to patients' sexuality. It was not so much the behavior that they were interested in understanding as the origins of the behavior. In other words, this research focused on "why" but not so much "what." This was despite them noticing a wide range of deviant sexual behaviors (see Gley, 1884), most of which were not necessarily considered crimes but sexual perversions. For the most part, patients were assessed in asylums and did not commit sex crimes. They were assessed because their behaviors were perceived as unnatural, bizarre, atypical, intensified, or abnormal (e.g., compulsive masturbation, erotomania, nymphomania). According to their clinical observations, the specific nature of the deviant sexual behavior was not informative of the underlying issues (Gley, 1884; Magnan, 1885). Put differently, physicians believed that the root cause was more important than the specific type of behavior that manifested and the multiplicity of deviant sexual behavior was reflective of the numerous factors that could influence sexual instincts and behaviors.

Physicians believed that sexual deviance was caused by physical and/or mental health problems (Gley, 1884; Prince, 1889). A detailed account of a patient's life history leading up to the onset of sexual deviance was a relatively common practice. However, this was always done retrospectively, with little attempt to build a developmental theory of deviant sexual behavior. Instead, the goal was to examine the antecedents of physical and mental health problems of these individuals and their family. Accordingly, the leading hypothesis was that these health problems impacted their sexual instincts or made them unable to express their sexual instinct in ways that complied with social norms such as neurosis, psychosis, degeneration, mental disabilities, and psychopathy (see Krafft-Ebing, 1886; 1895). Because the underlying causes of sexual deviance were non-sexual health problems, it was expected that these patients would present other abnormal behaviors that were not necessarily sexual in nature (e.g., obsessions, rituals, impulsive behaviors, pyromania, kleptomania). Consequently, the focus of their investigation was not so much on understanding the behavioral development of sexual deviance, but rather the development of their mental health problems and the mechanisms by which such problems influenced sexually deviant behavior. As Magnan (1885) observed, the development of mental health problems could either be sudden with an irregular progression or more chronic, repetitive, and increasingly serious over time, and so were sexual deviance manifestations. Many physicians believed that these mental health problems were inherited. Thus, case studies focused on the presence of similar problems among the patient's family members.

The investigation of developmental antecedents was not so much oriented toward those that influenced deviant sexual behaviors, but rather those that could lead to brain abnormalities. One explanation that was widely endorsed by physicians was degeneration theory. Degeneration is a broad term described by Morel (1857) as an unhealthy deviation of the human species. For some, degeneration was hereditary and evidence of an inferior species (e.g., atavism). For others, environmental factors led to brain degeneration (e.g., alcohol abuse, brain trauma, poisoning, sexually transmitted disease). Magnan (1885) and Lombroso (1887), who wrote about deviant sexual behaviors and sex criminals, respectively, espoused the degeneration theory. In fact, the application of degeneration theory to criminal behavior led to a new field of research referred to as criminal anthropology (Ellis, 1890). This focused on the anomalies of offenders' physique and psychological functioning. Magnan (1885) even suggested a link between specific brain impairments and different types of deviant sexual behaviors, including sexually inappropriate behaviors resulting from cognitive impairments (e.g., masturbating in front of strangers); inability to control sexual urges due to impulsivity; inability to cope with obsessive or overwhelming deviant sexual interests; and finally, those that result from a psychosis-related disorder. While physicians of the time did not establish a developmental model of sexual deviance, they were clearly aware of the first stream of developmental research; that is, that a variety of developmental pathways lead to sexual deviance.

"Sexual Deviants" in Psychiatric Hospitals (1930s–1960s)

In the 1930s, the study of the developmental antecedents of deviant sexual behavior emerged in North America, most commonly in psychiatric wards and hospitals. Rather than the degeneration and underlying brain impairments represented in a leading theory of earlier writings that emphasized sexual deviance as a fixed state, possibly even inherited, this next generation of theorizing focused on environmental factors that affected human behavior. The psychoanalytic approach (also called dynamic psychiatry at that time) to sexual deviance was predominant during this period (East, 1946; Hammer & Glueck, 1957). Early experiences of trauma and abuse became a focal point. The presentation of single cases, albeit criminal, but also extreme, bizarre, and eccentric, were used to make broader generalizations about individuals involved in sexual deviant behavior. At that time, the emergence of Sexual Psychopath Laws (SPL) in the USA (and Canada) contributed, in part, to the development of a clinical perspective on sexual deviance. The term "sexual psychopath" did not refer to any particular psychiatric nosology but instead was used to create a legal disposition for a subgroup of individuals convicted of a sex crime (Karpman, 1951).[2] Those characterized by the SPL legal disposition were not especially sexually violent and dangerous individuals but rather showed potential for rehabilitation (see Cormier & Simons, 1969). To be clear, this group included individuals having perpetrated homosexual acts, acts of exhibitionism and other sexually obscene acts committed in public, sexual touching of a minor, and rape. Clinical research during this period, therefore, remained extremely biased as it focused on a small group of convicted offenders who showed a reasonable potential for rehabilitation.

There was a developmental component underlying the dynamic psychiatry movement as it applied to psychiatrists' research on sexual offending. However, instead of a focus on the behavior, interest lay in the emotional processes and mechanisms that led to sexual deviancy. The lack of research on the behavior itself was driven by a belief that such behaviors resulted from irrational emotions, unconscious and overpowering forces (Abrahamsen, 1950).

This effectively pigeonholed researchers of the time to believe that it was not possible for the nature of the manifestation to be of importance. Of course, half a century later, such questions formed the second stream of developmentalists' research on antisocial and criminal behavior. In contrast, scientific writings during the middle of the 20th century were limited to clinical judgment, opinions, and impressions rather than a systematic examination of life history information using a rigorous, standardized and transparent methodology. Karpman's writings proposed various influential hypotheses about the causes of sexual offending. Acknowledging the limited scientific knowledge about the development antecedents of perpetrators of sexual offenses, Karpman (1951) supported the idea that sexual offending was not the result of an abnormal sexual upbringing or poor sexual education.[3]

Drs. Abrahamsen and Glueck sought to move beyond clinical impressions by systematically collecting and analyzing personal information about perpetrators who had been subjected to SPL. Abrahamsen (1950) observed some commonalities in the clinical profiles of these individuals. They tended to have: some form of mental disorder (mainly a form of neurosis), a rebellious and hostile attitude toward authority (though such rebellion did not necessarily emerge during childhood), alcohol issues, and poor records of employment, including problems getting along with colleagues. Abrahamsen believed that these individuals suffered from emotional deprivation because of their exposure in childhood to a "*destructive familial environment*" that included a sadistic and domineering parent. In effect, although only describing a single pathway, Abrahamsen's perspective recognized the "stepping-stone" concept discussed several decades later by developmental criminologists. Exposure to negative circumstances, especially early in the life course, can have cascading effects on later development through a process often referred to as cumulative disadvantage.

While Karpman and Abrahamsen's writings described a single developmental pathway, others eventually espoused the idea of multiple developmental pathways. To be clear, researchers of the time did not speak of development pathways or developmental processes, but their writings aligned with such ideas. They argued that individuals found in sex offender treatment programs were a heterogenous group and that such heterogeneity could be traced back to childhood experiences. Typologies were constructed to try to explain this heterogeneity. These typologies were the first concrete clinical articulation of developmental pathways of sexual offending and were based on clinical interpretations of the motives and the root causes of such motives.[4] Researchers such as Hammer and Glueck (1957) recognized important methodological limitations to their work: namely, they were based on information collected retrospectively from individuals in a hospital setting after the perpetration of the offense. As such, their clinical observations often reflected the perpetrator's and society's reactions (e.g., low self-esteem, shame, guilt, anxiety) to their sexual offense as opposed to its cause. While they were cautious about the generalizability of their conclusions, these ideas became popular interpretations of the underlying developmental pathways to sexual deviance among all offenders, and not just those under the purview of SPL.

The Search for the "Sex Offender" in the Community (1970s–1990s)

The search for the developmental antecedents of perpetrators of sexual offenses split into two main lines of research. The first continued the tradition of studying antecedents to sexual offending among offenders placed in prisons, psychiatric wards, and hospitals using a different frame of reference. Specifically, the psychodynamic perspective was gradually abandoned in favor of behavioral and/or cognitive-based models. In line with the growing popularity of behaviorally-oriented theoretical models, clinical research in psychiatric hospitals focused on measurable and observable factors like sexuality, sexual desire, and sexual arousal, which had been an afterthought in prior research (Abel & Blanchard, 1974; Marshall & Barbaree, 1990; McGuire et al., 1964). The search for developmental antecedents of sexual offending moved toward deviant sexual interests and preferences (e.g., rape, pedophilia, sadism, exhibitionism)—the deviant sexual preference hypothesis. They suggested that deviant sexual behaviors were manifestations of preferred sexual interests. Sexual fantasies and masturbation, as suggested by McGuire et al. (1964), became two key components of a conditioning mechanism, by which deviant sexual fantasies were rewarded and reinforced through masturbation in a way that ultimately paired deviant behaviors with pleasure. Understanding the role of (deviant) sexual arousal in sexual offending and its origins became a focal point. Marshall and Barbaree's writings (1984, 1990) presented one of the first developmentally-informed models of sexual offending. The model proposed a single pathway built around the presence of age-graded risk factors. Marshall and colleagues' writings were framed around the idea of psychosocial vulnerabilities that resulted from being exposed to childhood adversities. Their focus on developmental antecedents and underlying mechanisms leading to sexual offending was unique at the time and paved the way for a developmental approach to sexual offending, but subsequent research did not follow through using prospective longitudinal data.

The second line was fueled by the second wave of the feminist movement of the 1970s that led to important rape law reforms. While the former group of scholars continued their predecessors' focus and focused almost exclusively on sexual aggression against women. This group felt that sexual offending was much more common and not limited to individuals involved in bizarre, atypical, physically violent or eccentric forms of sexual behavior that necessarily was a product of an underlying pathology. The branching out of the search for developmental antecedents is important because it favored a greater diversity of theoretical perspectives, which expanded the search for possible explanatory factors. It also broke the mold of examining sexual deviance strictly from a psychiatric-medical standpoint. This period witnessed the emergence of social learning, sociocultural (e.g., rape myths), and media-related factors (e.g., pornography) as potential explanations for sexual offending. In that context, the portrayal of developmental pathways to sexual offending changed dramatically.

Community-based research focused on sexual offending, especially rape and sexual assault perpetrated by young adults (Briere & Malamuth, 1983; Koss et al., 1987). This research was, therefore, centered on more common manifestations of sexual offending that did not necessarily result in incarceration and hospitalization. The prevailing research model suggested that sexual deviance research was conducted in psychiatric wards and hospitals where convicted offenders were being clinically assessed and treated. With the impact of the second-wave feminism movement and the significant increase in women attending college and university, attitudes and perceptions about women and their sexuality became a focal point for research. Although community-based research on sexual offending was initially seen as somewhat unorthodox, researchers would later propose elaborate theoretical models that required revisiting commonly held beliefs about the study of sexual offending. Thus, contrary to clinical pathway models that emphasized the role of deviant sexual preferences, community-based research focused on beliefs, norms, and values, especially attitudes toward women and perceptions of gender norms, and how these factors related to sexual arousal and sexual offending. These models, such as the confluence model by Dr. Neil Malamuth (1998), portrayed the developmental pathway of sexual offending, especially rape and sexual assault, as characterized by sociocultural factors, namely, patriarchal values, perpetuation of gender inequalities, and the endorsement of violence and rape myths.

This line of research did not require potential sexual pathogenic experiences (e.g., sexual victimization) nor some form of trauma and abuse. In fact, it suggested that commonly held ideas and stereotypes about women and sexuality (e.g., rape myths), if endorsed, could provide the cognitive basis for the perpetration of a sexual offense. This implied that sexual offending was more common than previously observed based on police data and the prevalence of "sex offenders" in psychiatric hospitals and prison settings. It also implied that sexual offending was more "in the open" as perpetrators included middle-class young males with no readily apparent form of mental disorder or abnormal sexual preference. The development, testing, and use of self-reported measures of sexual offending perpetration and victimization was a pivotal scientific contribution during this period and contributed to the broadening of the study of the developmental pathways of sexual offending (Koss et al., 1987). Indeed, community-based research represented one of the very first efforts to systematically measure sexual offending as opposed to waiting for courts, corrections, and legal systems to define a behavior as being in violation of a particular section of a criminal code. Community-based researchers had to think about how to create surveys and instruments that would measure whether a person had a history of perpetrating sexual offenses. This new line of research was a key stepping-stone toward the second stream of developmental research concerning the measurement of sequences of sexual offending.[5]

The "Sexual Recidivist" in Prison (1990s–2010s)

The combination of victims' rights movements, conservative ideology, and new trends in corrections led to an increased focus on convicted offenders returning to the community. While prior research had long recognized the heterogeneity characterizing perpetrators of sexual offenses, during this period this heterogeneity was approached in terms of risk of sexual recidivism. From a developmental perspective, this period was significant in numerous ways. It saw the emergence of research that required longitudinal designs, which are pivotal from a developmental and life course viewpoint. While longitudinal studies on sexual recidivism sporadically appeared in the scientific literature since the 1950s, they increased and became more sophisticated in the 1990s (Quinsey et al., 1995). The longitudinal examination of sexual offending using a cohort of individuals examined at two different time points progressively favored the emergence of a more dynamic outlook on sexual offending, which, until this point, was considered a rather fixed and stable predisposition (Lussier et al., 2010). From a developmental perspective, recidivism studies were still limited because they involved examining offenders *after* their perpetration of a sexual offense, sometimes decades after the onset (Lussier & Mathesius, 2012). This makes it difficult to uncover the origins of the behavior because temporal order cannot be established and errors in memory recall bias retrospective reports.

This period also saw the formalization of the measurement of risk factors, that is, the development of standardized risk assessment tools that had both strengths and limitations (Hanson & Thornton, 2000). This was in sharp contrast with the prior work of clinical researchers who relied on broadly defined concepts and ideas about the contributing factors of sexual offending (e.g., intimacy, insecure attachment, cognitive deconstruction). While these concepts were accepted at face value, their empirical value in terms of explaining sexual offending was relatively unknown. This highlights the third key aspect of this period; namely, the accurate estimation of probabilities of sexual recidivism as a hallmark of correctional and risk management practices. Empirical testing using prospective longitudinal data became paramount to judge the value of research hypotheses.

Because clinicians, judges, and correctional officials were now primarily concerned with assessing risk and predicting sexual recidivism, research on developmental antecedents relevant to the origins of sexual offending became somewhat of an afterthought. Indeed, the focus shifted away from understanding pathways to the onset of sexual offending and increasingly toward prediction of repeat sexual offending. This is reflected by the focus on atheoretical factors that predict sexual recidivism (e.g., having a male victim) and the lack of attention given to developmental and age-graded factors. It is of interest that efforts to conceptualize the risk factors predicting sexual recidivism led to the identification of two dimensions of risk for sexual recidivism open to interpretation with respect to their meaning (see Brouillette-Alarie et al., 2018; Roberts et al., 2002). The first factor, often labeled as sexual deviance, refers to characteristics of a person's past sexual offenses, their victim's characteristics, and sexual offending parameters. The second dimension, often referred to as antisociality, refers to a person's past involvement with the criminal justice system for non-sexual offenses, such as their frequency of past convictions and involvement in non-sexual violence (see Lussier et al., 2005).[6] While the goal of this line of research was to predict sexual recidivism as accurately as possible, these two dimensions cannot be ignored as possible developmental pathways leading to the emergence of a first sexual offense. While these could have been seen as two complimentary dimensions and perspectives, they were often framed as a sexuality/antisociality dichotomy. The former implies that specific theories of sexual offending are needed, and the latter implies that theories of offending more broadly can also be generalized to sexual offending (Lussier et al., 2005).

Charting a Course for Integrating a Developmental Perspective into Sexual Deviance Research

While the scientific literature on sexual offending has helped to answer questions relevant to developmental principles, there have been few explicit attempts to define, describe, and explain sexual offending onset, continuity and discontinuity, as well as the heterotypic continuity of behavior over time (Lussier & Blokland, 2014; Lussier et al., 2007). That is, empirical testing of behavioral pathways to sexual offending is largely missing from the literature. The work conducted thus far has been mostly anecdotal, based on clinical impressions and opinions from a single source of information, and relies on single case studies or small, biased samples from psychiatric wards, hospitals, and prison-based sex offender treatment programs. Importantly, most of the information on developmental antecedents was collected retrospectively. This meant these antecedents were reported after the offender was detected, convicted, and possibly after they had participated in a treatment program, clinical sessions, and had learned from others in group therapy about their reasons for sexual offending. In effect, after 100 years of research on sexual deviance, this field continues to struggle with basic methodological problems that limit conclusions that can be made about the developmental course of sexual offending and the risk factors for sexual offending. Also, while familial environment and childhood life adversities are important, they offer only a limited understanding of developmental and life course patterns of sexual offending. Developmental and life course research is far more diverse when it comes to the measurement of different risk factors at different ages. This field of research has shown the presence of key in utero, perinatal, infancy as well as genetic, neuropsychological, individual, familial, school, peer, neighborhood, and sociocultural risk factors associated with general offending and antisocial behavior (Morizot & Kazemian, 2014). Furthermore, although there are some notable exceptions, such as the work of Dr. Freund on courtship disorders (Freund & Seto, 1998), there has been little effort invested in examining the behavioral development of sexual deviance (McCuish et al., 2015).

There are some consistent findings within the literature that can be used to help structure the incorporation of a developmental perspective into sexual offending research. As clinical and community-based research grew, some general trends emerged, including suggestions that there are meta-pathways to sexual offending. These pathways were sometimes described in different ways and resembled the sexual/antisocial dimensions found in risk assessment tools described earlier. Furthermore, they tend to be included in at least one of the following three domains of functioning: (a) inadequate drive, arousal, and motivation; (b) low or dysfunctional self-control; and (c) the presence of unconventional values, norms, and beliefs. Regarding the first domain, some researchers (Knight, 2010; Proulx & Beauregard, 2009) stressed that an inadequate drive and motivation (e.g., sexual arousal, anger) can be too overwhelming to control and regulate, which leads to sexual offending. The same researchers stressed that low self-control can lead someone to seek immediate gratification without thinking about more long-term consequences. Such persons may seek immediate sexual gratification without a person's consent or without consideration of long-term consequences. Finally, the third domain refers to deviant values, norms, and beliefs (e.g., justifications, rationalizations) that may lead someone to pursue goals that are socially inappropriate (Bachman et al., 1992; Locke & Mahalik, 2005). Values, norms, beliefs, and self-standards also provide a cognitive basis for behavioral inhibition while orienting a person's behavior toward certain goals and objectives. These mechanisms are key underlying components of self-regulation, which are associated with specific developmental tasks during infancy, childhood, and adolescence (e.g., modulation of state, being responsive to warning signs, internalization of social norms, adoption of contingency rules) (Kopp, 1982). Most importantly, these self-regulatory components have been referred to in the context of two potentially important developmental pathways leading to sexual offending.

The first meta-pathway is focused on sexual regulation and the role of a person's sexual functioning in sexual offending. Researchers have proposed various concepts and risk factors that can impede the development of a person's sexual functioning in such a way as to impact a person's life course trajectory. Inappropriate sexual urges and hypersexuality (e.g., Kafka, 2010), using sex as a coping mechanism (Cortoni & Marshall, 2001), limited and/or dysfunctional control over sexual urges (e.g., Lussier et al., 2005), and distorted beliefs/myths about sexuality (Malamuth, 1981) are key underlying concepts characterizing this meta-pathway. These themes, however, have not been examined from a developmental pathway perspective. For example, when does sex as a coping mechanism start and how does it develop over time? What are the first signs and manifestations? Is there a longitudinal sequence of development? What are the contributing factors at each stage of development? More broadly, researchers have pointed to biological factors, childhood experiences, and sociocultural factors to explain the development of this meta-pathway. One central set of developmental factors is exposure to deviant sexual behaviors, sexual promiscuity within the familial environment, and experiences of sexual victimization (Cale & Lussier, 2017). Others have also stressed the role of repeated exposure to cultural messages from media sources that directly (presenting women as secretly desiring to be raped) or indirectly (depicting women as sex objects) support deviant sexual behavior (Kingston et al., 2008). It remains unclear how these factors develop (e.g., whether they co-occur with deviant sexual fantasies or psychopathy; Williams et al., 2009), at what stage of development they emerge, and how they operate to increase the risk of sexual offending. Historically, researchers have stressed puberty as a critical developmental period for this pathway (Marshall & Barbaree, 1990). However, clinical research indicates that the onset of normative and non-normative sexual behavior begins much earlier (Lussier et al., 2018).

The second meta-pathway is focused on self-regulation and the role of social functioning in the perpetration of a sexual offense. Researchers have proposed various concepts and risk factors that can impede the development of a person's social functioning in a way that impacts a person's life course trajectory. Research focused on the link between early trauma and abuse, intimacy deficits, low self-esteem, and sexual offending (Smallbone & Dadds, 1998). The most comprehensive presentation of this meta-pathway involves criminogenic factors that are responsible for the development of a broad range of antisocial and criminal behaviors, including sexual offenses (for a review, see Lussier & Mathesius, 2018). More importantly, this meta-pathway suggests a development characterized by three key elements: (a) emotional dysregulation and difficulties coping with negative moods and emotions (e.g., anger, frustration, depression); (b) poor self-control, limited behavioral inhibitions and a tendency to seek immediate gratification; and (c) social information processing biases and antisocial values, norms, and beliefs (e.g., self-centeredness, acceptance of aggression). Theoretical models for antisocial and criminal behaviors have distinguished two main developmental patterns of risk: (a) state-dependent (transitory, malleable, influenced by period-specific and age-graded factors); and (b) population heterogeneity (stable and fixed propensity, life-course persistent, cumulative deficits) (Nagin & Paternoster, 1991). These two processes, therefore, suggest the presence of multiple longitudinal patterns of sexual offending. Due to the nature of this meta-pathway, some have stressed that individuals will also be aggressive in non-sexual ways (e.g., intimate partner violence, child abuse, gang fight), while others suggest that behavior along this meta-pathway is broader, including a myriad of antisocial, rule-breaking, reckless, aggressive and violent behaviors. In other words, sexual offending is one of many antisocial behavior manifestations of this meta-pathway.

The two meta-pathways highlight possible developmental routes by which individuals may not develop adequate self-regulation over their sexual interests and preferences. These developmental pathways offer hypotheses regarding why someone may fail to regulate their thoughts, emotions, and behavior, potentially leading to sexually deviant behaviors. Sexual and self-regulation mechanisms may provide information about the strength of sexual desire, the regulation of such desire, and when and where the expression of one's sexual desire is socially adequate. The *sexual functioning* meta-pathway offers possible clues about the nature, strength, and ability to regulate sexual desire, urges, and behavior, while the *social functioning* meta-pathway offers possible clues about the nature, strength, and ability to regulate social behavior and how sexual desire, urges, and behaviors are expressed in a social, interpersonal context. Sexual interests and preferences exist irrespective of the ability to regulate the sexual and social aspects of their behavioral manifestations. Considering that deviant sexual fantasies are more common in the general population than previously thought (Ahlers et al., 2011; Joyal & Carpentier, 2017), sexual and self-regulation mechanisms can operate in ways that ensure these fantasies are expressed in a socially appropriate way. In other words, sexual and social functioning pathways are more informative about sexual offending than they are about sexual interests and sexual preferences. Of importance is that the scientific knowledge being built from retrospective data leads to a problem of retrospective biases (Lussier & Blokland, 2014; McCuish & Lussier, 2017). These findings based on clinical observations with perpetrators of sex crimes suggest that sexual offending is almost inevitable in the presence of some of these pathway characteristics. In contrast, the literature on the development of antisocial and criminal behavior suggests otherwise. In fact, the plasticity of human development in the context of sexual deviance and sexual offending is relatively unknown.

While these two meta-pathways are focused on developmental pathways leading to sexual offending, it remains unclear how they are associated with the development of deviant sexual interests and preferences. Although some researchers have emphasized conditioning and social learning processes (Laws & Marshall, 1990), the developmental process remains highly speculative. The introduction of penile plethysmography (PPG) in the 1960s was a major step in the measurement of men's sexual interests (Freund et al., 1965). However, it has been mainly used as a clinical research tool to examine the presence and prevalence of deviant sexual interests among convicted offenders. Thus, these studies cannot elucidate whether deviant sexual interests influence sexual offending or vice-versa. PPG has been underused as a clinical research instrument to address more fundamental questions about the origins and development of deviant sexual interests and preferences (Briere & Runtz, 1989; Lussier et al., 2005; Murphy et al., 2001). Using PPG data, the developmental correlates of deviant sexual interests examined have been limited and the findings somewhat inconsistent across studies. Notably, these findings suggest that early life adversities and neurodevelopmental factors could be evidence of multiple pathways leading to the development of pedophilic interests (Blanchard et al., 2002; Lussier et al., 2005), which is consistent with the findings of taxometric studies using phallometric data (McPhail et al., 2018; Michaud & Proulx, 2009). The overlap in risk factors for deviant sexual interests and the risk factors for the two meta-pathways could explain why some individuals are more prone to acting out their deviant sexual interests compared to others.

To move forward with the developmental approach and the identification of pathways to sexual deviance, researchers need to examine the development of sexual behavior (i.e., not just sexual offending or sexual behavior *problems*) from its onset and onward. Research initiated by Dr. William Friedrich (Friedrich et al., 2001) with clinical samples of children that had been sexually abused led to the implementation of epidemiological studies with population-based samples of children. The findings highlighted the need to examine the developmental process by which deviant and non-deviant sexual behavior develops prior to puberty. While the disentangling of normative and non-normative manifestations during that period remains a challenge for researchers, the study of intrusive, coercive, repetitive, and age-inappropriate sexual behavior during childhood has grown in recent years (Lussier et al., 2018). Some children experienced persistent difficulties regulating their sexual behavior in a social context, leading to the emergence of sexual behavioral problems (SBP). During that developmental stage, there was evidence of the co-occurrence of childhood SBP and other behavioral problems (e.g., aggression, antisocial behavior) on one hand, and childhood SBP, poly-victimization, and exposure to multiple life adversities (e.g., parental neglect, physical abuse) on the other. To be clear, it is not believed that all individuals having perpetrated a sex crime have self-regulation problems and difficulties that *originate from childhood*. Until pathways to sexual deviance are examined using a prospective longitudinal age-graded approach across multiple developmental stages, questions about the developmental origins and continuity of sexual offending will remain poorly understood. It would be fruitful to examine more closely the developmental processes by which individuals develop the ability to regulate their sexual desire and sexual interests, and ensure that such factors are expressed in age-appropriate ways. This research should also include examining, at each stage of development, the factors that may impede, temporarily or more permanently, the ability to regulate sexual desires and interests.

Notes

1. For example, a difficult infant may be more at risk of developing a bad temper in early childhood and later more prone to experiencing negative emotional states. That child may have more problems coping with rules and frustrations at home and might be more prone to being rebellious and defiant at school. Being a difficult infant with a bad temper may create negative and hostile reactions from the environment that reinforce rebellious and defiant behaviors. From a developmentalist and life course perspective, humans are active participants in their life course; they are able to make rational choices and act on certain preferences. However, these abilities and tendencies are not equal across persons. As one example, the aging process provides individuals with increased agency over their own development. Aging affords the opportunity to choose social circles, activities to take part in, etc. that in turn can have reciprocal effects on development.

2. Although more contemporary definitions of psychopathy tend to engender beliefs about the lack of efficacy of treatment, SPL were driven by the idea that rehabilitation, not punishment, would better serve perpetrators of sex crimes.
3. While Karpman conceded that some offenders had brain impairments, his theory focused on the role of the familial and social environment in childhood. Karpman believed that parents' unhealthy and repressive attitude (e.g., masturbation can lead to insanity) toward a child's expression of sexuality (e.g., playing doctor, masturbation) could lead to the child's expression of sexuality through aberrant channels.
4. Hammer and Glueck (1957) provided one early typology composed of four risk factor profiles: (a) unconscious fear and anxiety towards women; (b) low self-esteem combined with feelings of being unappreciated and not respected by others; (c) low self-control; and (d) the lack of a capacity for sublimation of sexual impulses (also see Turner, 1961).
5. Community-based research stressed that societal leniency toward rape and sexual assault (e.g., marital rape, sexual assaulting an intoxicated victim unable to consent) limited the detection of such behaviors and therefore, from a research standpoint, the inability to recognize developmental pathways to sexual offending. This framed research on sexual offending in prisons and hospitals as something that came from how society chose to punish certain sexual offenses versus others as opposed to being most relevant or important to understanding sexual offending more broadly. Some felt that this focus on community-based research swung the pendulum too far from research on the clinical profile of incarcerated adult offenders presenting deviant sexual fantasies, especially violent sexual fantasies (Knight & Sims-Knight, 2003; see also Lussier et al., 2005).
6. Other dimensions have been alluded to, such as a history of mental health problems, reminiscent of the early work conducted in psychiatric wards and hospitals.

References

Abel, G. G., & Blanchard, E. B. (1974). The role of fantasy in the treatment of sexual deviation. *Archives of General Psychiatry, 30*(4), 467–475. doi: 10.1001/archpsyc.1974.01760100035007

Abrahamsen, D. (1950). Study of 102 sex offenders at Sing Sing. *Federal Probation, 14*, 26–32.

Ahlers, C. J., Schaefer, G. A., Mundt, I. A., Roll, S., Englert, H., Willich, S. N., & Beier, K. M. (2011). How unusual are the contents of paraphilias? Paraphilia-associated sexual arousal patterns in a community-based sample of men. *The Journal of Sexual Medicine, 8*(5), 1362–1370. https://doi.org/10.1111/j.1743-6109.2009.01597.x

Bachman, R., Paternoster, R., & Ward, S. (1992). The rationality of sexual offending: Testing a deterrence/rational choice conception of sexual assault. *Law and Society Review*, 343–372. https://doi.org/10.2307/3053901

Blanchard, R., Christensen, B. K., Strong, S. M., Cantor, J. M., Kuban, M. E., Klassen, P., Dickey, R., & Blak, T. (2002). Retrospective self-reports of childhood accidents causing unconsciousness in phallometrically diagnosed pedophiles. *Archives of Sexual Behavior, 31*(6), 511–526. https://doi.org/10.1023/A:1020659331965

Briere, J., & Malamuth, N. M. (1983). Self-reported likelihood of sexually aggressive behavior: Attitudinal versus sexual explanations. *Journal of Research in Personality, 17*(3), 315–323. https://doi.org/10.1016/0092-6566(83)90023-5

Briere, J., & Runtz, M. (1989). University males' sexual interest in children: Predicting potential indices of "pedophilia" in a nonforensic sample. *Child Abuse & Neglect, 13*(1), 65–75. https://doi.org/10.1016/0145-2134(89)90030-6

Brouillette-Alarie, S., Proulx, J., & Hanson, R. K. (2018). Three central dimensions of sexual recidivism risk: Understanding the latent constructs of Static-99R and Static-2002R. *Sexual Abuse, 30*(6), 676–704. https://doi.org/10.1177/1079063217691965

Cale, J., & Lussier, P. (2017). Sexual behaviour in preschool children in the context of intra-parental violence and sexual coercion. *Criminal Behaviour and Mental Health, 27*(2), 176–190. https://doi.org/10.1002/cbm.1996

Caspi, A. (2000). The child is father of the man: Personality continuities from childhood to adulthood. *Journal of Personality and Social Psychology, 78*(1), 158–172. https://doi.org/10.1037/0022-3514.78.1.158

Chaffin, M. (2008). Our minds are made up—Don't confuse us with the facts: Commentary on policies concerning children with sexual behavior problems and juvenile sex offenders. *Child Maltreatment, 13*(2), 110–121. https://doi.org/10.1177/1077559508314510

Cormier, B. M., & Simons, S. P. (1969). The problem of the dangerous sexual offender. *Canadian Psychiatric Association Journal, 14*(4), 329–335.

Cortoni, F., & Marshall, W. L. (2001). Sex as a coping strategy and its relationship to juvenile sexual history and intimacy in sexual offenders. *Sexual Abuse: A Journal of Research and Treatment, 13*(1), 27–43. https://doi.org/10.1023/A:1009562312658

Cullen, F. T. (2011). Beyond adolescence-limited criminology: Choosing our future—the American Society of Criminology 2010 Sutherland address. Criminology, *49*(2), 287–330. https://doi.org/10.1111/j.1745-9125.2011.00224.x

East, W. N. (1946). Sexual offenders. *The Journal of Nervous and Mental Disease, 103*(6), 626–666.

Elkovitch, N., Latzman, R. D., Hansen, D. J., & Flood, M. F. (2009). Understanding child sexual behavior problems: A developmental psychopathology framework. *Clinical Psychology Review, 29*(7), 586–598. https://doi.org/10.1016/j.cpr.2009.06.006

Ellis, H. (1896). Criminal Anthropology. *Journal of Mental Science, 42*(179), 849–859.

Farrington, D. P. (2003). Developmental and life-course criminology: Key theoretical and empirical issues-the 2002 Sutherland award address. *Criminology, 41*(2), 221–225. https://doi.org/10.1111/j.1745-9125.2003.tb00987.x

Freund, K., Sedlacek, F., & Knob, K. (1965). A simple transducer for mechanical plethysmography of the male genital. *Journal of the Experimental Analysis of Behavior, 8*(3), 169–170. doi: 10.1901/jeab.1965.8-169

Freund, K., & Seto, M. C. (1998). Preferential rape in the theory of courtship disorder. *Archives of Sexual Behavior, 27*(5), 433–443. https://doi.org/10.1023/A:1018796312289

Friedrich, W. N., Fisher, J. L., Dittner, C. A., Acton, R., Berliner, L., Butler, J., Damon, L., Davies, W. H., Gray, A., & Wright, J. (2001). Child sexual behavior inventory: Normative, psychiatric, and sexual abuse comparisons. *Child Maltreatment, 6*(1), 37–49. https://doi.org/10.1177/1077559501006001004

Gley, E. (1884). Les aberrations de l'instinct sexuel: D'après Des travaux récentş. *Revue Philosophique de la France et de l'Étranger, 17*, 66–92.

Glueck, S., & Glueck, E. T. (1930). *500 criminal careers*. AA Knopf.

Hammer, E. F., & Glueck, B. C. (1957). Psychodynamic patterns in sex offenders: A four-factor theory. *The Psychiatric Quarterly, 31*(1–4), 325–345. https://doi.org/10.1007/BF01568731

Hanson, R. K., & Thornton, D. (2000). Improving risk assessments for sex offenders: A comparison of three actuarial scales. *Law and Human Behavior, 24*(1), 119–136. https://doi.org/10.1023/A:1005482921333

Hunter, J. A., Goodwin, D. W., & Becker, J. V. (1994). The relationship between phallometrically measured deviant sexual arousal and clinical characteristics in juvenile sexual offenders. *Behaviour Research and Therapy, 32*(5), 533–538. https://doi.org/10.1016/0005-7967(94)90142-2

Joyal, C. C., & Carpentier, J. (2017). The prevalence of paraphilic interests and behaviors in the general population: A provincial survey. *The Journal of Sex Research, 54*(2), 161–171. https://doi.org/10.1080/00224499.2016.1139034

Kafka, M. P. (2010). Hypersexual disorder: A proposed diagnosis for DSM-V. *Archives of Sexual Behavior, 39*(2), 377–400. https://doi.org/10.1007/s10508-009-9574-7

Karpman, B. (1951). The sexual psychopath. *The Journal of Criminal Law, Criminology, and Police Science, 42*(2), 184–198.

Kingston, D. A., Fedoroff, P., Firestone, P., Curry, S., & Bradford, J. M. (2008). Pornography use and sexual aggression: The impact of frequency and type of pornography use on recidivism among sexual offenders. *Aggressive Behavior: Official Journal of the International Society for Research on Aggression, 34*(4), 341–351. https://doi.org/10.1002/ab.20250

Knight, R. A. (2010). Typologies for rapists: The generation of a new structural model. In A. Schlank (Ed.), *The sexual predator* (Vol. 4, pp. 17–28). Civic Research Institute.

Knight, R. A., & Sims-Knight, J. E. (2003). The developmental antecedents of sexual coercion against women: Testing alternative hypotheses with structural equation modeling. *Annals of the New York Academy of Sciences, 989*(1), 72–85. https://doi.org/10.1111/j.1749-6632.2003.tb07294.x

Kopp, C. B. (1982). Antecedents of self-regulation: A developmental perspective. *Developmental Psychology, 18*(2), 199–214. https://doi.org/10.1037/0012-1649.18.2.199

Koss, M. P., Gidycz, C. A., & Wisniewski, N. (1987). The scope of rape: Incidence and prevalence of sexual aggression and victimization in a national sample of higher education students. *Journal of Consulting and Clinical Psychology, 55*(2), 162-170. https://doi.org/10.1037/0022-006X.55.2.162

Krafft-Ebing, R. V. (1886; 1895). *Psychopathy sexualis: Étude médico-légale*. George Carré.

Laws, D. R., & Marshall, W. L. (1990). A conditioning theory of the etiology and maintenance of deviant sexual preference and behavior. In W. L. Marshall, D. R. Laws, & H. E. Barbaree (Eds.), *Handbook of sexual assault* (pp. 209–229). Springer.

Le Blanc, M., & Fréchette, M. (1989). *Male criminal activity from childhood through youth*. Springer-Verlag.

Locke, B. D., & Mahalik, J. R. (2005). Examining masculinity norms, problem drinking, and athletic involvement as predictors of sexual aggression in college men. *Journal of Counseling Psychology, 52*(3), 279–283. https://doi.org/10.1037/0022-0167.52.3.279

Loeber, R., & Farrington, D. P. (Eds.). (1998). *Serious and violent juvenile offenders: Risk factors and successful interventions*. Sage Publications.

Loeber, R., & Le Blanc, M. (1990). Toward a developmental criminology. *Crime and Justice, 12*, 375–473.

Loeber, R., Wung, P., Keenan, K., Giroux, B., Stouthamer-Loeber, M., Van Kammen, W. B., & Maugham, B. (1993). Developmental pathways in disruptive child behavior. *Development and Psychopathology, 5*(1–2), 103–133. https://doi.org/10.1017/S0954579400004296

Lombroso, C. (1887). *L'homme criminel: criminel-né, fou moral, épileptique: Étude anthropologique et médico-légale*. Germer Baillière.

Lussier, P. (2005). The criminal activity of sexual offenders in adulthood: Revisiting the specialization debate. *Sexual Abuse: A Journal of Research and Treatment, 17*(3), 269–292. https://doi.org/10.1007/s11194-005-5057-0

Lussier, P. (2017). Juvenile sex offending through a developmental life course criminology perspective: An agenda for policy and research. *Sexual Abuse: A Journal of Research and Treatment, 29*(1), 51–80. https://doi.org/10.1177/1079063215580966

Lussier, P., Beauregard, E., Proulx, J., & Nicole, A. (2005). Developmental factors related to deviant sexual preferences in child molesters. *Journal of Interpersonal Violence, 20*(9), 999–1017. https://doi.org/10.1177/0886260505278024

Lussier, P., & Blokland, A. (2014). The adolescence-adulthood transition and Robins's continuity paradox: Criminal career patterns of juvenile and adult sex offenders in a prospective longitudinal birth cohort study. *Journal of Criminal Justice, 42*(2), 153–163. https://doi.org/10.1016/j.jcrimjus.2013.07.004

Lussier, P., Leclerc, B., Cale, J., & Proulx, J. (2007). Developmental pathways of deviance in sexual aggressors. *Criminal Justice and Behavior, 34*(11), 1441–1462. https://doi.org/10.1177/0093854807306350

Lussier, P., & Mathesius, J. (2012). Criminal achievement, criminal career initiation, and detection avoidance: The onset of successful sex offending. *Journal of Crime and Justice, 35*(3), 376–394. https://doi.org/10.1080/0735648X.2012.666842

Lussier, P., & Mathesius, J. (2018). Integrating general and specific theories of sex offending: A path breaking perspective. In P. Lussier & Beauregard, E. (eds.), *Sexual offeding: A criminological perspective* (pp. 12–43). Routledge.

Lussier, P., McCuish, E., Mathesius, J., Corrado, R., & Nadeau, D. (2018). Developmental trajectories of child sexual behaviors on the path of sexual behavioral problems: Evidence from a prospective longitudinal study. *Sexual Abuse, 30*(6), 622–658. https://doi.org/10.1177/1079063217691963

Lussier, P., Tzoumakis, S., Cale, J., & Amirault, J. (2010). Criminal trajectories of adult sex offenders and the age effect: Examining the dynamic aspect of offending in adulthood. *International Criminal Justice Review, 20*(2), 147–168. https://doi.org/10.1177/1057567710368360

Magnan, V. (1885). *Des anomalies, des aberrations et des perversions sexuelles.* Progrès médical.

Malamuth, N. M. (1981). Rape proclivity among males. *Journal of Social Issues, 37*(4), 138–157. https://doi.org/10.1111/j.1540-4560.1981.tb01075.x

Malamuth, N. M. (1998). The confluence model as an organizing framework for research on sexually aggressive men: Risk moderators, imagined aggression, and pornography consumption. In *Human aggression* (pp. 229–245). Academic Press.

Marshall, W. L., & Barbaree, H. E. (1984). A behavioral view of rape. *International Journal of Law and Psychiatry, 7*(1), 51–77. https://doi.org/10.1016/0160-2527(84)90006-2

Marshall, W. L., & Barbaree, H. E. (1990). An integrated theory of the etiology of sexual offending. In W. L. Marshall, D. R. Laws, & H. E. Barbaree (Eds.), *Handbook of sexual assault* (pp. 257–275). Springer.

Maruna, S. (2001). *Making good.* American Psychological Association.

McCuish, E. C., & Lussier, P. (2017). Unfinished stories: From juvenile sex offenders to juvenile sex offending through a developmental life course perspective. *Aggression and Violent Behavior, 37,* 71–82. https://doi.org/10.1016/j.avb.2017.09.004

McCuish, E. C., Lussier, P., & Corrado, R. R. (2015). Examining antisocial behavioral antecedents of juvenile sexual offenders and juvenile non-sexual offenders. *Sexual Abuse, 27*(4), 414–438. doi:10.1177/1079063213517268

McGuire, R. J., Carlisle, J. U., & Young, B. G. (1964). Sexual deviations as conditioned behaviour: A hypothesis. *Behaviour Research and Therapy, 2*(2–4), 185–190.

McPhail, I. V., Olver, M. E., Brouillette-Alarie, S., & Looman, J. (2018). Taxometric analysis of the latent structure of pedophilic interest. *Archives of Sexual Behavior, 47*(8), 2223–2240. https://doi.org/10.1007/s10508-018-1225-4

Michaud, P., & Proulx, J. (2009). Penile-response profiles of sexual aggressors during phallometric testing. *Sexual Abuse, 21*(3), 308–334. https://doi.org/10.1177/1079063209342073

Moffitt, T. (1993). Adolescence-limited and life-course-persistent antisocial behavior: A developmental taxonomy. *Psychological Review, 100*(4), 674–701. https://doi.org/10.1037/0033-295X.100.4.674

Moreau, J. J. (1859). *La psychologie morbide dans ses rapports avec la philosophie de l'histoire: ou, De l'influence des névropathies sur le dynamisme intellectuel.* Masson.

Morel, B. A. (1857). *Traite des dégénérescences physiques, intellectuelles et morales de l'espèce humaine et des causes qui produisent ces variétés maladives par le Docteur BA Morel*. J.-B. Bailliere.

Morizot, J., & Kazemian, L. (2014). *The development of criminal and antisocial behavior*. Springer.

Murphy, W. D., DiLillo, D., Haynes, M. R., & Steere, E. (2001). An exploration of factors related to deviant sexual arousal among juvenile sex offenders. *Sexual Abuse: A Journal of Research and Treatment, 13*(2), 91–103. doi.org/10.1023/A:1026648220419

Nagin, D. S., Farrington, D. P., & Moffitt, T. E. (1995). Life-course trajectories of different types of offenders. *Criminology, 33*(1), 111–139. https://doi.org/10.1111/j.1745-9125.1995.tb01173.x

Nagin, D. S., & Paternoster, R. (1991). On the relationship of past to future participation in delinquency. *Criminology, 29*(2), 163–189. https://doi.org/10.1111/j.1745-9125.1991.tb01063.x

Patterson, G. R., & Yoerger, K. (1993). Developmental models for delinquent behavior. In S. Hodgins (Ed.), *Mental disorder and crime* (pp. 140–172). Sage.

Piquero, A. R., Farrington, D. P., & Blumstein, A. (2003). The criminal career paradigm. *Crime and Justice, 30*, 359–506.

Prince, M. (1898). Sexual perversion or vice? A pathological and therapeutic inquiry. *The Journal of Nervous and Mental Disease, 25*(4), 237–256.

Proulx, J., & Beauregard, E. (2009). Decision making during the offending process: An assessment among subtypes of sexual aggressors of women. In A. R. Beech, L. A. Craig, & K. D. Browne (Eds.), *Assessment and treatment of sex offenders: A handbook* (pp. 181–197). John Wiley & Sons.

Quinsey, V. L., Rice, M. E., & Harris, G. T. (1995). Actuarial prediction of sexual recidivism. *Journal of Interpersonal Violence, 10*(1), 85–105. https://doi.org/10.1177/088626095010001006

Robins, L. N. (1978). Sturdy childhood predictors of adult antisocial behaviour: Replications from longitudinal studies. *Psychological Medicine, 8*(4), 611–622. https://doi.org/10.1017/S0033291700018821

Sampson, R. J., & Laub, J. H. (2003). Life-course desisters? Trajectories of crime among delinquent boys followed to age 70. *Criminology, 41*(3), 555–592. https://doi.org/10.1111/j.1745-9125.2003.tb00997.x

Smallbone, S. W., & Dadds, M. R. (1998). Childhood attachment and adult attachment in incarcerated adult male sex offenders. *Journal of Interpersonal Violence, 13*(5), 555–573. https://doi.org/10.1177/088626098013005001

Tonry, M., Ohlin, L. E., & Farrington, D. P. (1991). *Human development and criminal behavior: New ways of advancing knowledge*. Springer.

Turner, R. E. (1961). The group treatment of sexual deviations. *Canadian Journal of Corrections, 3*(4), 485–491. https://doi.org/10.3138/cjcor.3.4.485

West, D. J., & Farrington, D. P. (1973). *Who becomes delinquent? Second report of the Cambridge study in delinquent development* (Vol. 34). Heinemann Educational.

Williams, K. M., Cooper, B. S., Howell, T. M., Yuille, J. C., & Paulhus, D. L. (2009). Inferring sexually deviant behavior from corresponding fantasies: The role of personality and pornography consumption. *Criminal Justice and Behavior, 36*(2), 198–222. https://doi.org/10.1177/0093854808327277

3

Toward a Theory of Chronophilic Sexual Orientation in Heterosexual Men

Alexander F. Schmidt[1] *and Roland Imhoff*[2]

[1,2] *Department of Psychology, Social & Legal Psychology, Johannes Gutenberg-University Mainz, Germany*

Sexual Interest and Sexual Deviance

Sexual interests are diverse. Humans are almost universally experiencing a vast amount of idiosyncratic sexual fantasies (Leitenberg & Henning, 1995) and there is a virtually endless repertoire of lived sexual behaviors, as a quick unsystematic internet search will immediately reveal. Although sexual interest is a fundamental part of every sexually reproducing species, it remains, to a large extent, an enigma. To this day, a general theory of sexual interest is lacking from a behavioral science perspective, specifically in terms of a causal theory on how sexual interests are developed (Bailey et al., 2016). The proposed causal factors stem from a nature (i.e., biological factors, such as genetics, hormone exposition, etc.) vs. nurture (i.e., learned sexual interests) framework (Bailey et al., 2016; Quinsey, 2003; Walters, 1997), but are difficult to test in rigorous research designs for obvious ethical reasons (Bailey et al., 2016; Pfaus et al., 2020).

The lack of a theoretical framework to explain sexual interest as an everyday phenomenon is exacerbated, from an applied point of view, when it comes to the forensic domain, where deviant sexual interests are: (a) empirically established as a prime recidivism risk factor for sexual reoffending (Mann et al., 2010); and (b) regarded as a focal precipitating factor to explain the onset of deviant sexual behavior (e.g., Seto, 2019). According to the so-called "sexual-preference hypothesis"—a widely-held view among lay people and professionals alike—sexually deviant behaviors result from respective underlying deviant sexual interests.

In this chapter we will argue that theories of sexual deviance suffer from a crucial problem due to an inherent confounding of two related but empirically distinguishable phenomena, namely, deviant sexual interest and offending behavior. This hinders focusing on the *sexual* etiology of sexual offending and runs the risk of resembling theories of general offending. Indeed, the history of sexual deviance theories is largely a history of known general crime correlates and, to a much lesser degree, based on a detailed understanding of the underlying sexual inclinations. Although we certainly will not be able to close this theoretical gap, we suggest that the field will profit from a better understanding of how sexual orientations and motivations are related to sexual behaviors. This will form a necessary step to explaining sexual deviation from the empirical average of socially adjusted sexual behavior. This will also be scientifically more parsimonious than developing specific theories for every sexual kink or deviation itself (Imhoff et al., 2017). We will exemplify an attempt at this effort by reporting preliminary data from an empirically testable evolutionary psychologically-informed theory. We propose this as a building block in solving the puzzle of chronophilias (Seto, 2017) in heterosexual males' sexual interest in females across varying age levels (Imhoff et al., 2017).[1]

Sexual Deviance: Understanding and Managing Deviant Sexual Interests and Paraphilic Disorders, First Edition. Edited by Leam A. Craig and Ross M. Bartels.
© 2021 John Wiley & Sons, Ltd. Published 2021 by John Wiley & Sons, Ltd.

The Confound in Theories of Sexual Deviance

For the ease of following our arguments in the remainder of the chapter, sexual deviance is defined as sexually criminal behavior (i.e., behavior involving sexual offenses), which is distinguished from deviant sexual interests (i.e., [mostly paraphilic] sexual fantasies that only if acted out constitute a sexual crime). Note that, according to the sexual-preference hypothesis, there should be a strong fantasy-behavior link. Thus, reverse inferences from offending behavior are often used as a proxy for sexual interest assessments (Lehmann et al., 2018). However, not every person who has sexually offended shows marked deviant sexual interests or even preferences (i.e., relatively stronger deviant interests than normatively unproblematic sexual interests; e.g., Schmidt et al., 2013). Also, not every individual with deviant sexual interests acts on these interests, as research involving non-offending community members has revealed (e.g., Dombert et al., 2016).

The following reasoning is largely informed by the seminal paper from Smid and Wever (2019). Numerous theories of sexual deviance have been proposed (see Ward et al., 2006 for the most comprehensive outlook to date) seeking to explain sexual offending. The common core that unites all these theories is a simple underlying structure that has been best exemplified in Seto's (2019) recent Motivation-Facilitation Model of sexual offending. Basically, two types of factors are postulated as driving sexual offending: (a) sexually motivating forces in the narrow sense, such as sexual interests in behaviors that are legally problematic (i.e., illegal paraphilic behaviors considered to be crimes in most Western jurisdictions, such as sex with children, animals, or corpses), or dispositionally high mating effort (i.e., sex drive); and (b) facilitating factors (not necessarily of a sexual nature) that lower the individual threshold to commit respective crimes. These forms of disinhibition can be classified as either temporary states, such as acute intoxication or sexual arousal (Imhoff & Schmidt, 2014; Seto, 2019), or stable traits, such as dispositions of high impulsivity and antisociality (Klein et al., 2015; Mann et al., 2010; Ward & Beech, 2006).

The confounding relationship between facilitating facets and common risk factors for non-sexual criminality (i.e., impulsivity, self-regulation problems, antisociality) is particularly problematic as it renders these models unspecific. This is reflected in the fact that only the deviant sexual interest (motivating) factor is specific for sexual reoffending, whereas the (non-sexual) disinhibiting factors predict general (non-sexual) reoffending (Brouillette-Alarie et al., 2018) in people who have sexually offended. While drawing largely upon research based on studies comparing people who have offended with those who have not offended, sexual offending is treated as just another subcategory of general offending (Smid & Wever, 2019). Hence, it is difficult to distinguish between sexual interests and factors linked to general crime-proneness (i.e., antisociality) as causal drivers of sexual deviance. This is corroborated, for example, by recent findings showing that child sexual offending was specifically related to reduced executive functioning (instead of pedophilic interest) only when non-offending pedophilic control groups had been sampled concurrently (Massau et al., 2017). Only recently has research started to disentangle deviant sexual interest and general risk factors for criminality in designs that incorporate non-institutionalized individuals with deviant sexual interests from the community (Jahnke et al., 2020). Utilizing such a design, Gerwinn et al. (2018) found "many of the factors reported as being related to paedophilia may [...] actually be associated with committing child sex offences and vice versa" (p. 75).

Distinguishing delinquency that is driven by sexual factors in the narrow sense from delinquency that is just another form of general crime-proneness (i.e., antisociality) is important for understanding vexing conundrums. These include, on the one hand, why so many people who have sexually offended desist from further sexual offending even without treatment (Mews et al., 2017) and, on the other hand, why so many relatively well-adjusted community men admit coercive sexual acts (Anderson et al., 2019). Instead of focusing on sexual offending as another form of general delinquency, Smid and Wever (2019) argue that "enrichment of sex offender theory can be found in the description of sexual offending behavior as *sexual* behavior, especially if we aim to clarify possible mechanisms behind the development of sexual deviance" (p. 735).

In part, there have been attempts to fill this theoretical gap by evolutionary psychological accounts of men's sexual offending (Camilleri, 2012; Quinsey & Lalumière, 1995), which postulate sexual offending to be adaptations or by-products of male strategies to increase their reproductive success under certain boundary conditions. However, these approaches have been much more convincing when applied to the victimization of post-pubescent females compared to decidedly non-adaptive victim selections, such as children. In the following section, we outline our theoretical approach for heterosexual males' chronophilic[2] interest. This approach has been informed by the notion that sexual orientations are fueled by evolutionary-adaptive mechanisms, whereas sexual motivations are acquired from gratifying sexual experiences.

Sexual Orientations and Sexual Motivations

Theories of human sexual interests need to be able to deal with the fact that human sexual interest comes in all shapes and forms. Instead of responding to this huge variety with a multi-dimensional array of sexual orientations to do justice to mostly all walks of (male) human sexuality (Seto, 2017), we propose that the larger share of variance in sexual interests stems from sexual experiences in the sense of learned behavior (Imhoff et al., 2017). Theoretically, an endless set of sexual behaviors and fantasies can be acquired through sexual learning (i.e., classical and operant conditioning, model learning; Hoffmann et al., 2004; Pfaus et al., 2020). Regardless of the exact processes of how these sexual tastes (or sexual motivations as we will refer to them) are acquired, we suppose that there is no critical developmental phase for these highly idiosyncratic associations to be formed. Rather, they are subject to life-long learning. Consequently, such sexual motivations are, in principle, flexible and even reversible (Imhoff et al., 2017). Sexual motivations, in the sense of sexual fantasies related to sexual activities or modes, are frequently refined and may become increasingly sophisticated as long as individuals are sexually active. However, the acquisition process of sexual motivations is restricted and certain necessary boundary conditions need to be met in order for sexual fantasies and behaviors to become competent sexual stimuli that may be "loaded" or associated with sexual incentives (see Smid & Wever, 2019 for an intriguingly rich—but in its entirety hard to test—theory of sexual deviance and its associated phenomena). These boundaries are largely a function of sexual orientations.

In opposition to sexual motivations, we propose to use the term sexual orientation for deeply engrained sexual inclinations that are not amenable (or exceedingly difficult) to change (Imhoff et al., 2017). Prototypical sexual orientations are highly typified gender (hetero- vs. homosexual) or sexual maturity (pedophilic vs. teleiophilic) orientations. Empirically, these can be best understood as discrete classes (or taxa) rather than dimensional continuums (McPhail et al., 2018; Norris et al., 2015; Schmidt et al., 2013). Further, most scholars agree that sexual orientations: (a) have an early onset preceding the start of sexual activities as a form of "sexual awakening" (Bailey et al., 2016; McPhail, 2018); and (b) cannot be changed effectively later in life. As sexual orientations are bound to general object features, such as gender or pre-, peri,- or postpubescent sexual maturity status, they form the frame within which sexual motivations may develop. This can be seen in analogy to vegetarian vs. meat food "orientations" that represent in each category a plethora of different dishes and cooking recipes. Based on this notion, it is likely that a heterosexual teleiophilic man, for instance, may develop a sexual motivation for high heels associated with his general sexual targets. However, it is unlikely that his fetish will generalize to elegant Italian men's shoes (Imhoff et al., 2017).

Importantly, sexual motivations and orientations should not only differ descriptively (flexible vs. inflexible, late vs. early onset, highly vs. less detailed in terms of modes and forms of desired sexual behavior) but should also be caused by different psychological mechanisms. Furthermore, such a theory has not only to be able to explain sexual deviations from the norm but also the most frequent type of sexuality. It is unlikely that we will understand why some men become pedophilic or hebephilic until we understand why most men become teleiophilic (Imhoff et al., 2017).

A Sexual Orientation Theory of Heterosexual Male Chronophilias

Hitherto, evolutionary-psychological theories of sexual orientations have failed to convincingly explain the sexual victimization of prepubescent children, and the origins of pedophilic interest are as yet unknown (Quinsey, 2003). Inspired by the fact that men's mate selection strategies are highly dependent on visible cues (e.g., Ogas & Gaddam, 2012) and Seto's (2008) idea that pedophilic interest results from a malfunction of males' sexual preference for youthfulness, we hypothesize that sexual target identification in heterosexual males is a function of the interplay of several modules that are sensitive to differential visual target features (Imhoff et al., 2017). Accordingly, if it was an evolutionary successful strategy to detect females' ability to become pregnant, modules that direct sexual attraction to visible indicators of reproductive maturity and fertility should have been adaptive to men's reproductive fitness. Youth and sexual maturity are, to a large degree, culture-dependent social constructs rather than perceivable features of potential mating partners. Therefore, these mate detection modules need to be sensitive to visible target characteristics that are easily accessible in everyday life. From Seto's (2017, Table 2) list of hypothetical features that are of interest to heterosexual men, breast size might be such a candidate signaling reproductive ability. Waist-to-hip ratio (WHR) might be another one, as wide enough hips are associated with reproductive ability, while small enough waists indicate the absence of pregnancy and menopause. Finally, neotenous facial features and smoothness of skin signal youth and health. This list is not definitive, as other features, such as eye size and head-to-shoulder ratio, are also conceivable. All these characteristics carry important information concerning the reproductive potential (e.g., years of reproductive life left), fertility (i.e., physical maturity of reproductive apparatus), and health status (i.e., genetic fitness) of female mates.

Importantly, these indicators have differential distributions over the female age span and, thus, cannot all be maximized at the same time. Smooth skin and neotenous facial features peak in early childhood, while breast development starts later with the onset of puberty and continues throughout adulthood. Similarly, the WHR of newborns is roughly 1 but decreases to the ideal of 0.75 for 16- to 21-year olds (Fredriks et al., 2005) only to slowly increase again thereafter (Shimokata et al., 1989). Hence, a trade-off needs to be found in order to arrive at the choice of an optimal mating partner. Within a system of checks and balances between these modules, seeking an equilibrium between or an optimal combination of these features will arrive at young adult women (minimal WHR, fully developed breasts, still sufficiently smooth skin and neotenous facial features). This combination explains normative teleiophilic heterosexual mate preferences (Imhoff et al., 2017).

How can other heterosexual chronophilic orientations be modeled based on this theoretical account? For whatever reasons (that must remain another open part of the puzzle of chronophilias and currently are hypothesized to be neurodevelopmental perturbations) it is conceivable that men differ in their module's sensitivity to parse information about breast size and WHR. Such decreased skills will maximize sexual attractiveness of mates with smooth skin and facial neoteny (i.e., prepubescent children) leading to a pedophilic orientation (potentially even relatively indifferent toward target gender). In contrast, males with a sole insensitivity to breast size will determine their optimal mating partners between youth indicators and WHR, likely resulting in a hebephilic orientation, predominantly toward female adolescents. Notably, men who do not take into account WHR, skin smoothness, or neoteny might be likely to end up with a mesophilic preference (i.e., sexual interest in middle-aged females), as breast size continues to grow at least slightly in postpubescence.

In summary, this account is able to explain various chronophilic orientations with the exception of a preference for elderly women (i.e., gerontophilia). Strikingly, no single combination of these modules will produce a strong attraction to the body schemas of elderly women. Certainly, this does not mean that such an attraction does not exist (which the internet will readily prove). Rather, such sexual inclinations might better be framed as sexual motivations that are, in principle, flexible and only develop in later stages of life (as opposed to the rigid sexual orientations that have an early onset). An empirically testable question derived from this is whether there is a sizeable number (better a majority) of self-identified men who describe themselves as gerontophilic and report an early onset of these sexual interests in puberty or preferably before they started to become sexually active. Not expecting to find this, we hypothesize that gerontophilic interest is better understood as an acquired, transient sexual motivation that is likely to be co-shaped via the compromising of sexual youth preferences and aging males' success in attracting sexual partners (Imhoff et al., 2017). As our proposed list of modules certainly might not be exhaustive, it is conceivable that the mate detection system also is attuned to indicators of child caregiving experience—an indicator whose sole overfunction might increase the age of the ideal mate to be in the gerontophilic realm. This, again, is an empirically testable prediction.

Finally, further empirically accessible predictions can be derived from this model. A mate detection system based on the modules described above should be highly sensitive to a maximization of all relevant characteristics at the same time. Hence, a super-ideal of the corresponding features should provoke the strongest response of this system (i.e., strongest perceived sexual attractiveness). As these super-combinations of features are not common or even possible in the natural human environment, turning to fictitious characters inspired by the hentai genre[3] might pose a way of creating relevant stimuli. This economically thriving cultural subgenre depicts fully fictitious sexual targets that represent a highly idealized combination of extremely smooth skin, overly neotenous facial features, enormous breast sizes, and excessively low WHR. Notably, an unsystematic internet search did not turn up super-ideals in the gerontophilic range, although some mesophilic hentai pictures were found. This anecdotal evidence challenges the idea that upper-end chronophilic interest could be construed as a genuine gerontophilic sexual orientation, as proposed by Seto (2017).

More importantly, however, these super-ideals point to a feasible empirical testing strategy. Stimuli characters could be construed along orthogonally manipulated experimental factors representing variations of the postulated mate detection modules. In such a full factorial design, teleiophilic men should report the strongest attraction to the unrealistically super-idealized character. In contrast, pedophilic men should be most sensitive to the youth indicators, particularly those that are associated with affective endearment responses, such as eye size and head-to-shoulder ratio (Ponseti et al., 2018; Smid & Wever, 2019). Breast size and WHR should have either no or even opposite effects for pedophilic men, whereas hebephilic men should show increased sexual attractiveness perception on these factors. Finally, if our framework is corroborated, mesophilic men should reveal a strong attraction to large breasts (as well as a lack of sexual attraction to flat-chested middle-aged women). Notably, such a research design will not only be restricted to self-reports but is, in principle, open to physiological and other more objective measures of sexual interest. For example, viewing time measures are particularly easy to incorporate into such a design (Imhoff et al., 2010, 2012; Schmidt et al., 2017).

Feasibility Exploration

Can this basic assumption of a modular system, in which different markers pull attraction in different directions but that typically settles for an ideal compromise, be tested? In a pilot study, we used the hentai manga images described above as inspirations and created two stimulus sets that orthogonally manipulated four dimensions (Imhoff et al., 2020). Two of these images were expected to signal maturity (pronounced WHR, breast size), and two were expected to signal youthfulness (large eyes in relation to face size; large head in relation to shoulder):

- Waist-to-Hip-Ratio (5 steps: 0.6, 0.7, 0.8, 0.9, 1.0)
- Breast size (5 steps: none, only nipples, small, medium, large)
- Eye size (3 steps: small, regular, large)
- Head size (relative to shoulders; 3 steps: regular, large, extra-large)

The orthogonal combination of these factors, thus, yielded 225 images per stimulus set (450 in total; see Figure 3.1 for examples). The first two factors signal maturity and, therefore, pull

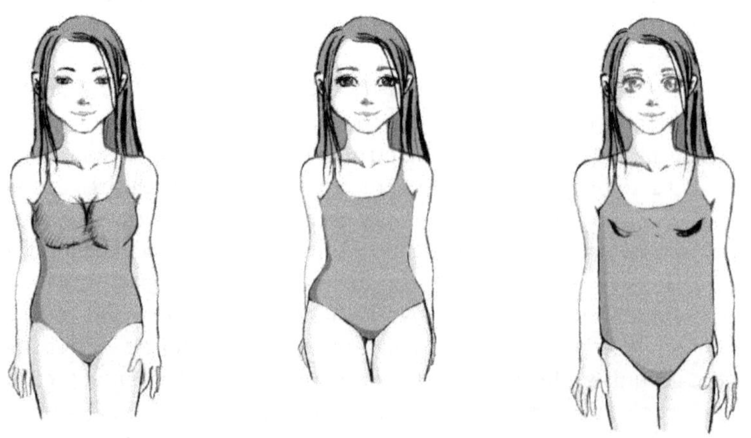

Figure 3.1 Example stimuli from one of the picture sets.

attractiveness impressions in the direction of a pronounced (i.e., small) WHR and large breasts. The last two factors signal youthfulness and, hence, should create impressions of attractiveness for large eyes and large heads (in relation to shoulder). Our modular model now allows a few testable and falsifiable predictions. First, all factors should have an effect on attractiveness ratings in teleiophilic heterosexual men (H1). Second, in an idealized world liberated from physical constraints, attractiveness in the eyes of heterosexual teleiophilic men should peak at the "ideal" combination of maximal youthfulness and maximal maturity (H2, akin to Figure 3.3).

Further predictions follow the "module dysfunction" explanation of chronophilias described above. If sexual interest in mature women (mesophilia) can be understood by a dysfunctional youthfulness module (and hence a lack of a force pulling in the opposite direction of maturity), only the first two factors should play a role (H3). On the contrary, for men sexually interested in minors (pedohebephilia), only the last two factors should influence attractiveness (H4). Their interest in young children would, thus, result from a perfectly normal preference for youthfulness combined with a lack of an antagonistic force pulling in the direction of maturity. It might also be that such men are repulsed by maturity indicators. As such, they would exert an effect but in the opposite direction. This would challenge our mechanistic model of defect modules and, thus, require a less parsimonious adaptation of the theory. Importantly, however, these predictions are testable and falsifiable.

We conducted a very first, preliminary feasibility exploration by having these images rated on sexual attractiveness. Although participation in this study was not restricted to them, here we only report results for (predominantly) heterosexual teleiophilic men ($n = 25$). Each participant rated all 225 pictures resulting from the orthogonal combination of the four factors ($5 \times 5 \times 3 \times 3$) on sexual attractiveness (from 1 to 7) in random order. Subjecting these ratings to a WHR × Breast Size × Eye Size × Head Size rmANOVA yielded significant main effects of all four factors. Specifically, WHR was the strongest predictor of attractiveness ratings with $F(1.97, 47.29) = 46.60, p < .001, \eta_p^2 = .66$, with strong evidence for a linear contrast of increasing attractiveness with increasingly pronounced WHR, $F(1, 24) = 72.54, p < .001, \eta_p^2 = .75$ (see Figure 3.2a).

Likewise, but in a less pronounced fashion, increasing breast size increased impressions of attractiveness, $F(1.67, 40.12) = 8.94, p = .001, \eta_p^2 = .27$, in a mostly linear fashion, $F(1, 24) = 12.49, p < .001, \eta_p^2 = .34$ (with a small dip for the images that only showed nipples; see Figure 3.2b). For both youthfulness indicators, however, the effects were smaller and more compatible with quadratic than with linear effects (see Figure 3.2c and 3.2d). The effects of eye size, $F(1.54, 36.90) = 11.59, p < .001, \eta_p^2 = .32$, were composed of both a linear, $F(1, 24) = 8.25, p = .008, \eta_p^2 = .26$, as well as a quadratic contrast, $F(1, 24) = 15.20, p = .001, \eta_p^2 = .39$. The effect of head size, however, $F(2, 23) = 5.09, p = .015, \eta_p^2 = .31$, was only due to a quadratic effect, $F(1, 24) = 9.24, p = .006, \eta_p^2 = .28$.

In total, the data (see Figure 3.2) do not fully conform to our hypotheses. Nevertheless, it might be too early to give up on the idea. Specifically, the large eyes were not just large, but also less dark and so might not have signaled youthfulness. Instead, they may have made the image appear uncanny. The same issue of uncanniness might constitute an issue for physically impossible or rare combinations of, for instance, large breasts on an otherwise child-like figure. Looking in an isolated fashion at which image received the highest ratings, it becomes apparent that this almost fully corroborates H2. The most attractively rated image maximizes breast size, minimizes WHR, maximizes head size, and has "regular" (but admittedly still large) eyes (see Figure 3.3). It is also noteworthy that WHR had by far the strongest influence, which seems compatible with our general reasoning. As WHR signals maturity and youthfulness at the same time and exhibits a maximally pronounced pattern for early adulthood, a parsimonious approach would be to rely mostly on this feature (i.e., if one could process only one signal, this

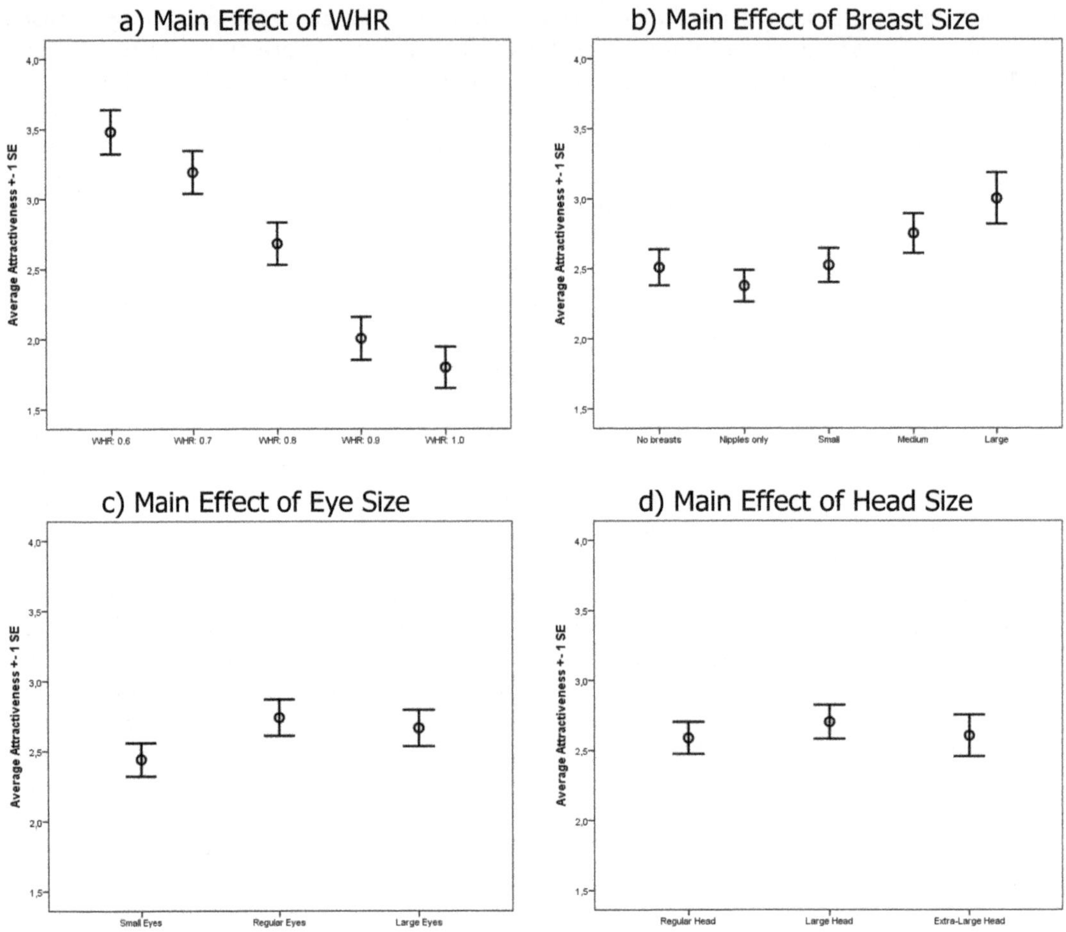

Figure 3.2 Main effects of manipulated factors.

would be most diagnostic). Certainly, this research approach needs to be further developed and validated before the more interesting hypotheses about deviant sexual interest (H3, H4) can be reliably tackled.

Conclusion and Outlook

We see a major advantage in providing a model of not only testable, but most importantly falsifiable predictions. At present, the very idea is speculative at best. Also, our preliminary data provide little more than a clichéd image of male heterosexual preferences (wasp waist, large breasts, young appearance) and it may very well be that we will never move beyond this (and thus let dust settle on this speculation). If, however, we succeed in corroborating the idea (or rather failing to falsify its predictions), including deviant chronophilic sexual interests, it might provide a step forward in deriving a model of deviant sexual orientations that does not rely on general crime risk factors but instead stems from mechanisms that explain normative sexual interests.

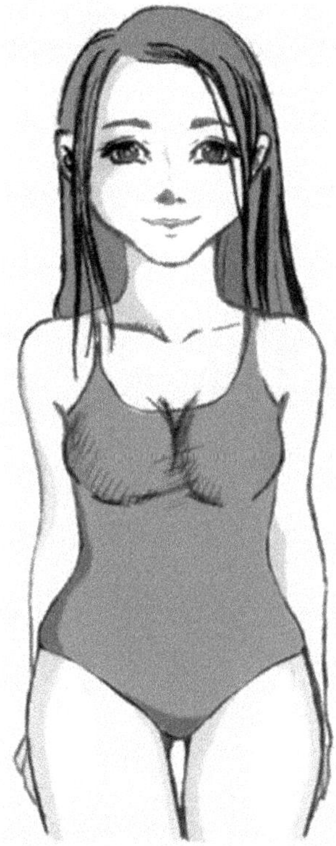

Figure 3.3 Most attractively rated image.

Although our model at present seems artificially and painfully restricted to heterosexual chronophilias, it might actually also provide a lead as to why homosexual pedohebephilia is so much more frequent than homosexual teleiophilia among men who have sexually abused children (Freund & Watson, 1992). The (admittedly oversimplified) reliance on visual cues creates an asymmetric situation when it comes to sex typicality. While the maturity indicators do not just signal maturity, but also femaleness (as breast and pronounced WHRs are typical for women but not men), the youthfulness indicators do not point to a specific sex (i.e., neotenous features are exhibited by young males and females). Taking the notion seriously that pedophilic men have dysfunctional maturity indicators would actually lead to the strong prediction that they should *not* have a greater preference for female over male body shapes (but only for smooth skin and neotenous features).

In summary, we propose to take up the challenge implied in our firm conviction that an explanation for the development of deviant sexual interest will remain out of reach unless we have a better understanding of the development of normative sexual interest and how it relates to sexual gratification. Until we can explain why a man who has sexually offended finds a specific sexual target attractive (or whether there are other [co-occurring] reasons that are related to his sexual offending), it will be difficult to understand his specific sexual needs and the specific risk factors that are relevant for specific predictions regarding his (future) sexual offending pattern. Interestingly, when deviant sexual preferences (i.e., the relative stronger reaction to deviant target categories over normative ones) are referred to, most clinicians tend to focus on sexual overreactions to the preferred deviant categories, neglecting the implications that stem from the deficiency to get aroused by normative sexual targets. Smid and Wever

(2019) postulate intriguing ways of how particularly this deficit in normative arousability might relate to sexual offending in circumstances when deviant sexual interest is used as a sexual coping mechanism to upregulate erectile deficiencies. Literally speaking, much can be gained from putting the sexual component back into sexual offending.

Notes

1. The much less specific sexual orientation of heterosexual women calls for a different theory of sexual interest (Bailey, 2009). For the same reasons as outlined in Seto (2017) we will restrict our reasoning to heterosexual males' development of deviant sexual interests.
2. Chronophilia is a term used by Seto (2017) to refer to (paraphilic) sexual interests directed at different sexual maturity and age levels (i.e., pedophilia, hebephilia, teleiophilia, mesophilia, gerontophilia).
3. Hentai (Japanese for "abnormity, perversion"). Outside of Japanese culture this usually refers to pornographic media such as comics (manga) or films (anime).

References

Further reading recommendations are marked with an (*)

Anderson, R. E., Silver, K. E., Ciampaglia, A. M., Vitale, A. M., & Delahanty, D. L. (2019). The frequency of sexual perpetration in college men: A systematic review of reported prevalence rates from 2000 to 2017. *Trauma, Violence, & Abuse*, 1524838019860619. https://doi.org/10.1177%2F1524838019860619

Bailey, J. M. (2009). What is sexual orientation and do women have one? In D. A. Hope (Ed.), *Contemporary perspectives on lesbian, gay, and bisexual identities* (pp. 43–63). Springer. https://doi.org/10.1007/978-0-387-09556-1_3

Bailey, J. M., Vasey, P. L., Diamond, L. M., Breedlove, S. M., Vilain, E., & Epprecht, M. (2016). Sexual orientation, controversy, and science. *Psychological Science in the Public Interest*, 17(2), 45–101. https://doi.org/10.1177%2F1529100616637616

Brouillette-Alarie, S., Proulx, J., & Hanson, R. K. (2018). Three central dimensions of sexual recidivism risk: Understanding the latent constructs of Static-99R and Static-2002R. *Sexual Abuse*, 30(6), 676–704. https://doi.org/10.1177%2F1079063217691965

Camilleri, J. A. (2012). Evolutionary psychological perspectives on sexual offending: From etiology to intervention. In T. K. Shackelford, & V. A. Weekes-Shackelford (Eds.), *Oxford library of psychology. The Oxford handbook of evolutionary perspectives on violence, homicide, and war* (pp. 173–196). Oxford University Press.

Dombert, B., Schmidt, A. F., Banse, R., Briken, P., Hoyer, J., Neutze, J., & Osterheider, M. (2016). How common is men's self-reported sexual interest in prepubescent children? *The Journal of Sex Research*, 53(2), 214–223. https://doi.org/10.1080/00224499.2015.1020108

Fredriks, A. M., van Buuren, S., Fekkes, M., Verloove-Vanhorick, S. P., & Wit, J. M. (2005). Are age references for waist circumference, hip circumference and waist-hip ratio in Dutch children useful in clinical practice? *European Journal of Pediatrics*, 164(4), 216–222. https://doi.org/10.1007/s00431-004-1586-7

Freund, K., & Watson, R. J. (1992). The proportions of heterosexual and homosexual pedophiles among sex offenders against children: An exploratory study. *Journal of Sex & Marital Therapy*, 18(1), 34–43. https://doi.org/10.1080/00926239208404356

(*) Gerwinn, H., Weiß, S., Tenbergen, G., Amelung, T., Födisch, C., Pohl, A., Massau, C., Kneer, J., Mohnke, S., Kärgel, C., & Wittfoth, M. (2018). Clinical characteristics associated with paedophilia and child sex offending – Differentiating sexual preference from offence status. *European Psychiatry*, 51, 74–85. https://doi.org/10.1016/j.eurpsy.2018.02.002

Hoffmann, H., Janssen, E., & Turner, S. L. (2004). Classical conditioning of sexual arousal in women and men: Effects of varying awareness and biological relevance of the conditioned stimulus. *Archives of Sexual Behavior*, 33(1), 43–53. https://doi.org/10.1023/B:ASEB.0000007461.59019.d3

(*) Imhoff, R., Banse, R., & Schmidt, A. F. (2017). Toward a theoretical understanding of sexual orientation and sexual motivation. *Archives of Sexual Behavior*, 46(1), 29–33. https://doi.org/10.1007/s10508-016-0881-5

Imhoff, R., Posselt, M., & Walter, M. (2020). [Pilot Study Manga Project]. Unpublished raw data.

Imhoff, R., & Schmidt, A. F. (2014). Sexual disinhibition under sexual arousal: Evidence for domain specificity in men and women. *Archives of Sexual Behavior*, 43(6), 1123–1136. https://doi.org/10.1007/s10508-014-0329-8

Imhoff, R., Schmidt, A. F., Nordsiek, U., Luzar, C., Young, A. W., & Banse, R. (2010). Viewing time revisited: Prolonged response latencies for sexually attractive targets under restricted conditions. *Archives of Sexual Behavior*, 39(6), 1275–1288. https://doi.org/10.1007/s10508-009-9595-2

Imhoff, R., Schmidt, A. F., Weiß, S., Young, A. W., & Banse, R. (2012). Vicarious viewing time: Prolonged response latencies for sexually attractive targets as a function of task- or stimulus-specific processing. *Archives of Sexual Behavior*, 41(6), 1389–1401. https://doi.org/10.1007/s10508-011-9879-1

Jahnke, S., Schmidt, A. F., Klöckner, A., & Hoyer, J. (2020). *Disentangling neurodevelopmental differences, sexual offending, and pedophilia: Findings from two online surveys.* Manuscript submitted for publication.

Klein, V., Schmidt, A. F., Turner, D., & Briken, P. (2015). Are sex drive and hypersexuality associated with pedophilic interest and child sexual abuse in a male community sample? *PloS One*, 10(7), e0129730. https://doi.org/10.1371/journal.pone.0129730

Lehmann, R. J. B., Dahle, K.-P., & Schmidt, A. F. (2018). Primer on the contribution of crime scene behavior to the forensic assessment of sexual offenders. *European Psychologist*, 23(2), 154–166. https://doi.org/10.1027/1016-9040/a000324

Leitenberg, H., & Henning, K. (1995). Sexual fantasy. *Psychological Bulletin*, 117(3), 469–496. https://psycnet.apa.org/doi/10.1037/0033-2909.117.3.469

Mann, R. E., Hanson, R. K., & Thornton, D. (2010). Assessing risk for sexual recidivism: Some proposals on the nature of psychologically meaningful risk factors. *Sexual Abuse: A Journal of Research and Treatment*, 22(2), 191–217. https://doi.org/10.1177%2F1079063210366039

Massau, C., Tenbergen, G., Kärgel, C., Weiß, S., Gerwinn, H., Pohl, A., Amelung, T., Mohnke, S., Kneer, J., Wittfoth, M., & Ristow, I. (2017). Executive functioning in pedophilia and child sexual offending. *Journal of the International Neuropsychological Society: JINS*, 23(6), 460–470. https://doi.org/10.1017/s1355617717000315

McPhail, I. V. (2018). Age of onset in pedohebephilic interests. *Archives of Sexual Behavior*, 47(5), 1313–1317. https://doi.org/10.1007/s10508-018-1198-3

McPhail, I. V., Olver, M. E., Brouillette-Alarie, S., & Looman, J. (2018). Taxometric analysis of the latent structure of pedophilic interest. *Archives of Sexual Behavior*, 47(8), 2223–2 240. https://doi.org/10.1007/s10508-018-1225-4

Mews, A., Di Bella, L., & Purver, M. (2017). *Impact evaluation of the prison-based core sex offender treatment programme.* Ministry of Justice. https://www.go.uk/government/uploads/system/attachment_data/file/623877/sotp-report-print.pdf

Norris, A. L., Marcus, D. K., & Green, B. A. (2015). Homosexuality as a discrete class. *Psychological Science*, 26(12), 1843–1853. https://doi.org/10.1177%2F0956797615598617

Ogas, O., & Gaddam, S. (2012). *A billion wicked thoughts: What the internet tells us about sexual relationships*. Plume.

Pfaus, J. G., Quintana, G. R., Mac Cionnaith, C. E., Gerson, C. A., Dubé, S., & Coria-Avila, G. A. (2020). Conditioning of sexual interests and paraphilias in humans is difficult to see, virtually impossible to test, and probably exactly how it happens: A comment on Hsu and Bailey (2020). *Archives of Sexual Behavior*, 49(5), 1403–1407. https://doi.org/10.1007/s10508-020-01739-2

Ponseti, J., Bruhn, D., Nolting, J., Gerwinn, H., Pohl, A., Stirn, A., Granert, O., Laufs, H., Deuschl, G., Wolff, S., & Jansen, O. (2018). Decoding pedophilia: Increased anterior insula response to infant animal pictures. *Frontiers in Human Neuroscience*, 11, 645. https://doi.org/10.3389/fnhum.2017.00645

Quinsey, V. L. (2003). The etiology of anomalous sexual preferences in men. *Annals of the New York Academy of Sciences*, 989(1), 105–117. https://doi.org/10.1111/j.1749-6632.2003.tb07297.x

Quinsey, V. L., & Lalumière, M. L. (1995). Evolutionary perspectives on sexual offending. *Sexual Abuse: A Journal of Research and Treatment*, 7(4), 301–315. https://doi.org/10.1177%2F107906329500700406

Schmidt, A. F., Babchishin, K. M., & Lehmann, R. J. (2017). A meta-analysis of viewing time measures of sexual interest in children. *Archives of Sexual Behavior*, 46(1), 287–300. https://doi.org/10.1007/s10508-016-0806-3

Schmidt, A. F., Mokros, A., & Banse, R. (2013). Is pedophilic sexual preference continuous? A taxometric analysis based on direct and indirect measures. *Psychological Assessment*, 25(4), 1146–1153. https://psycnet.apa.org/doi/10.1037/a0033326

Seto, M. C. (2008). *Pedophilia and sexual offending against children: Theory, assessment, and intervention*. American Psychological Association. https://psycnet.apa.org/doi/10.1037/11639-000

Seto, M. C. (2017). The puzzle of male chronophilias. *Archives of Sexual Behavior*, 46(1), 3–22. https://doi.org/10.1007/s10508–016–0799–y

Seto, M. C. (2019). The motivation-facilitation model of sexual offending. *Sexual Abuse*, 31(1), 3–24. https://doi.org/10.1177%2F1079063217720919

Shimokata, H., Tobin, J. D., Muller, D. C., Elahi, D., Coon, P. J., & Andres, R. (1989). Studies in the distribution of body fat: I. effects of age, sex, and obesity. *Journal of Gerontology*, 44(2), M66–M73. https://doi.org/10.1093/geronj/44.2.M66

(*) Smid, W. J., & Wever, E. C. (2019). Mixed emotions: An incentive motivational model of sexual deviance. *Sexual Abuse*, 31(7), 731–764. https://doi.org/10.1177%2F1079063218775972

Walters, G. D. (1997). The paraphilias: A dialectically informed review of etiology, development, and process. *Sexual Addiction & Compulsivity: The Journal of Treatment and Prevention*, 4(3), 221–243. https://doi.org/10.1080/10720169708404229

Ward, T., & Beech, A. (2006). An integrated theory of sexual offending. *Aggression and Violent Behavior*, 11(1), 44–63. https://doi.org/10.1016/j.avb.2005.05.002

Ward, T., Polaschek, D., & Beech, A. R. (2006). *Theories of sexual offending*. John Wiley & Sons.

4

Understanding Sexual Thoughts and Sexual Fantasizing

The Dual-Process Model of Sexual Thinking

Ross M. Bartels[1], Anthony R. Beech[2], and Leigh Harkins[3]

[1] School of Psychology, University of Lincoln, UK
[2] Centre for Applied Psychology, University of Birmingham, UK
[3] University of Ontario Institute of Technology, Canada

Introduction

Sexual interest and sexual fantasy are intricately linked. The target of someone's sexual interest (whether a person, object, or behavior) is typically represented within the content of their sexual fantasies (Noorishad et al., 2019). As such, sexual fantasies provide a source of sexual arousal (Gee et al., 2003). In addition, conditioning-based theories propose that the repeated pairing of sexual arousal (via masturbation) with a sexual fantasy can produce a sexual interest (Laws & Marshall, 1990; McGuire et al., 1964; Storms, 1981). While this is unlikely to be the case for broad categories of sexual orientation, it is conceivable that specific targets/behaviors can acquire erotic value via conditioning processes, especially considering the range of sexual interests, fetishes, and kinks that people report (Imhoff et al., 2017; Smid & Wever, 2019).

It is crucial, therefore, to have a clear understanding of sexual fantasy. However, there is little to no theoretical work on sexual fantasy. Fortunately, a plethora of research exists on the topic, covering the content (Arndt et al., 1985; Rokach, 1990), frequency (Harvey & Jeglic, 2020; Joyal et al., 2015), function (Davidson & Hoffman, 1986; Gee et al., 2003), and appraisal of sexual fantasies (Renaud & Byers, 2001), along with its link to other factors, such as personality (Baughman et al., 2014), attachment (Birnbaum, 2007), attitudes/beliefs (Zurbriggen & Yost, 2004), and corresponding behavior (Bouchard et al., 2017; Noorishad et al., 2019). In addition, there is a vast literature base on mental imagery and episodic simulation that provides valuable insight into human thought. Synthesizing key aspects of this literature, we recently developed a theoretical account of sexual thoughts and fantasizing termed the *Dual-Process Model of Sexual Thinking* (DPM-ST). This theory was first presented at professional conferences (Bartels et al., 2014), before being outlined in a book chapter on theories of deviant sexual fantasy (Bartels & Beech, 2016). In the present chapter, we provide a more focused and updated account of the DPM-ST. First, however, we must have a clear conceptualization of sexual thinking.

Definitions of Sexual Fantasy

Historically, the literature lacked a consistent definition of sexual fantasy. Either no definition was provided, or they varied from study to study (Renaud & Byers, 1999). For example, Purifoy et al. (1992) stated that "the content of sexual fantasies is always fantastic or unreal" (p. 370). Yet research found that "previous sexual experience" is often used as fantasy content (Crepault & Couture, 1980; Davidson, 1985; Ellis & Symons, 1990; Hariton & Singer, 1974). Others, drawing upon Singer's (1966) work on daydreaming, defined sexual fantasy as internally

Sexual Deviance: Understanding and Managing Deviant Sexual Interests and Paraphilic Disorders,
First Edition. Edited by Leam A. Craig and Ross M. Bartels.
© 2021 John Wiley & Sons, Ltd. Published 2021 by John Wiley & Sons, Ltd.

generated thought that is unrelated to environmental stimuli (e.g., Jones & Barlow, 1990). However, sexual fantasies are often related to the environment, such as during intercourse (Crepault & Couture, 1980; Davidson, 1985; Hariton & Singer, 1974; Knafo & Jaffe, 1984).

Due to these varied findings, researchers were left to draw broad conclusions. For example, Wilson (1978) asserted that a sexual fantasy can be spontaneous or deliberate; fleeting or elaborate; a previous experience or purely imagined; and realistic or bizarre. This led to considerably broad definitions of sexual fantasy. Leitenberg and Henning (1995), for example, defined sexual fantasy as "almost any mental imagery that is sexually arousing to the individual" (p. 470). This is still the most widely used definition. However, broad definitions like this essentially render "sexual fantasy" as an umbrella term for nearly all forms of sexual cognition (Bartels & Gannon, 2011; Renaud & Byers, 2001). This is limiting, both theoretically and practically. In order to address this, we must unpack the various features of sexual thought that have been conflated.

Separating Content from Process

Broad definitions of sexual fantasy conflate content-based features (e.g., previously experienced vs. imagined content) and process-based features of thought (e.g., fleeting vs. prolonged thoughts). For these features to be conflated, they must have a unifying element. Based on Leitenberg and Henning's (1995) definition, this appears to be their erotic connotation. However, a thought process in and of itself is unlikely to be sexually appealing. This leaves the fantasy content. Indeed, if someone reports a specific sexual fantasy (e.g., about rape), it does not matter if it is fleeting, prolonged, spontaneous, or deliberate; the content remains constant. This means that broad definitions of sexual fantasy are ultimately focused on *what* someone thinks, not *how* they think about it.

This highlights an important point that has received little attention. Namely, "having" a sexual fantasy is not the same as "engaging in" a sexual fantasy (i.e., sexual fantasizing). A sexual fantasy is essentially a cognitive structure containing information about what someone finds sexually appealing (whether enduring or transient). Sexual fantasizing involves envisaging mental imagery and so is more akin to a cognitive process (Carlson & Coleman, 1977; MacInnis & Price, 1987). Thus, not only do sexual fantasy and sexual fantasizing differ semantically (i.e., one is a noun and one is a verb, respectively), they are also conceptually distinct. This means that an individual can sexually fantasize about a sexual fantasy.

This distinction between structure and process is rarely considered by researchers. Yet it needs to be. Reporting a specific sexual fantasy may indicate the presence of a sexual interest but provides no insight into how often the sexual fantasy is fantasized about (if at all). As such, it offers no indication of how strong the potential sexual interest is. Imagine that John and David both share the same sexual fantasy (noun) of choking their partner. Arguably, both men find this act sexually appealing. Now imagine that they are asked to report how often they fantasize (verb) about this sexual fantasy. For John, it is twice a week, while for David it is twice a year. This extra information is clearly crucial. It shows that, although both men share the same sexual fantasy, John fantasizes about it more often, potentially indicating a stronger interest.

A Closer Look at Thought Processes

Although content and process are conflated within sexual fantasy definitions, most studies *do* typically assess how frequently people fantasize about specific content. However, a key issue pervading nearly all of these studies is that they *do not* distinguish between different dimensions of thought (e.g., Hicks & Leitenberg, 2001; O'Donohue et al., 1997). This is an issue because, between and within studies, researchers "may be examining different variables" (Jones & Barlow, 1990, p. 270). For example, people can experience "fleeting sexual thoughts" or "more elaborate and ongoing sexual fantasies," as well as "sexual thoughts that are experienced as intrusive" versus "sexual thoughts and fantasies that are engaged in deliberately" (Renaud & Byers, 2001, p. 253). Put simply, sexual thoughts can differ in terms of *duration* and *intention*.

Duration: Fleeting vs. Prolonged Sexual Thoughts

In 1890, William James stated that the stream of human thought is "Like a bird's life, it seems to be made of an alternation of flights and perchings". That is, it involves numerous transitions ("flights") between different thoughts ("perchings"). Klinger (1978) found that, in a 16-hour day, people experience approximately 4,000 distinct thoughts, each with a median duration of five seconds. Thus, rapid "flights" and fleeting "perchings" seems to be the norm (Klinger, 1996; Mildner & Tamir, 2019). However, some thoughts can become fixed upon a specific subject (e.g., rumination, planning), meaning that some "perchings" can have a longer duration (Mildner & Tamir, 2019). Based on this, we can argue for a distinction between fleeting and prolonged *sexual* thoughts, with the former occurring more often. Indeed, Cameron and Biber (1973) found that "in-passing" (fleeting) sexual thoughts generally occurred more frequently than "focal" (prolonged) sexual thoughts. Unfortunately, most research has not distinguished fleeting and prolonged sexual thoughts, since broad definitions state that sexual fantasies "can be an elaborate story, or [...] a fleeting thought" (Hicks & Leitenberg, 2001, p. 45).

This conflation should be avoided, especially when measuring the frequency of sexual thoughts. There are two reasons for this. The first is that assessing frequency provides no information about the nature of the thought. Imagine that John experiences frequent fleeting sexual thoughts about children, while David regularly envisions longer sexual scenarios involving children. On a typical sexual fantasy questionnaire (defining sexual fantasy as "any sexual thought"), both men will report that they fantasize frequently about children. In other words, the fact that they experience a different type of sexual thought is missed. The second reason pertains to the fact that thought frequency is confounded with thought duration (Lambert et al., 2014). For example, following treatment, David and John report experiencing only a single sexual thought in the last 24 hours. However, for David, this was a prolonged sexual thought lasting a few hours, while for John it was a fleeting sexual thought lasting a few seconds. Again, important information has gone undetected. This information is important because it may indicate a difference in the strength of their sexual interest or a difference in their self-regulation skills. Furthermore, the effect of their sexual thoughts may differ. For example, offense scripts are thought to be created by the repeated use of sexual fantasies (Gee et al., 2003; Ward & Hudson, 2000). As noted by Bartels and Gannon (2011), this is conceivable if someone envisions "an elaborate sexual script, but less likely if they only experience brief lustful thoughts" (p. 553). Thus, it is important that we differentiate fleeting and prolonged sexual thoughts.

Intention: Spontaneous vs. Deliberate Sexual Thoughts

Some researchers have stated that sexual fantasies occur spontaneously (Jones & Barlow, 1990), while others viewed them as being deliberate (Purifoy et al., 1992). Later, Leitenberg and Henning (1995) stated that sexual fantasies can be either spontaneously or deliberately imagined. This raises the question of whether spontaneous and deliberate sexual thoughts should be treated as equal. Recent work on human thought would suggest not. For example, Andrews-Hanna et al. (2018) state that "thoughts arising in a spontaneous or unintentional fashion should not be equated with thoughts arising deliberately, even when such thoughts have similar [...] contents" (p. 145). This is because they are underpinned by different processes (Christoff et al., 2016).

Spontaneous thought is defined as "a mental state [...] that arises relatively freely due to an absence of strong constraints on the contents [...] and on the transitions from one mental state to another" (Christoff et al., 2016, p. 719). In other words, for a thought to be entirely spontaneous, the contents should arise involuntarily and effortlessly, and must not be deliberately directed by the thinker (Christoff, 2012). Thus, truly spontaneous thoughts transition quickly from topic to topic (Andrews-Hanna et al., 2018). These thoughts most likely arise from the spreading activation of complex associative networks, triggered by an external or internal cue (Christoff et al., 2016; Jordão et al., 2019; Kavanagh et al., 2005; Mace, 2010; Mildner & Tamir, 2019).

In contrast, thoughts that remain fixed upon a specific topic for a prolonged time are not regarded as fully spontaneous. According to Christoff et al. (2016), these include automatically constrained and deliberately constrained thoughts. *Automatically constrained thoughts* arise unintentionally but then remain automatically restricted or biased toward the thought's content due to its affective or sensory salience. This is driven by "a family of mechanisms that operate outside of cognitive control to hold attention on a restricted set of information" (Christoff et al., 2016, p. 719). It can be argued, therefore, that the bottom-up (non-conscious) processing of an unintentional salient sexual thought may automatically constrain a person's attention, leading to a longer duration of thought. The saliency of the thought will be influenced by the level of sexual arousal it elicits (Smid & Wever, 2019), and/or the positive evaluation of its content (Little & Byers, 2000). Indeed, Little and Byers (2000) proposed that, if an unintentional sexual thought is sexually arousing and positive, a person may keep thinking about it. A sexual thought will also be automatically constrained if its content reflects a person's current concerns or needs (Klinger, 1971). Also, in the same way that individuals suffering from depression become "stuck" on negative ruminative thoughts due to strong automatic constraints (Christoff et al., 2016), hypersexual individuals, and those with high sexual excitation, are likely to find themselves automatically constrained (preoccupied) with sexual thought content (Walton & Bhullar, 2018).

Conversely, *deliberately constrained thoughts* are intentionally confined to a specific topic. They are prolonged, goal-directed, and consciously guided by top-down (controlled) processes (Christoff et al., 2016). This would include prolonged sexual thoughts that are deliberately evoked to induce sexual arousal (Davidson, 1985; Gee et al., 2003; Lunde et al., 1991), as well as those used to mentally plan or rehearse a future sexual experience (Gee et al., 2003; MacCulloch et al., 1983). Deliberate sexual thoughts also tend to be positively appraised (Little & Byers, 2000; Renaud & Byers, 2001). This likely due to the individual being able to guide them to fit their own purpose. As Leitenberg and Henning (1995) note, "the essential element of a deliberate sexual fantasy is the ability to control in imagination exactly what takes place" (p. 470). Deliberately constrained thoughts may be directly evoked, or they may follow on from an initial spontaneous sexual thought. For example, Little and Byers (2000) proposed that an unintentional sexual thought may be deliberately used to "create a continued positive sexual fantasy" that is longer in duration (p. 177). The idea of an initial intrusive thought being deliberately elaborated upon also underpins Kavanagh et al.'s Elaborated-Intrusion Theory of desire (Kavanagh et al., 2005).

A New Conceptualization

Drawing upon the above literature on human thought and sexual fantasies, we propose a conceptual distinction between fleeting sexual thoughts and prolonged sexual fantasizing. A "fleeting sexual thought" is defined as *a passing internal mental event involving visual and/or verbal sexual content that arises unintentionally during the dynamic flow of thought.* The defining feature here is the nature in which the thought arises, not just its sexual content. That is, it spontaneously "pops" into mind before freely moving on to a new topic. Thus, the content is not strongly constrained and so lasts only a few seconds.

"Sexual fantasizing" is defined as *the intentional or unintentional prolonged act of mentally simulating an ongoing sexual scenario.* Again, the defining feature is the nature of the thought process. That is, regardless of it arising spontaneously or deliberately, the thought is more strongly constrained (i.e., to a sexual scenario) and so is more elaborate in content and longer in duration. When the content is automatically constrained due to its saliency, the thought will unfold in an automatic manner, influenced by one's affective state and/or current needs. When the content is deliberately evoked and constrained, it will be consciously guided in a top-down, goal-directed manner (see Table 4.1 for examples of different types of sexual thought).

Dual-Process Model of Sexual Thinking

Having conceptually distinguished fleeting sexual thoughts from sexual fantasizing, we now turn our attention to the *Dual-Process Model of Sexual Thinking* (DPM-ST). This theory was developed by knitting together the literature on sexual fantasies with relevant literature on human cognition (e.g., dual-process theories, mental imagery, working memory, episodic simulation, and thought appraisal). As such, it can help explain existing findings, while also providing new avenues for future research. Note, the DPM-ST does not aim to explain the emergence of sexual interest, but rather the mechanisms that give rise to and underpin sexual thoughts and sexual fantasizing irrespective of their content. Thus, the DPM-ST applies to sexual thinking that involves both typical and atypical sexual content (see Figure 4.1).

Redressing the Theoretical Foundation

Most dual-process theories are based on the idea that human cognition is driven by processes that operate automatically (i.e., unintentionally, unknowingly, uncontrollably, and effortlessly) or in a controlled manner (i.e., intentionally, knowingly, controllably, and effortfully; Gawronski & Creighton, 2013). This framework was applied to sexual thinking in the DPM-ST. Inspired by Kavanagh et al.'s theory of desire (Kavanagh et al., 2005), we initially proposed that spontaneous, fleeting sexual thoughts are underpinned by associative processes that operate automatically, while prolonged sexual fantasizing is underpinned by controlled, elaborative processes (Bartels & Beech, 2016). However, as discussed earlier, the content of prolonged thinking can be automatically constrained (Christoff et al., 2016). This seemed to introduce the contradiction that a controlled process can operate automatically.

The issue is that *operating principles* (what a given process does) and *operating conditions* (when a given process operates) were treated as synonymous, when they should not have been (Gawronski & Bodenhausen, 2011). For example, Gawronski and Bodenhausen (2011) noted that the associative and propositional processes involved in attitudinal evaluations (operating principles) both have automatic and controlled aspects (operating conditions). In consideration of this, we have amended the core foundation of the DPM-ST. We now do not assume that the associative processes (underpinning fleeting sexual thoughts) and elaborative processes (underpinning sexual fantasizing) are exclusively automatic and controlled, respectively. Instead, the DPM-ST is now based on an associative-elaborative dichotomy. This duality refers to what the two processes do (i.e., activation and mental simulation, respectively), which can operate under both automatic and controlled conditions.

Table 4.1 Types of sexual thought

	FleetingSexual Thought	**Sexual Fantasizing**	
	No Constraints	*AutomaticallyConstrained*	*Deliberately Constrained(Goal-Directed)*
Internally Triggered	On the train home from work, an individual suddenly recalls a sexual experience involving their partner. Their thoughts then quickly and freely change to the topic of a meeting they have in the morning.	On the train home from work, an individual suddenly recalls a sexual experience they once had with their partner. This thought is highly arousing, and they find themself envisioning the sexual scenario for a prolonged length of time.	While on the train home, a person suddenly thinks of a sexual experience they once had with their partner. In response to this, they deliberately evoke and visualize the various sexual behaviors they plan to enact with their partner that night.
	During her daily workout, a woman randomly thinks about a sexual behavior that interests her. A few seconds later, the woman's thought content randomly and freely transitions to a funny scene she saw in a recent movie.	One evening, a man was writing an important piece of work. However, despite his best efforts to concentrate, the man kept finding himself mentally envisioning a prolonged arousing sexual scenario that he wishes to enact one day.	After a stressful day, a person struggles to relax. They decide to deliberately create and envision a sexual scenario to help alleviate their stress. They consciously guide the imagery so that it sexually arouses them and then begin to masturbate to it.
Externally Triggered	While sat in a coffee shop, a man sees a young child. He then suddenly and unintentionally experiences an inappropriate sexual thought involving the child, before switching freely to thoughts about what to have for their dinner.	In a coffee shop, a man sees a child and suddenly experiences an unintentional sexual thought about the child. The thought is sexually arousing, and the man finds himself envisaging a prolonged sexual scenario involving the child.	While sat in a coffee shop, a man sees a young child and experiences an unintentional sexual thought about them, which arouses him. Later at home, the man deliberately evokes and elaborates upon the thought in the form of a prolonged scenario.
	While taking a walk down the street, a person notices someone they find sexually attractive. They then involuntarily think "I wonder what they look like naked." Their thoughts then freely change to how nice the weather is.	During a movie, a person sees an attractive actor and suddenly thinks "I'd like to see them naked." A while later, they notice they have lost track of the film as they had been envisioning a sexual scenario involving the character.	While engaging in sexual intercourse with their partner, an individual deliberately evokes and envisions various sexual scenarios involving their partner, consciously switching between scenarios to maintain sexual arousal and facilitate orgasm.

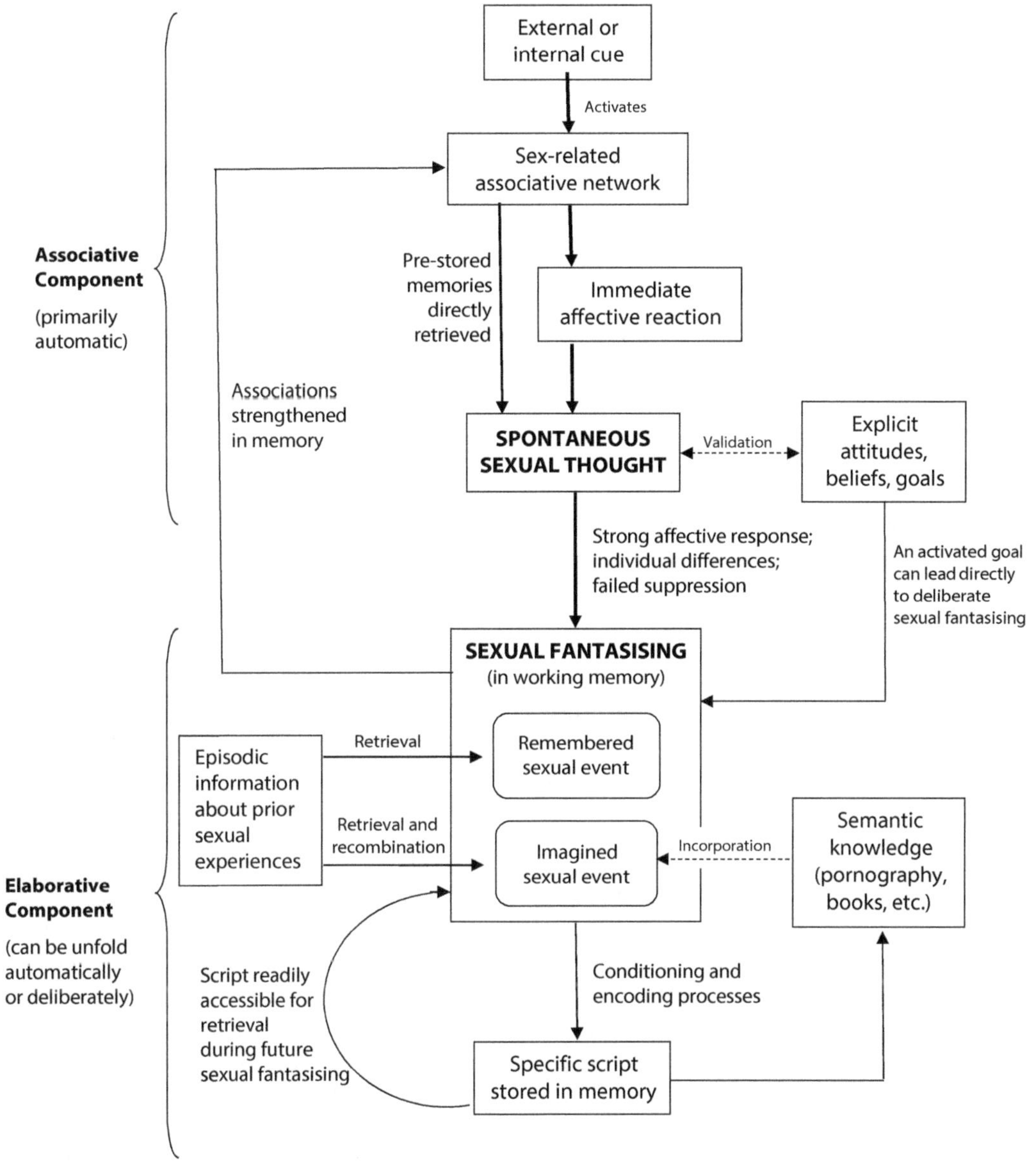

Figure 4.1 Schematic representation of the Dual-Process Model of Sexual Thinking (DPM-ST).

Fleeting Sexual Thoughts (Associative Processes)

Spontaneous, fleeting sexual thoughts are the result of associative processes that involve the activation of mental associations. People hold associative networks in memory, which can consist of associations between sex and other concepts. These include people (children, ex-partner), behaviors (submission, spanking), objects (fetishes), affective states (joy, stress), and needs (intimacy, power). These associations are formed from prior sexual experiences and/or through acquired semantic knowledge (e.g., pornography). The pre-existing structure of these associations in memory influence the pattern of activation elicited by a specific external trigger (e.g., a person, object, behavior) or internal trigger (e.g., emotion, goal, thought), as does the context in which they are activated (Gawronski & Bodenhausen, 2006). For example, when a person sees an attractive person during the day, no sex-related associations are activated. However, when they see them again in a nightclub, sex-related associations may be activated. Associative networks also include episodic memories that are pre-stored as "event representations". These memories can be directly retrieved in an involuntary manner (Uzer et al., 2012). The same applies to "pre-made" memories of a future event (Cole & Kvavilashvili, 2019), which we extend to include pre-made "fantasy events" (i.e., sexual events that are not expected to occur in the future).

The continuous input from external and internal cues causes a transitory pattern of activation that continually rises and dissipates within in one's associative network (Conway et al., 2019). If sex-related associations are activated, it will lead to an automatic affective reaction that immediately translates into a spontaneous visual or verbal sexual thought, including evaluative judgments (e.g., "I am sexually attracted to X"). The memory of a prior sexual experience, a planned future sexual experience, or a stored fantasy sequence may also directly enter conscious awareness as a spontaneous thought following its activation. All spontaneous thoughts will feel completely random if the person is unable to connect the thought to its cue (Mace, 2010). They will also be short-lived if no constraints are imposed upon them.

Responding to a Sexual Thought

Not all sexual thoughts will be fleeting. That is, some thoughts will grab an individual's attention due to eliciting a strong affective response (Kavanagh et al., 2005). Typically, this will be a strong feeling of sexual arousal (Little & Byers, 2000). However, it can also include positive affect, such as nostalgia (Muise et al., 2020), or negative affect, such as guilt or disgust (Little & Byers, 2000). Attention may also be captured if a sexual thought reflects the current needs of a person (Rummel & Nied, 2017).

Once attention is directed toward a sexual thought, it will undergo a validation or appraisal process. A sexual thought will be validated if it is congruent with explicit attitudes and/or other momentarily considered propositions (Gawronski & Bodenhausen, 2006), such as when a sexual thought about a child is consistent with the belief that children enjoy sex with adults. If validated, the thought may be elaborated upon. Conversely, if a sexual thought is inconsistent with one's beliefs or other considered propositions (e.g., "Sex with children is wrong"), it will be rejected and negatively appraised. As a result, the person may try to dismiss it from conscious awareness. The dismal or suppression of a sexual thought will be difficult, however, if it elicits strong sexual arousal (Clark et al., 2000; Johnston et al., 1997). Thought suppression may also be attempted if a sexual thought does not match one's current goals. For example, a person trying to abstain from sexually reoffending may try to suppress an offence-related sexual thought (Pithers et al., 1988).

Sexual Fantasizing (Elaborative Processes)

If a spontaneous sexual thought is positively appraised (or is unsuccessfully suppressed), it may be elaborated upon in the form of a prolonged mental simulation (i.e., sexual fantasizing). This elaborative process involves mental imagery, which is defined as the "mental invention or recreation of an experience that, in at least some respects, resembles the experience of actually perceiving an object or an event" (Finke, 1989, p. 2). Mental imagery involves several cognitive mechanisms working together (Kosslyn, 1995), which includes retrieving episodic information from memory in order to reconstruct a prior experience or construct a future sexual scenario, whether it is planned or pure fantasy (Schacter et al., 2008). It can also involve drawing upon semantic sexual knowledge acquired via external stimuli such as pornography (Gee et al., 2006). This retrieved information must be held in mind so that the mental simulation of the sexual scenario can be sufficiently (re)constructed. Thus, the elaborative process also requires the resources of working memory[1] (Baddeley & Andrade, 2000; Bartels et al., 2018; Moulton & Kosslyn, 2009). In short, the elaborative process involves the cognitive search for target-relevant information in long-term memory, which is then mentally represented, held, and manipulated in working memory in the form of a mental simulation (Kavanagh et al., 2005; MacInnis & Price, 1987).

If an individual's thoughts become automatically constrained, the prolonged experience of sexual fantasizing will unfold in a non-deliberate manner. Here, the elaborative process is not deliberately guided by the individual. Instead, its direction is influenced by existing preferences, current needs, and/or the present context. Thus, the search for relevant target information (e.g., a preferred sexual target or behavior) will unfold in a non-conscious manner, while still drawing upon the resources of working memory (Hassin, 2005). Conversely, if the initial spontaneous sexual thought reflects a specific goal, an individual may *intentionally* engage in sexual fantasizing. Here, the elaborative process will involve a more controlled search for target-relevant information (Kavanagh et al., 2005). This information will be deliberately directed, resulting in the construction of a sexual mental simulation in working memory. In short, the content is deliberately constrained and consciously directed in order to achieve one's goal. This includes planning a future sexual experience or inducing/increasing sexual arousal (Gee et al., 2003). Deliberate sexual fantasizing can also occur without the prompt of an initial spontaneous sexual thought, such as when a specific goal is directly activated (see Table 4.1 and Figure 4.1).

The likelihood and duration of sexual fantasizing will also be affected by various individual differences. For example, it may be more likely to occur (and for longer) if someone has a greater working memory capacity, and/or can readily form vivid mental imagery (Smith & Over, 1987). Similarly, people that are generally "fantasy prone" are more likely to engage in sexual fantasizing (Bartels et al., 2020). Also, the more that someone is sexually interested in a specific behavior, the more frequently they will fantasize about that behavior (Noorishad et al., 2019). People with greater levels of sexual excitation (who are more easily sexually aroused by stimuli) will also participate in sexual fantasizing more frequently (Walton & Bhullar, 2018). Contextual factors will also affect sexual fantasizing. For instance, sexual thoughts are deemed positive if they are deliberate and occur in public contexts (Little & Byers, 2000). Also, deliberate sexual fantasizing that is accompanied by masturbation will likely have a longer duration, as the sexual content must be kept in mind until climax is reached.

Two final key points are also worth noting. The first is that frequent sexual fantasizing will strengthen associations that are represented within the imagery, as well as lead to the formation of new associations (Blair et al., 2001). Second, frequent sexual fantasizing will lead a sexual scenario itself to be stored as a knowledge structure or "cognitive script" (Ward & Hudson, 2000). This specific script can then be retrieved during future sexual fantasizing.

Conclusions

The DPM-ST offers exciting new hypotheses to be tested. Not only will this add to the literature, but it will help to corroborate the DPM-ST and enable further theoretical developments. The DPM-ST also has practical implications. For example, the differentiation between fleeting and prolonged sexual thoughts can increase the efficacy of sexual fantasy assessment. This will provide a more refined understanding of the relationship between an individual's sexual interest and corresponding sexual thoughts (e.g., whether they are frequent but fleeting, or frequent and prolonged). This can inform case formulations and help identify appropriate lines of treatment (e.g., mindfulness, Acceptance and Commitment Therapy). Given that the DPM-ST is the only theoretical account for how sexual thoughts and fantasizing operate, we hope that researchers and clinicians find it useful.

Note

1. Working memory is a limited-capacity system where task-relevant information is retained and manipulated during a cognitive task (Baddeley & Hitch, 1974).

References

Andrews-Hanna, J. R., Irving, Z. C., Fox, K. C., Spreng, R. N., & Christoff, K. (2018). The neuroscience of spontaneous thought: An evolving interdisciplinary field. In K. C. Fox, & K. Christoff (Eds.), *The Oxford handbook of spontaneous thought: Mind-wandering, creativity, and dreaming*. Oxford University Press. https://doi.org/10.1093/oxfordhb/9780190464745.013.33

Arndt, W. B., Foehl, J. C., & Good, F. E. (1985). Specific sexual fantasy themes: A multidimensional study. *Journal of Personality and Social Psychology, 48*(2), 472–480. https://doi.org/10.1037/0022-3514.48.2.472

Baddeley, A. D., & Andrade, J. (2000). Working memory and the vividness of imagery. *Journal of Experimental Psychology: General, 129*(1), 126–145. https://doi.org/10.1037/0096-3445.129.1.126

Baddeley, A. D., & Hitch, G. J. (1974). Working memory. In G. H. Bower (Ed.), *The psychology of learning and motivation, Vol.* 8 (pp. 47–89). Academic Press.

Bartels, R., & Beech, A. (2016). Theories of deviant sexual fantasy. In A. R. Beech, & T. Ward (Eds.), *The Wiley handbook on the theories, assessment and treatment of sexual offending* (pp. 165–186). Wiley Blackwell. https://doi.org/10.1002/9781118574003.wattso008

Bartels, R. M., Beech, A. R., & Harkins, L. (2014, September). *Reacting fast, imagining slow: The dual-process model of sexual thinking. Paper presented at the 13th Annual Conference of the International Association for the Treatment of Sexual Offenders*, Porto, Portugal.

Bartels, R. M., & Gannon, T. A. (2011). Understanding the sexual fantasies of sex offenders and their correlates. *Aggression and Violent Behavior, 16*(6), 551–561. https://doi.org/10.1016/j.avb.2011.08.002

Bartels, R. M., Harkins, L., & Beech, A. R. (2020). The influence of fantasy proneness, dissociation, and vividness of mental imagery on male's aggressive sexual fantasies. *Journal of Interpersonal Violence, 35*(3–4), 964–987. https://doi.org/10.1177/0886260517691523

Bartels, R. M., Harkins, L., Harrison, S. C., Beard, N., & Beech, A. R. (2018). The effect of bilateral eye-movements versus no eye-movements on sexual fantasies. *Journal of Behavior Therapy and Experimental Psychiatry, 59*, 107–114. https://doi.org/10.1016/j.jbtep.2018.01.001

Baughman, H. M., Jonason, P. K., Veselka, L., & Vernon, P. A. (2014). Four shades of sexual fantasies linked to the Dark Triad. *Personality and Individual Differences, 67*, 47–51. https://doi.org/10.1016/j.paid.2014.01.034

Birnbaum, G. E. (2007). Beyond the borders of reality: Attachment orientations and sexual fantasies. *Personal Relationships, 14*(2), 321–342. https://doi.org/10.1111/j.1475-6811.2007.00157.x

Blair, I. V., Ma, J. E., & Lenton, A. P. (2001). Imagining stereotypes away: The moderation of implicit stereotypes through mental imagery. *Journal of Personality and Social Psychology, 81*(5), 828–841. https://doi.org/10.1037/0022-3514.81.5.828

Bouchard, K. N., Dawson, S. J., & Lalumière, M. L. (2017). The effects of sex drive and paraphilic interests on paraphilic behaviours in a nonclinical sample of men and women. *The Canadian Journal of Human Sexuality, 26*(2), 97–111. https://doi.org/10.3138/cjhs.262-a8

Cameron, P., & Biber, H. (1973). Sexual thought throughout the life-span. *The Gerontologist, 13*(2), 144–147. https://doi.org/10.1093/geront/13.2.144

Carlson, E. R., & Coleman, C. E. (1977). Experiential and motivational determinants of the richness of an induced sexual fantasy. *Journal of Personality, 45*(4), 528–542. https://doi.org/10.1111/j.1467-6494.1977.tb00169.x

Christoff, K. (2012). Undirected thought: Neural determinants and correlates. *Brain Research, 1428*, 51–59. https://doi.org/10.1016/j.brainres.2011.09.060

Christoff, K., Irving, Z. C., Fox, K. C., Spreng, R. N., & Andrews-Hanna, J. R. (2016). Mind-wandering as spontaneous thought: A dynamic framework. *Nature Reviews Neuroscience, 17*(11), 718–731. https://doi.org/10.1038/nrn.2016.113

Clark, D. A., Purdon, C., & Byers, E. S. (2000). Appraisal and control of sexual and non-sexual intrusive thoughts in university students. *Behaviour Research and Therapy, 38*(5), 439–455. https://doi.org/10.1016/S0005-7967(99)00047-9

Cole, S., & Kvavilashvili, L. (2019). Spontaneous and deliberate future thinking: A dual process account. *Psychological Research*, 1–16. https://doi.org/10.1007/s00426-019-01262-7

Conway, M. A., Justice, L., & D'Argembeau, A. (2019). The Self-memory system revisited: Past, present, and future. In J. H. Mace (Ed.), *The organization and structure of autobiographical memory*. Oxford University Press.

Crepault, C., & Couture, M. (1980). Men's erotic fantasies. *Archives of Sexual Behavior, 9*(6), 565–581. https://doi.org/10.1007/BF01542159

Davidson, S. J. K. (1985). The utilization of sexual fantasies by sexually experienced university students. *Journal of American College Health, 34*, 24–32. https://doi.org/10.1080/07448481.1985.9939614

Davidson, S. J. K., & Hoffman, L. E. (1986). Sexual fantasies and sexual satisfaction: An empirical analysis of erotic thought. *Journal of Sex Research, 22*(2), 184–205. https://doi.org/10.1080/00224498609551299

Ellis, B. J., & Symons, D. (1990). Sex differences in sexual fantasy: An evolutionary psychological approach. *Journal of Sex Research, 27*(4), 527–555. https://doi.org/10.1080/00224499009551579

Finke, R. A. (1989). *Principles of mental imagery*. MIT Press.

Gawronski, B., & Bodenhausen, G. V. (2006). Associative and propositional processes in evaluation: An integrative review of implicit and explicit attitude change. *Psychological Bulletin, 132*(5), 692–731. https://doi.org/10.1037/0033-2909.132.5.692

Gawronski, B., & Bodenhausen, G. V. (2011). The associative-propositional evaluation model: Theory, evidence, and open questions. In M. Zanna, & J. M. Olson (Eds.), *Advances in experimental social psychology* (Vol. 44, pp. 59–127). Elsevier. https://doi.org/10.1016/B978-0-12-385522-0.00002-0

Gawronski, B., & Creighton, L. A. (2013). Dual process theories. In D. E. Carlston (Ed.), *The Oxford handbook of social cognition* (pp. 282–312). American Psychologist Association. https://doi.org/10.1093/oxfordhb/9780199730018.013.0014

Gee, D., Ward, T., Belofastov, A., & Beech, A. (2006). The structural properties of sexual fantasies for sexual offenders: A preliminary model. *Journal of Sexual Aggression, 12*(3), 213–226. https://doi.org/10.1080/13552600601009956

Gee, D., Ward, T., & Eccleston, L. (2003). The function of sexual fantasies for sexual offenders: A preliminary model. *Behaviour Change, 20*(1), 44–60. https://doi.org/10.1375/bech.20.1.44.24846

Hariton, E. B., & Singer, J. L. (1974). Women's fantasies during sexual intercourse: Normative and theoretical implications. *Journal of Consulting and Clinical Psychology, 42*(3), 313–322. https://doi.org/10.1037/h0036669

Harvey, T. A., & Jeglic, E. L. (2020). Attenuation of deviant sexual fantasy across the lifespan in US adult males. *Psychiatry, Psychology and Law, 27*(2), 246–264. https://doi.org/10.1080/13218719.2020.1719376

Hassin, R. R. (2005). Nonconscious control and implicit working memory. In R. R. Hassin, J. S. Uleman, & J. A. Bargh (Eds.), *The new unconscious* (pp. 196–222). Oxford University Press.

Hicks, T. V., & Leitenberg, H. (2001). Sexual fantasies about one's partner versus someone else: Gender differences in incidence and frequency. *Journal of Sex Research, 38*(1), 43–50. https://doi.org/10.1080/00224490109552069

Imhoff, R., Banse, R., & Schmidt, A. F. (2017). Toward a theoretical understanding of sexual orientation and sexual motivation. *Archives of Sexual Behavior, 46*(1), 29–33. https://doi.org/10.1007/s10508-016-0881-5

Johnston, L., Ward, T., & Hudson, S. M. (1997). Deviant sexual thoughts: Mental control and the treatment of sexual offenders. *Journal of Sex Research, 34*(2), 121–130. https://doi.org/10.1080/00224499709551876

Jones, J. C., & Barlow, D. H. (1990). Self-reported frequency of sexual urges, fantasies, and masturbatory fantasies in heterosexual males and females. *Archives of Sexual Behavior, 19*(3), 269–279. https://doi.org/10.1007/BF0154155

Jordão, M., Pinho, M. S., & Jacques, P. L. S. (2019). Inducing spontaneous future thoughts in younger and older adults by priming future-oriented personal goals. *Psychological Research, 83*(4), 710–726. https://doi.org/10.1007/s00426-019-01146-w

Joyal, C. C., Cossette, A., & Lapierre, V. (2015). What exactly is an unusual sexual fantasy? *The Journal of Sexual Medicine, 12*(2), 328–340. https://doi.org/10.1111/jsm.12734

Kavanagh, D. J., Andrade, J., & May, J. (2005). Imaginary relish and exquisite torture: The elaborated intrusion theory of desire. *Psychological Review, 112*(2), 446–467. https://doi.org/10.1037/0033-295X.112.2.446

Klinger, E. (1971). *Structure and functions of fantasy.* Wiley Interscience.

Klinger, E. (1978). Modes of normal conscious flow. In K. S. Pope, & J. L. Singer (Eds.), *The stream of consciousness: Scientific investigations into the flow of human experience* (pp. 225–258). Plenum.

Klinger, E. (1996). The contents of thoughts: Interference as the downside of adaptive normal mechanisms in thought flow. In I. G. Sarason, G. R. Pierce, & B. R. Sarason (Eds.), *Cognitive interference: Theories, methods, and findings* (pp. 3–23). Erlbaum.

Knafo, D., & Jaffe, Y. (1984). Sexual fantasizing in males and females. *Journal of Research in Personality, 18*(4), 451–462. https://doi.org/10.1016/0092-6566(84)90004-7

Kosslyn, S. M. (1995). Mental imagery. In S. M. Kosslyn, & D. N. Osherson (Eds.), *Visual cognition: An invitation to cognitive science* (Vol. 2, pp. 267–296). MIT Press.

Lambert, A. E., Hu, Y., Magee, J. C., Beadel, J. R., & Teachman, B. A. (2014). Thought suppression across time: Change in frequency and duration of thought recurrence. *Journal of Obsessive-Compulsive and Related Disorders, 3*(1), 21–28. https://doi.org/10.1016/j.jocrd.2013.11.004

Laws, D. R., & Marshall, W. L. (1990). A conditioning theory of the etiology and Maintenance of deviant sexual preferences and behaviour. In W. L. Marshall, D. R. Laws, & H. E. Barbaree (Eds.), *Handbook of sexual assault: Issues, theories, and treatment of the offender* (pp. 209–230). Plenum Press.

Leitenberg, H., & Henning, K. (1995). Sexual fantasy. *Psychological Bulletin, 117*(3), 469–496. https://doi.org/10.1037/0033-2909.117.3.469

Little, C. A., & Byers, E. S. (2000). Differences between positive and negative sexual cognitions. *Canadian Journal of Human Sexuality, 9*(3), 167–179.

Lunde, I., Larsen, G. K., Fog, E., & Garde, K. (1991). Sexual desire, orgasm, and sexual fantasies: A study of 625 Danish women born in 1910, 1936, and 1958. *Journal of Sex Education and Therapy, 17*(2), 111–115. https://doi.org/10.1080/01614576.1991.11074012

MacCulloch, M. J., Snowden, P. R., Wood, P. J. W., & Mills, H. E. (1983). Sadistic fantasy, sadistic behaviour and offending. *The British Journal of Psychiatry, 143*(1), 20–29. https://doi.org/10.1192/bjp.143.1.20

Mace, J. H. (2010). Involuntary remembering and voluntary remembering: How different are they? In J. H. Mace (Ed.), *The act of remembering: Toward an understanding of how we recall the past* (pp. 43 55). Wiley-Blackwell.

MacInnis, D. J., & Price, L. L. (1987). The role of imagery in information processing: Review and extensions. *Journal of Consumer Research, 13*(4), 473–491. https://doi.org/10.1086/209082

McGuire, R. J., Carlisle, J. U., & Young, B. G. (1964). Sexual deviations as conditioned behaviour: A hypothesis. *Behaviour Research and Therapy, 2*(2–4), 185–190. https://doi.org/10.1016/0005-7967(64)90014-2

Mildner, J. N., & Tamir, D. I. (2019). Spontaneous thought as an unconstrained memory process. *Trends in Neurosciences, 42*(11), 763–777. https://doi.org/10.1016/j.tins.2019.09.001

Moulton, S. T., & Kosslyn, S. M. (2009). Imagining predictions: Mental imagery as mental emulation. *Philosophical Transactions of the Royal Society B: Biological Sciences, 364*(1521), 1273–1280. https://doi.org/10.1098/rstb.2008.0314

Muise, A., Kim, J. J., Debrot, A., Impett, E. A., & MacDonald, G. (2020). Sexual nostalgia as a response to unmet sexual and relational needs: The role of attachment avoidance. *Personality and Social Psychology Bulletin.* https://doi.org/10.1177/0146167220907468

Noorishad, P. G., Levaque, E., Byers, E. S., & Shaughnessy, K. (2019). More than one flavour: University students' specific sexual fantasies, interests, and experiences. *Canadian Journal of Human Sexuality, 28*(2), 143–158. https://doi.org/10.3138/cjhs.2019-0024

O'Donohue, W., Letourneau, E. J., & Dowling, H. (1997). Development and preliminary validation of a paraphilic sexual fantasy questionnaire. *Sexual Abuse, 9*(3), 167–178. https://doi.org/10.1007/BF02675062

Pithers, W. D., Kashima, K. M., Cummings, G. S., & Beal, L. S. (1988). Relapse prevention: A method of enhancing change in sex offender. In A. C. Salter (Ed.), *Treating child sex offenders and victims: A practical guide* (pp. 131–170). Sage.

Purifoy, F. E., Grodsky, A., & Giambra, L. M. (1992). The relationship of sexual daydreaming to sexual activity, sexual drive, and sexual attitudes for women across the life-span. *Archives of Sexual Behavior, 21*(4), 369–385. https://doi.org/10.1007/BF01542026

Renaud, C., & Byers, E. S. (1999). Exploring the frequency, diversity and content of university students' positive and negative sexual cognitions. *Canadian Journal of Human Sexuality, 8*(1), 17–30.

Renaud, C. A., & Byers, E. S. (2001). Positive and negative sexual cognitions: Subjective experience and relationships to sexual adjustment. *Journal of Sex Research, 38*(3), 252–262. https://doi.org/https://doi.org/10.1080/00224490109552094

Rokach, A. (1990). Content analysis of sexual fantasies of males and females. *The Journal of Psychology, 124*(4), 427–436. https://doi.org/10.1080/00223980.1990.10543238

Rummel, J., & Nied, L. (2017). Do drives drive the train of thought? Effects of hunger and sexual arousal on mind-wandering behavior. *Consciousness and Cognition, 55*, 179–187. https://doi.org/10.1016/j.concog.2017.08.013

Schacter, D. L., Addis, D. R., & Buckner, R. L. (2008). Episodic simulation of future events. In A. Kingstone & M. B. Miller (Eds.), *Annals of the New York Academy of Sciences, 1124, The year in cognitive neuroscience* (pp. 39–60). Blackwell Publishing. https://doi.org/10.1196/annals.1440.001

Singer, J. L. (1966). *Daydreaming: An introduction to the experimental study of inner experience.* Random House.

Smid, W. J., & Wever, E. C. (2019). Mixed emotions: An incentive motivational model of sexual deviance. *Sexual Abuse, 31*(7), 731–764. https://doi.org/10.1177/1079063218775972

Smith, D., & Over, R. (1987). Correlates of fantasy-induced and film-induced male sexual arousal. *Archives of Sexual Behavior, 16*(5), 395–409. https://doi.org/10.1007/BF01541422

Storms, M. D. (1981). A theory of erotic orientation development. *Psychological Review, 88*(4), 340–353. https://doi.org/10.1037/0033-295X.88.4.340

Uzer, T., Lee, P. J., & Brown, N. R. (2012). On the prevalence of directly retrieved autobiographical memories. *Journal of Experimental Psychology: Learning, Memory, and Cognition, 38*(5), 1296–1308. https://doi.org/10.1037/a0028142

Walton, M. T., & Bhullar, N. (2018). Hypersexuality, higher rates of intercourse, masturbation, sexual fantasy, and early sexual interest relate to higher sexual excitation/arousal. *Archives of Sexual Behavior, 47*(8), 2177–2183. https://doi.org/10.1007/s10508-018-1230-7

Ward, T., & Hudson, S. M. (2000). Sexual offenders' implicit planning: A conceptual model. *Sexual Abuse, 12*(3), 189–202. https://doi.org/10.1023/A:1009534109157

Wilson, G. D. (1978). *The secrets of sexual fantasy*. J. M. Dent.

Zurbriggen, E. L., & Yost, M. R. (2004). Power, desire, and pleasure in sexual fantasies. *Journal of Sex Research, 41*(3), 288–300. https://doi.org/10.1080/00224490409552236

5

Neurobiological Basis of Sexual Deviance

Tillmann H. C. Kruger[1] *and Jonas Kneer*[2]

[1,2] *Department of Psychiatry, Social Psychiatry and Psychotherapy, Division of Clinical Psychology and Sexual Medicine, Hannover Medical School, Carl-Neuberg-Str. 1, 30625 Hannover, Germany*

Introduction

There is reason to believe that sexual deviance—defined as attitudes, fantasies, urges or actions associated with sexual arousal for the affected person but condemned by society and/or social norms or causing suffering to the affected person or others—and acts of sexual violence, are grounded in an underlying neurobiological susceptibility that is just beginning to be understood (Siever, 2008). Neuroscience in general, and brain imaging methods in particular, are constantly developing and may provide useful tools for a better understanding of sexual deviance. Yet many methodological issues must be considered when interpreting results. In this chapter we will first provide an overview of the neurobiological foundations of *normal* sexual interest and behavior and provide some useful models that have been developed from these findings. This discussion will help to better evaluate findings that have evolved in the context of sexual deviance. We will conclude with a section on endocrinological and (epi-)genetic investigations and close with a critical conclusion.

Interpreting the Results of Neuroimaging

In the vast majority of studies, structural and functional magnetic resonance imaging (MRI) results are obtained from group analyses. However, the study design only allows for correlational interpretations at the group level, not the individual level. For a better understanding of the results obtained from a neuroimaging study, having a rudimentary background knowledge of the applied technique is crucial. A particular issue that emerges in MRI research is the control of confounders. These variables represent systematic differences between types of study groups, such as general intelligence, handedness, age or level of education, and, in the case of sexual deviance studies, variables such as substance abuse, sexual preference, medication, mental illness, incarceration, and former psychiatric treatment. These factors, if not controlled for, can lead the reader to wrong implications on the basis of spurious correlations. Therefore, an elaborated design is necessary to disentangle intermixed factors. Since deviant behavior, including

Sexual Deviance: Understanding and Managing Deviant Sexual Interests and Paraphilic Disorders,
First Edition. Edited by Leam A. Craig and Ross M. Bartels.
© 2021 John Wiley & Sons, Ltd. Published 2021 by John Wiley & Sons, Ltd.

child sexual offending (CSO) by someone with pedophilia, has been studied without clarity, one cannot say whether the driving factor is the sexual preference or the offensive act. Despite these restrictions, neurocognitive methods provide a potentially useful tool, especially if combined with a comprehensive psychological and/or psychiatric assessment of behavior or other objective parameters. For the interested reader, we recommend consulting Huettel et al. (2014).

What are the neurobiological correlates of *normal* sexual interest and behaviour?

The investigation of neurobiological underpinnings of normal sexual interest and arousal has some tradition. It began in the 1980s with measurements of hormonal parameters as a trait marker or during sexual activity. Brain imaging techniques then became equally important and were able to identify specific activations of brain areas during the processing of (mostly visual) sexual stimuli. Depending on the study paradigm and length of stimuli presentation, a variable degree of sexual arousal was evoked in most participants. Some studies even examined the effects of an orgasm. In summary, these studies revealed a distinct pattern of cortical and subcortical activation, including the occipitotemporal cortex, the precentral and cingulate gyrus, the superior and inferior parietal lobules, and parts of the frontal lobe during sexual stimuli processing. On a subcortical level, several (hypo)thalamic regions, the ventral striatum (VS), and the amygdala were identified (see Figures 5.1 and 5.2).

Comparative studies between homosexual and heterosexual men revealed that the visual presentation of a preferred sexual stimulus leads to activation of the neuronal structures listed

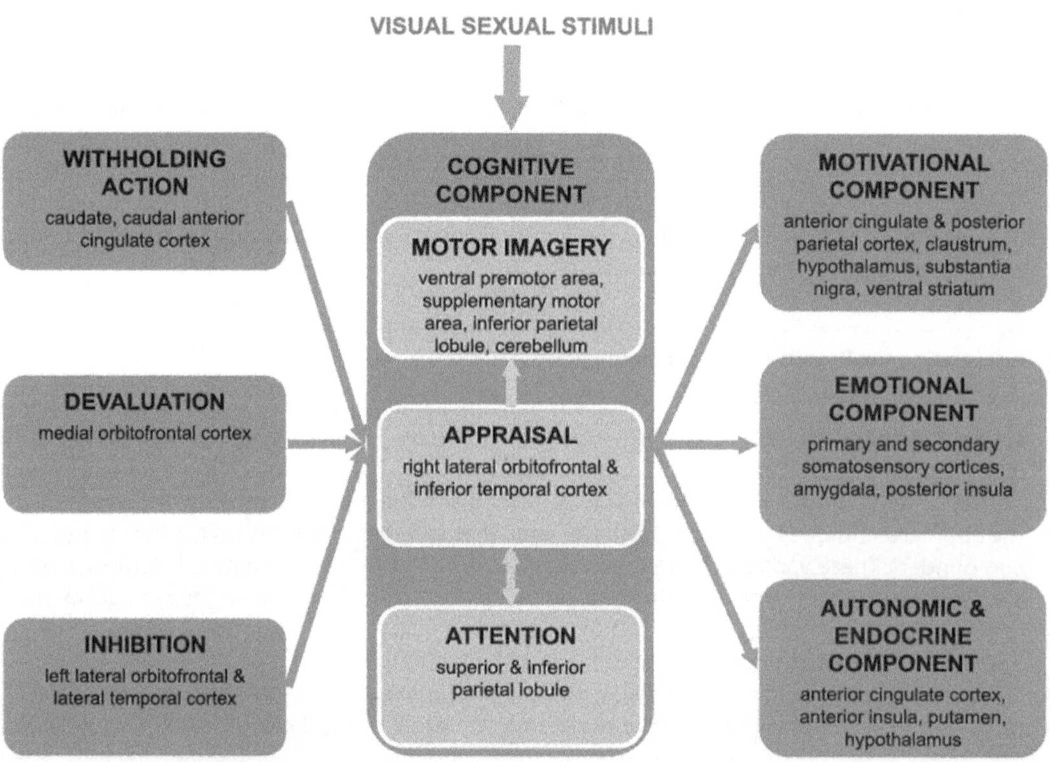

Figure 5.1 Neurophenomenological model of sexual arousal.
Adapted from Stoléru et al. (2012), with permission from Mohnke et al. (2014).

above. This activation pattern largely disappears during presentation of a non-preferred sexual stimulus (e.g., naked women for homosexual men) (Paul et al., 2008). Research demonstrated that activation of the hypothalamus (along with the VS) may best reflect the intensity of sexual stimuli: the stronger the hypothalamus activation, the higher the subjectively reported sexual arousal (Redouté et al., 2000). Further development of this approach allowed classification of participants regarding their sexual orientation and preference (in one case pedophilia; Ponseti et al., 2012). This classification was calculated according to cerebral reaction patterns in

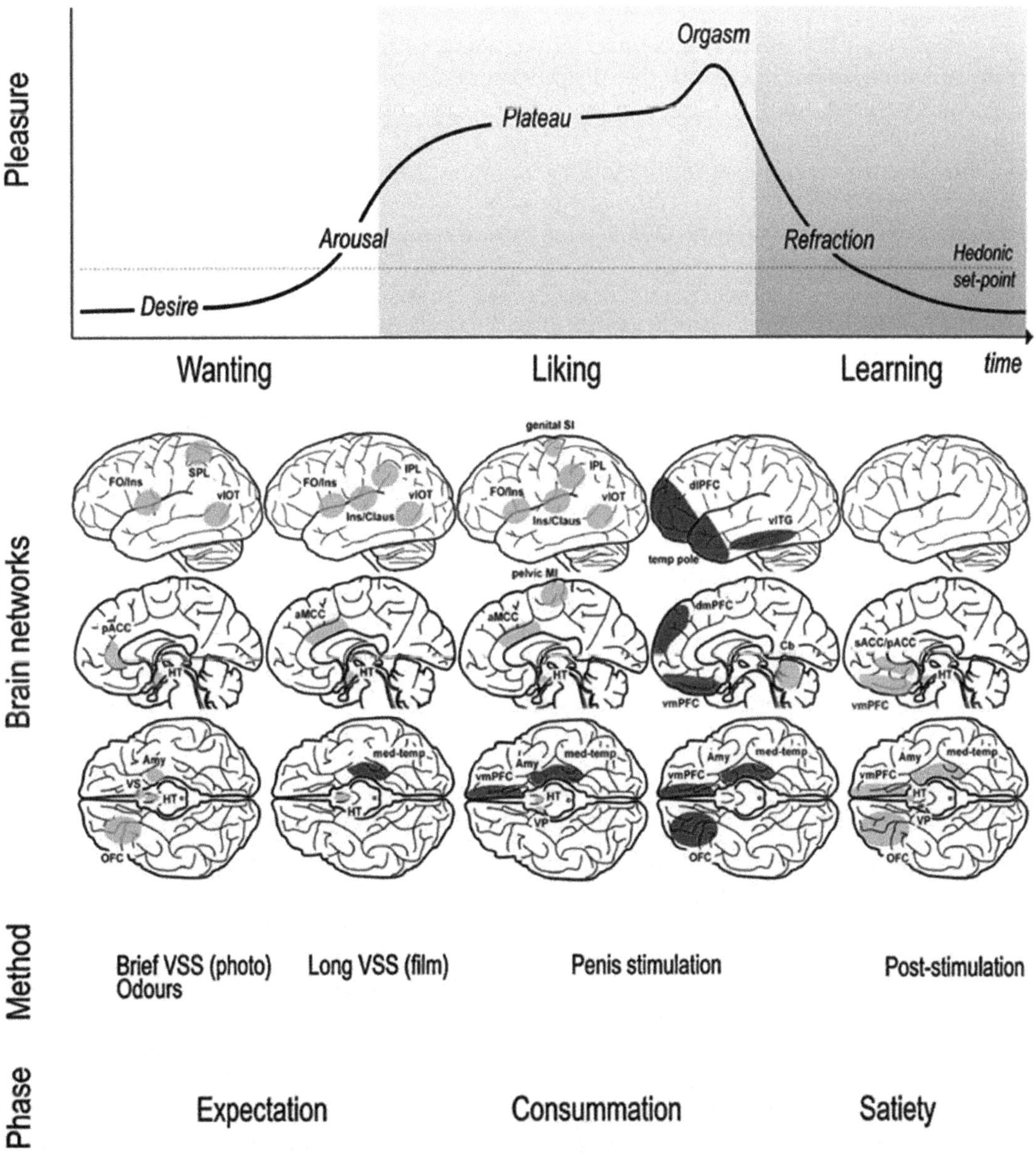

Figure 5.2 The functional neuroanatomy of the sexual response cycle in humans and its overlap with models of drug addiction. Note the fine balance between activated (orange) and inhibited (blue) brain areas during the different stages of sexual arousal. Abbreviation: VSS, visual sexual stimulus.
Reproduced with permission from Georgiadis and Kringelbach (2012).

response to sexual stimuli, with the highest classification accuracy achieved by Fisher linear discriminant analysis; the mean accuracy was 95% (100% specificity, 88% sensitivity). Future studies will determine whether this approach proves to be robust in detecting sexual orientation and preference, comparable (or superior) to personal exploration or other classification techniques, including penile plethysmography or viewing time paradigms.

Functional imaging also demonstrated aberrant central processing of sexually relevant stimuli in men and women suffering from sexual dysfunction (Bianchi-Demicheli et al., 2011; Cacioppo, 2017; Woodard et al., 2013). For instance, participants with hypoactive sexual desire disorder (HSDD) exhibit less activation of brain areas connected to the processing of sexually relevant stimuli. They also show greater activation of cortical brain areas connected to social and visual cognition, such as self-observation, along with stronger activation of prefrontal brain areas. These findings led to the assumption of a neurofunctional correlate of increased levels of observation and evaluation of individual sexual reactions in affected subjects.

Based on these studies, several models were developed in order to combine different aspects of sexual interest and arousal with specific brain areas. Neuroimaging results correspond to a behavioral neurobiological model initially proposed by Redouté et al. (2000) and adapted in subsequent years (Stoléru et al., 2012). This model assigns specific brain areas to cognitive, motivational, emotional, and autonomous components of central processing of sexual stimuli (for an overview, see Figure 5.1). A quantitative meta-analysis conducted by Poeppl et al. (2014) identified two distinct brain networks that underlie psychosexual arousal (i.e., a mental representation of arousal) and physiosexual arousal (i.e., lubrication, penile erection). Psychosexual arousal appears to be connected to neuronal structures linked to cognitive and affective evaluation of sexually relevant stimuli, top-down modulation of attention and stimulus processing, and the initiation of autonomous processes (i.e., multiple cortical areas, the amygdala, the hypothalamus and the basal ganglia). In contrast, physiosexual arousal is apparently connected to neuronal structures that are responsible for the regulation and monitoring of initiated autonomic processes and emotions, and for processing somatosensory inputs (where several areas are involved, including the cingulate gyrus, insula, and basal ganglia). Moreover, both neuronal sets seem to be subcortically interconnected via the claustrum and putamen, enabling information exchange between these areas. Finally, Georgiadis and Kringelbach (2012) provided a helpful review by forging a bridge between the classical sexual response cycle, as described by Masters and Johnson (1966), and the neurobiological correlates of sex and other pleasures such as intake of water and food or social contact (see Figure 5.2).

From Normal to Deviant Sexual Behavior: What Can We Learn from Research on "Sex Addiction"?

Besides evidence for functional and structural brain alterations in individuals with "sex addiction" or "compulsive sexual behavior" (CSB, new nomenclature in ICD-11 [World Health Organization, 2018]), studies indicate that affected individuals not only have increased levels of sexual drive but also elevated rates of sexual coercive fantasies and behaviors. In a recent online study ($N = 1{,}194$), 59% of men and 18% of women reported *fantasies* of sexual coercion, whereas 21% of men and 4% of women even reported *acts* of sexual coercion (Engel, Kessler et al., 2019). Findings from a controlled clinical study in men (Engel, Veit et al., 2019) support this observation. Compared to men without CSB, men with CSB had more paraphilias (47% vs. 3%), more often exhibited sexually violent behavior (70% vs. 21%), and more often viewed child abuse images (81% vs. 0%). The question arises as to whether, outside the margin of increased sexual drive, there exists an overlap with deviant fantasies and behaviors that might serve to further increase levels of sexual arousal.

What Are the Neurobiological Correlates of *Deviant* Sexual Interest and Behavior?

Structure

There are strong arguments that neurobiological processes, including prefrontal deficits, play a key role in the aetiology of deviant sexual behavior (Mills & Raine, 1994). Since the beginning of neurocognitive research, the neurobiological underpinnings of sexual offending have been continuously studied. A major challenge in research, however, has been differentiation between the effects of sexual preference (e.g., pedophilia) and the effects of offense status on brain structure. The majority of studies have not accounted for this important differentiation, and a number of false conclusions have probably been made. In the following section, we will therefore very cautiously discuss the implications of neurobiological findings for sexual deviance, and wherever the study design allows, we will carefully assign findings to sexual preference, behavior, or other factors. Moreover, we will distinguish between sexually deviant behavior against children and adults.

Sexual Deviant Behavior Against Children

One of the most important risk factors for sexual offending against children is the presence of a pedophilic preference, accounting for approximately 50% of cases (Seto, 2008). Therefore, while there are many other risk factors (e.g., impulsivity, emotion regulation problems, executive dysfunctions, and cognitive distortions), pedophilia is usually the main focus of research.

> **Early Days of Neuroimaging in Sexual Deviance**
>
> One of the first studies on structural brain abnormalities in pedophiles was published in 1982 by Graber, Hartmann, Coffman, Huey, and Golden using computed tomography (CT) scans. They observed reduced general brain density in three males who had sexually abused a child. Hendricks et al. (1988) then replicated Graber et al.'s (1982) results using data collected from 12 imprisoned non-pedophilic men who had sexually abused children or adolescents without cerebral abnormalities and 16 healthy controls. Unfortunately, their use of an inadequate control group (that included women) makes it difficult to correctly interpret these results. Subsequent research could not replicate these findings (Langevin et al., 1988, 1989; Wright et al., 1990). Other CT studies indicated greater brain asymmetry in pedophilic men for example, in terms of smaller left hemispheric widths mainly located in the temporal lobe (Wright et al., 1990). All these findings can not be said to be pedophilia-specific due to methodological limitations (Langevin et al., 1988).

Pedophilia as a neurodevelopmental disorder? For a relatively long time, the neurobiological underpinnings of pedophilia were discussed as being related to global deficits, such as decreased cognitive functioning and other signs of a neurodevelopmental disorder (Cantor et al., 2004). For instance, Cantor et al. (2004) showed a significant negative correlation between pedophilia and IQ, as well as deficits in recall memory. Consistent with some other experts in this field (Blanchard et al., 2007; Bogaert, 2001; Rahman & Symeonides, 2008), the idea of pedophilia being related to left-handedness was supported (Cantor et al., 2004, 2005). Subsequently, Cantor and colleagues concluded that pedophilia is related to cognitive deficits, and that frequent left-handedness is a clinical correlate of early neurodevelopmental perturbations.

Similar to Cantor et al. (2004), many other studies concentrated on neuropsychological characteristics of people who commit sexual offenses. However, only a few differentiated sexual preference from delinquent behavior (see Tenbergen et al., 2015, for an extensive review). For example, Suchy et al. (2009) found a general impairment in executive functions (EFs) as a specific dysfunction for non-pedophilic men with a history of child sexual offending (CSOs), whereas more distinct deficits occur in pedophilic CSOs. Overall, non-pedophilic CSOs show lower semantic knowledge, whilst slower speed of processing seems to be characteristic of CSOs with a primary sexual interest in children. Eastvold et al. (2011) reported similar results. They concluded that pedophilic CSOs appear to have no general EF impairment. Instead, they show a diverse pattern of differences in EFs, including a deficit in behavioral inhibition measures. Consistently, Schiffer and Vonlaufen (2011) found pedophilic CSOs are superior in abstract reasoning and planning measures compared to non-pedophilic CSOs and men with no history of sexual offending.

Recently, Suchy et al. (2014) replicated their findings and concluded that pedophilic CSOs show a distinct neurocognitive deficiency, with lower performance in inhibition and processing speeds. In contrast to these findings, Cohen et al. (2002) failed to find deficits in attention capacities or higher impulsivity but did reveal a lower IQ level in incarcerated pedophilic men when compared to controls. These data are consistent with Kruger and Schiffer (2011), who used a shortened IQ measure. Moreover, Cantor et al. (2005) not only observed lower IQ in pedophilic CSOs, but also showed that the lower their IQ, the younger the victim. Using a 2 × 2 factorial design (offense status vs. sexual preference), Massau et al. (2017) ($N = 158$, four groups) observed no broad EF deficits in pedophilic men, but having an offense was linked to having a worse response inhibition ability. Regarding set-shifting abilities, pedophilic CSOs demonstrated the best performance compared to the other groups. Notably, Kärgel et al. (2017) found that non-offending pedophiles performed significantly better on a Go/No-Go task. Furthermore, performance was functionally correlated with functional MRI (fMRI) results. Hence, the current data are heterogenous and many confounders (e.g., offense status, incarceration, comorbidities, etc) may have driven the results. Thus, there is no clear evidence from neuropsychological data that speaks to a neurodevelopmental disorder as a cause of pedophilia.

Besides neuropsychology, research has also focused on the potential role of brain structure alterations to provide additional answers for understanding sexual deviance. For a long time, a so-called "symptomatic" sexual deviance (including pedophilic behaviors) was reported after traumatic brain injury (e.g., Miller et al., 1986), brain tumors (e.g., Burns & Swerdlow, 2003; Lesniak et al., 1972), and immunological (multiple sclerosis) and neurodegenerative diseases (e.g., Mendez & Shapira, 2011) (for a systematic review, see Mohnke et al., 2014). These observations may not necessarily reflect a genuine change of sexual preference or a disclosure of a latent paraphilic disorder, but they may indicate the importance of intact brain function for controlling sexual behaviors, particularly temporal and frontal regions. Sexual disinhibition might explain a non-specific broadening of sexual interests and behaviors (like a disturbance of a sexual stimulus filter system) that may include deviant ones.

To investigate possible neurodevelopmental alterations that lead to pedophilia, many studies have concentrated on gray matter (GM) volume reductions, as well as white matter alterations (Cantor & Blanchard, 2012; Cantor et al., 2008; Schiffer et al., 2007; Schiltz et al., 2007). As carefully reviewed by Mohnke et al. (2014), the overall findings were inconsistent (i.e., differences in the orbitofrontal and prefrontal cortex, striatum, hypothalamus, and the temporal and limbic cortex), with the exception of a reduced right amygdala volume observed in several studies (Mendez et al., 2000; Poeppl et al., 2013; Schiffer et al., 2007; Schiltz et al., 2007). However, considering that pedophilia and child sexual abuse were frequently not differentiated, it is unclear whether a reduced amygdala volume is exclusively linked to sexual preference,

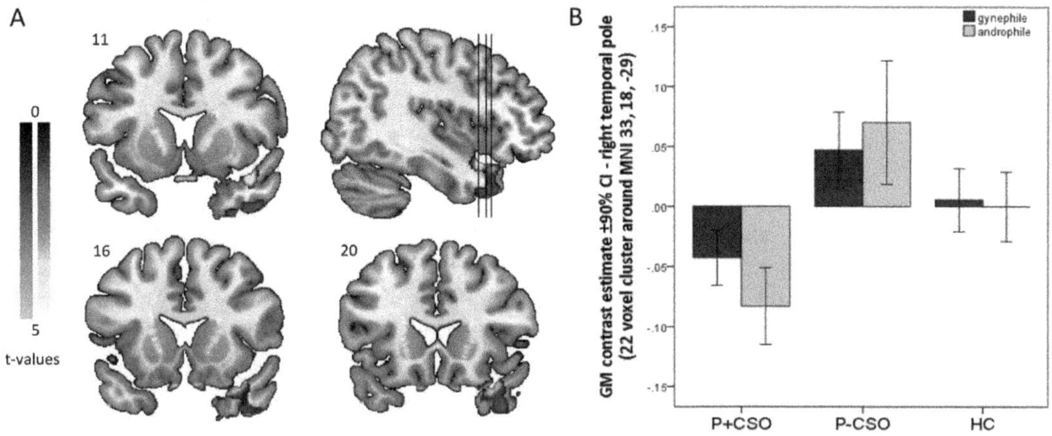

Figure 5.3 Alterations in brain volume (gray matter) in pedophiles with and without a history of child sexual offending. (A) Offense-related gray matter (GM) volume alterations were analysed using a whole-brain analysis of covariance (ANCOVA) model of the entire sample (red-colored overlay) and the matched sample (blue-colored overlay) in the right temporal pole. The color bars indicate *t*-statistic values. (B) The bar chart illustrates the contrast estimates of these relative GM volume differences at the single-group level (matched samples) and for the given subgroups attracted to girls/women (white) and boys/men (black). These distinctions had no significant impact on the GM volume anomalies in the right temporal pole. Abbreviations: P+CSO, men with pedophilia and a history of hands-on child sexual offenses; P-CSO, men with pedophilia and without history of hands-on child sexual offenses. Reprinted from Schiffer et al. (2017), with permission from Springer Nature.

the act of child sexual offending, or other factors. Indeed, in a follow-up study that used the above mentioned 2 × 2 factorial approach (offense status vs. sexual preference), Schiffer et al. (2017) were unable to corroborate this finding in a total sample of 219 men with and without pedophilia and/or child sexual abuse. In contrast, this study identified a highly significant and CSO-related alteration of above versus below normal gray matter volume of the right temporal pole, with non-offending pedophilic men exhibiting even larger volumes compared to pedophilic men who had offended (see Figure 5.3).

Additionally, regression analysis showed that a lower gray matter volume of the dorsomedial prefrontal or anterior cingulate cortex is associated with a higher risk of reoffending in pedophilic CSOs, an interesting finding that requires confirmation in future studies. Finally, Cantor et al. (2008) did not detect any gray matter volume differences in pedophilic CSOs(N = 65) compared to men with non-sexual offenses (N = 62). However, there was an impaired connectivity of diverse cortical and subcortical brain regions (superior fronto-occipital fasciculus and right arcuate fasciculus). This finding was interpreted as a disconnection problem within a network relevant for recognizing sexually relevant stimuli (see also Cantor & Blanchard, 2012 for additional white matter analyses). These findings were not observed by other groups when using the diffusion tensor imaging technique in 24 pedophilic men compared to 32 teleiophilic controls (Gerwinn et al., 2015). Using the 2 × 2 factorial design, a multimodal neuroimaging approach that included measures of cortical thickness, surface area (SA), and white matter fractional anisotropy (FA), as well as full scale IQ (FSIQ) performance, indicated aberrant neuroanatomy (i.e., reduced cortical thickness, reduced SA, and reduced FA in specific brain areas) and lower intelligence as being a potential core feature underlying child sexual abuse behavior in pedophilic men (Lett et al., 2018).

The Neurobiology of Pedophilia—A Critical Conclusion

Neuropsychological data does not allow one to definitively state that pedophilia can be explained by obvious neurodevelopmental perturbations, as seen in other diseases such as attention deficit hyperactivity disorder, autism spectrum disorder, or schizophrenia. The findings are relatively discrete, and when using proper research protocols, some of them may be offense-related (indicating problems with impulse control) or related to other factors such as incarceration, psychiatric comorbidities, medication, etc (for a further discussion, see Fazio, 2018; Joyal et al., 2019). Additionally, the reported structural brain alterations are inconclusive and there is no single robust finding that definitively accounts for pedophilia. Some authors state that pedophilia is another sexual orientation, but the lack of pronounced and consistent neurostructural data might, at least, suggest normal hardware in affected persons. This finding does not legitimize any offensive behavior towards children, and it remains to be investigated whether more subtle changes in specific nuclei or connectivity problems will be detected in the future by using more sophisticated methods.

Sexual Deviant Behavior Against Adults

There are myriad reasons for sexual deviant behavior towards adults, and there is no leading risk factor (such as pedophilia in case of child sexual offending). Therefore, various factors must be considered when interpreting neurostructural findings of sexual deviant behavior. As historical examples, in 1986, Miller et al. reported cases of people with orbitofrontal lesions who exhibited inappropriate sexual behaviors, such as public masturbation. A few years later, Langevin et al. (1988) observed a high prevalence of brain injuries and unconsciousness in a sample of 476 sexual offenders. Around the same time, Hucker et al. (1988) found anomalies in the right temporal horn in 41% of sadistic perpetrators by applying cerebral computed tomography (CCT), while only 11–13% of the subjects in the comparison group showed these alterations. In 1994, Mills and Raine analysed 20 brain imaging studies of violent and sexual offenders, which used CCT, MRI, and positron emission tomography (PET). They found nonsexual violent offending was associated with abnormalities in the frontal lobe. Comparatively, non-violent sexual offending (e.g., incest and pedophilia) more often occurred in individuals with temporal lobe abnormalities (Mills & Raine, 1994). Moreover, violent sexual offenses (acts combining both elements, such as rape) were associated with abnormalities in both brain regions. These early results clearly demonstrate that this "abnormal" behavior is concordant with the clinical picture of a frontal lobe disorder. Furthermore, any significant disturbance of frontal and temporal lobe structures may be the reason for disturbances in the control of sexual behavior and aggression.

More elaborate and recent studies on the neurobiological underpinnings of sexual deviance are limited. Eher et al. (1996) used MRI to investigate 17 sex offenders with structural brain changes and compared them to 21 sex offenders without brain changes. Within the group with brain changes, 76.5% had committed more violent sex crimes. However, in the control group, only 47.6% had committed such crimes. These data support the assumption made above. Aigner et al. (2000) compared 82 sex offenders who differed in terms of the extent of the violence exhibited (high versus low). In the highly violent group, 65.5% of the participants showed tangible changes in the structural integrity of the brain. These changes only occurred in 16.6% of the low-violence group cases. Similarly, Eher et al. (2000) used MRI to compare 17 participants (with structural anomalies) who had committed sex offenses against adults to 21 sex offenders without brain anomalies. Consistent with the previous findings, they concluded that the more severe the brain impairment, the more violent the sexual offenses.

In summary, there is evidence that the macroscopic integrity of temporal and frontal brain structure is highly important for the control of diverse cognitive functions and behaviors, including behavioral control, impulse control, sexual behavior, and aggression, among others. However, structural brain imaging has not yet successfully identified discrete brain areas responsible for specific types of sexual deviance. Overall, knowledge about the neurobiological underpinnings of sexual deviance is still in its infancy. Answering one question regularly raises several new ones. Even if there is a history of extensive research on the association between brain damage and neuropathology in the area of sexual offending and recidivism (see Fabian, 2012 for a review), no direct relationship between brain damage and sexual offending can be concluded. There is no evidence that brain damage actually causes genuine sexual deviancy. In the future, broad and multimodal research will be crucial to further our understanding of the mechanisms that underlie sexual deviance.

Functional Brain Correlates of Deviant Sexual Preference and Behavior

Although highly relevant, there is still little known about the functional correlates of deviant sexual preference and behavior. The lack of neuroimaging studies may reflect stigmatization and reluctance of affected individuals to volunteer for research, due to the risk of drawing attention to their sexual preferences and the potential risk for criminal behavior. While some paraphilias, like masochism and fetishism, have little to no potential to harm others, sexual sadism and pedophilia may lead individuals to harm others. In the following section, we focus on research that investigated the functional brain correlates of pedophilia, sexual sadism, and deviant sexual behavior.

Pedophilia Is Not the Same as Child Sexual Offending

Although pedophilia can be a central risk factor for sexually deviant behavior, pedophilia is neither a necessary nor sufficient condition for offensive sexual behavior. In fact, offensive sexual behavior and pedophilia are distinct phenomena. Pedophilia *per se* has long been perceived as a psychiatric disorder of high public concern. The DSM-5 (American Psychiatric Association, 2013) now differentiates between deviant sexual interests (i.e., paraphilia) that do not entail distress for the individual or an imminent risk of harming others and paraphilic disorders that are accompanied by distress and/or an immanent risk for offending/reoffending.

Functional Brain Correlates of Pedophilia

Are there pedophilia-specific functional brain correlates? For over a decade, functional neuroimaging techniques have been used to investigate the mechanisms of sexual attraction to children. To investigate the neurobiological mechanisms of pedophilia, the research focus must be broadened beyond sexual processing. Pedophilia has often been considered to be a consequence of disturbed sexual brain processing. However, current research lacks a more comprehensive understanding (Ponseti et al., 2018). For instance, by using pictures of infant animals (instead of human infants), Ponseti et al. (2018) aimed to examine a theory of elevated nurturing behavior in pedophilia without triggering sexual processing during an fMRI study. Group comparison of pedophilic and non-pedophilic participants revealed elevated brain responses to nurturing stimuli in the anterior insula in pedophiles—an area that was previously related to nurturing behaviors. In another recent study, Fonteille et al. (2019) used PET scans to investigate the brain responses of 15 male outpatients with a pedophilic disorder (mixed sample of those who had and had not offended). The group comparison revealed lower activation in the right inferior temporal cortex in response to visual sexual stimuli depicting children (VSSc) in patients compared to healthy controls. This level of activation in the right inferior temporal gyrus is positively correlated with ratings of sexual arousal elicited by VSSc. The authors concluded that the inferior temporal gyrus plays an important role in mediating sexual arousal in patients with pedophilic disorder. Stoleru et al. (1999) previously stressed the relevance of the inferior temporal gyrus and visually evoked sexual arousal in a non-clinical sample. Further research is needed to clarify the function of the inferior temporal gyrus in sexual processing in general and deviant sexual processing in particular.

Functional imaging as a technique to detect sexual preference? In 2012, Ponseti et al. successfully identified a pedophilic or teleiophilic preference on the basis of brain response to sexual stimuli. By measuring differences in the blood oxygen level-dependent (BoLD) response to child and adult sexual stimuli, they differentiated between men with a pedophilic or teleiophilic preference with high accuracy (100% specificity, 88% sensitivity). Hence, there appears to be a robust and specific brain response to preferred sexual stimuli that can be detected using fMRI. An automatic classification of these patterns might be a promising objective tool to clinically assess pedophilia and potentially other paraphilias. Nevertheless, a confirmation of this promising data is still pending. Poeppl et al. (2016) identified subcortical brain areas that might represent a possible neural structure that encodes sexual preference. This area was identified within small and phylogenetically old subcortical brain structures such as the (hypo)thalamus, septal area, and perirhinal parahippocampus (Poeppl et al., 2016).

What do we measure: sexual preference or delinquent behavior? Pedophilia has often been associated with significant neuropsychological, structural, and functional alterations (Tenbergen et al., 2015), and neurodevelopmental disorder theories have been discussed (see Fazio, 2018 for an overview). In an investigation of resting state functional connectivity, Cantor et al. (2016) found that pedophile CSOs showed significant differences in the functional connectivity of the brain compared to non-pedophilic controls, consistent with previously reported differences in structural connectivity.

Differentiating Between Sexual Preference and Delinquent Behavior

When paraphilic individuals with a history of sexual offending are analyzed, one can hardly detect whether the act of offending or the sexual preference is the variable that drives a certain effect. A 2 × 2 factorial design is necessary to differentiate between sexually deviant behavior and sexual preference, including pedophiles who already offended and pedophiles who never act out their urges. Additionally, a group of non-pedophilic CSOs and a group of teleiophilic controls should be included. The NeMUP-Consortium (NeMuP stands for Neuronal Mechanisms Underlying Paedodphilia and Child Sexual Abuse) was the first to differentiate between these two factors. They emphasized that the majority of alterations in structure and function are more related to the act of child sexual offending than to the pedophilic preference itself (e.g., Kärgel et al., 2017; Lett et al., 2018; Schiffer et al., 2017). For a detailed and extensive review of the history of pedophilia research using fMRI, see Mohnke et al. (2014) and Tenbergen et al. (2015).

An initial functional study by Walter et al. (2007) found differences in brain activity during sexual stimuli processing by showing images of naked adults to 13 pedophilic CSOs and 14 healthy controls. Pedophilic CSOs exhibited decreased activation of the hypothalamus and disrupted activity in the dorsolateral prefrontal cortex. This alteration correlated with the degree of cognitive impairment. These findings were interpreted as a functional correlate of decreased sexual interest in adults. However, because the study did not control sexual preference or the act of child sexual offending, and because non-preferred stimuli were used, interpretation of the results is difficult. More recent studies have found evidence that functional alterations in limbic and prefrontal regions may be related to delinquent behavior rather than sexual preference. For instance, Kärgel et al. (2015) studied resting state functional connectivity (RSFC) in 26 pedophilic men classified by offense status (14 participants with CSO, 12 without CSO) and 14 controls within (1) the default mode, and (2) the limbic network. Pedophilic men with CSO show diminished RSFC in both networks (specifically diminished RSFC between the left amygdala and orbitofrontal cortex, as well as in anterior prefrontal regions) compared to controls and pedophiles without a history of CSO. Kneer et al. (2019) compared non-pedophilic CSOs with healthy controls and found evidence for diminished functional connectivity between the amygdala and the dorsolateral prefrontal cortex (dlPFC). These data again indicate a relationship of the findings with delinquent behavior but not sexual preference.

While specific functional findings for a pedophilic preference are rather sparse or indicate some degree of dysfunction (e.g., Habermeyer et al., 2013), there is some evidence that pedophilic men without any hands-on offenses may perform better compared to their offending counterparts. Kärgel et al. (2017) first reported evidence for superior executive functioning in non-offending pedophiles using a Go/No-Go paradigm during fMRI (see Figure 5.4). Besides a lower error commission rate on the behavior levels, they found inhibition-related increased activation of the posterior cingulate (PCC) and frontal cortex while performing this task. Hence, heightened inhibition-related recruitment of these areas may be related to better inhibitory control in pedophilic men who successfully avoid committing hands-on sexual offenses against children. Assuming that these findings are true, an important question is whether the superior cognitive and neural function seen in these participants is inherent or learned and how it can be most effectively achieved during psychotherapeutic interventions.

Functional Brain Correlates of Rape and Sexual Sadism

Despite its crucial relevance, there is a lack of functional imaging studies using men who have committed rape offenses. The only fMRI study that exists focused on the neural correlates of pain observation in male sexual sadists (Harenski et al., 2012). By investigating 15 men who had committed violent sexual offenses against adults (eight sexual sadists and seven non-sadistic offenders), sadistic participants showed (as hypothesized) greater amygdala activation when viewing pain pictures. The authors concluded that sexual sadists show unusually heightened sensitivity to the pain of others. Particularly in males, amygdala activation is linked to sexual arousal (Hamann et al., 2004), data that might support the importance of this finding.

Hormones, Genes, and Epigenetic Regulation

There has long been great interest in identifying endocrine and genetic parameters that might explain sexual deviance and violent behavior. Androgens have been assigned a particularly crucial role in regulating sexual drive and function, as well as violent and aggressive behavior (Jordan et al., 2011a, 2011b; Mazur & Booth, 1998; Van Anders, 2013). Thus, we will primarily focus on androgens in this section. Efforts to better understand the role of androgens in sexual deviance are puzzling. With respect to a greater impact of contextual, cognitive, emotional, and

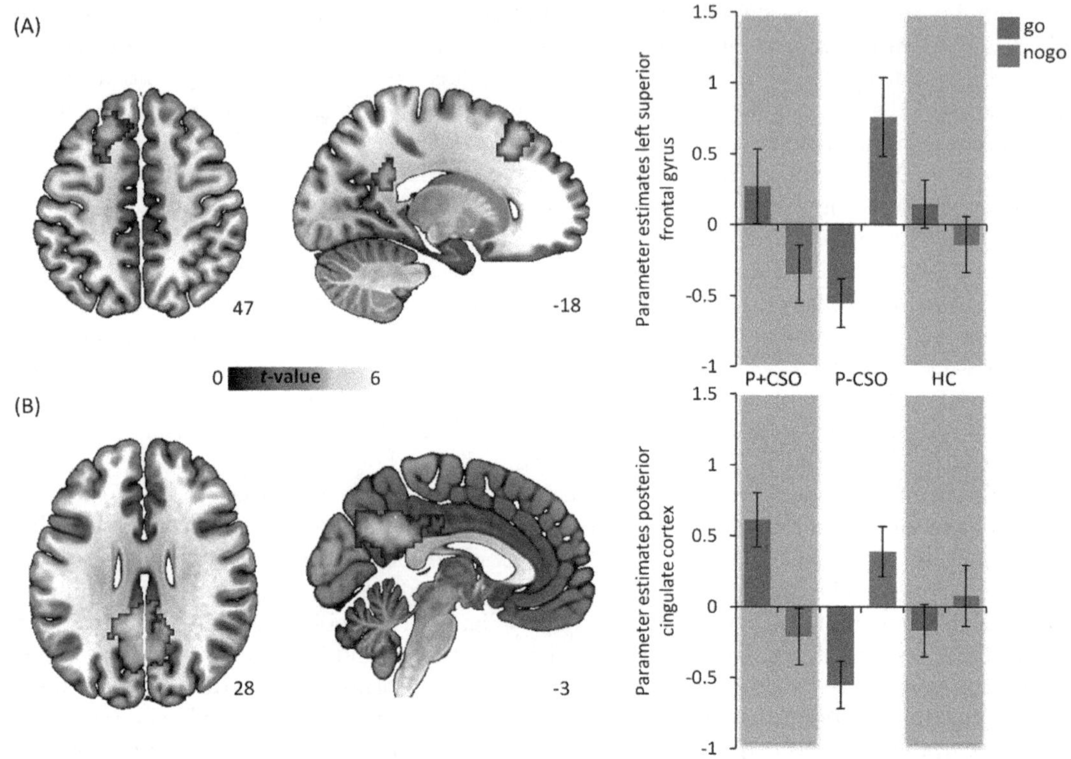

Figure 5.4 Differences in brain function (inhibitory control) in pedophilic men with and without child sexual offending (CSO) and healthy controls. Between group fMRI analysis. Post-hoc examination of a No-Go > Go paradigm contrast showed significantly increased activation in the (A) posterior cingulate gyrus and (B) left superior frontal gyrus in pedophiles without CSO (P-CSO) compared to pedophiles with CSO (P+CSO). Reprinted with permission from Kärgel et al. (2017).

social factors, the relationship between androgens and sexual behavior and aggression appears to be much more complex in humans compared to other animals. Although the majority of studies in this area have methodological flaws, some indicate a positive relationship between testosterone and/or gonadotropins and antisocial personality traits, novelty-seeking, self-reported hostility, sexual violence, sexual offense recidivism, and impulsive/aggressive behavior in men who have sexually offended against children and/or adults (for an overview, see Jordan et al., 2011a, b; Kingston et al., 2012; Studer et al., 2005). The relationship between androgens and behavior remains complex and may rely on different external factors, as well as the age of the respective organism. Different theories have been developed to explain the role of androgens under different circumstances:

- The **organizational–activational theory** is one of the most important and well-examined theories. It focuses on the effects of sex steroids during critical life periods, including the perinatal period and puberty. During this time, sex steroids lead to a sustained dimorphic differentiation of the brain (organizational effects). In contrast, activational effects occur when hormones induce acute, sex-specific behaviors in the adult organism by modulating specific brain areas (Lenz et al., 2012; Phoenix et al., 1959; Schulz, Molenda-Figueira et al., 2009; Schulz, Zehr et al., 2009).

- According to the **reciprocal model or challenge hypothesis**, testosterone levels depend on specific tasks and challenges. Testosterone levels increase after a successful event and decrease after failures.
- The **basal model** states that testosterone is a *trait marker* of a specific organism that determines behavior.
- According to the **status theory**, testosterone may facilitate the perception of social status and may even cause fair bargaining behavior for personal reasons in terms of status-seeking (Eisenegger et al., 2010; Mazur & Booth, 1998), as concluded in a study on women after administration of oral testosterone using an experimental paradigm (Eisenegger et al., 2010).

We have only rudimentary theories as to when and how sexual preference might develop (Bao & Swaab, 2010; Seto, 2008). According to some experts, such a determination might occur during fetal development (Bao & Swaab, 2010), at a time when organizational effects of sex steroids lead to sexual differentiation of the brain. As discussed by some authors (Bao & Swaab, 2010; Blanchard, 2010; Eisenegger et al., 2010; Jordan et al., 2011a, 2011b; Lenz et al., 2012; Mazur & Booth, 1998; O'Donohue, 2010; Phoenix et al., 1959; Schulz, Molenda-Figueira et al., 2009; Schulz, Zehr et al., 2009; Seto, 2012; Van Anders, 2013), sexual preference may also be categorized as a sexual orientation. With respect to the neurodevelopment of sexual orientation, studies indicate that androgens and an X chromosome-linked inheritance might explain some of the variance (Bao & Swaab, 2010; Rahman, 2005). In their emphasis on prenatal factors, Bao and Swaab (2010) go so far to say "There is no evidence that one's postnatal social environment plays a crucial role in gender identity or sexual orientation" (Bao & Swaab, 2010, p. 241). Clinically, pedophilia occurs almost exclusively in males, which may further corroborate the role of male sex steroids during brain maturation.

Preliminary, small-scale (and probably underpowered) studies on genetic variants in pedophiles ($N = 13$) (Alanko et al., 2016) and paraphilic sexual offenders ($N = 97$) (Jakubczyk et al., 2017) were unable to detect alterations in a specific neurotransmitter system. Earlier findings from a family study with small groups of inpatients with pedophilia ($N = 33$) and non-pedophilic paraphilias ($N = 21$) indicated elevated rates of pedophilia in the families of pedophiles, and other paraphilias in the families of people with non-pedophilic paraphilias (Gaffney et al., 1984). In a population-based Finnish cohort sample, male twins and their male siblings (aged 21–43 years) were analyzed regarding the occurrence of sexual interest in children and youth under age 16. The incidence of sexual interest in this age group was 3%, which is comparable to other investigations among men. Using a behavioral genetic model fitting (including genetic effects and non-shared environmental influences), the variance attributed to non-additive genetic influences was estimated to be almost 15% (Alanko et al., 2013). The largest genome-wide association study in almost 500,000 individuals found five autosomal loci were significantly associated with same-sex sexual behavior. All tested genetic variants accounted for 8–25% of variation in male and female same-sex sexual behavior (Ganna et al., 2019). Additional analyses of these loci suggest biological pathways linked to sex hormone regulation and olfaction. Although data is sparse regarding sexual preference and deviance, we can assume a genetic contribution to the developmental path towards pedophilia and possibly other paraphilias (see also Figure 5.5 for a working model).

Another relevant target has also been studied, namely, cysteine-adenine-guanine (CAG) repeat polymorphisms. Lower numbers of CAG codon repeats are related to elevated transactivational competence of the androgen receptor protein (Chamberlain et al., 1994; Kazemi-Esfarjani et al., 1995). Consequently, men with shorter CAG repeats may have larger physiological androgen-driven effects than men with longer repeats. Studies have revealed a relationship between shorter CAG repeats and various externalizing behaviors, as well as male violent criminal behavior (Cheng et al., 2006; Rajender et al., 2008).

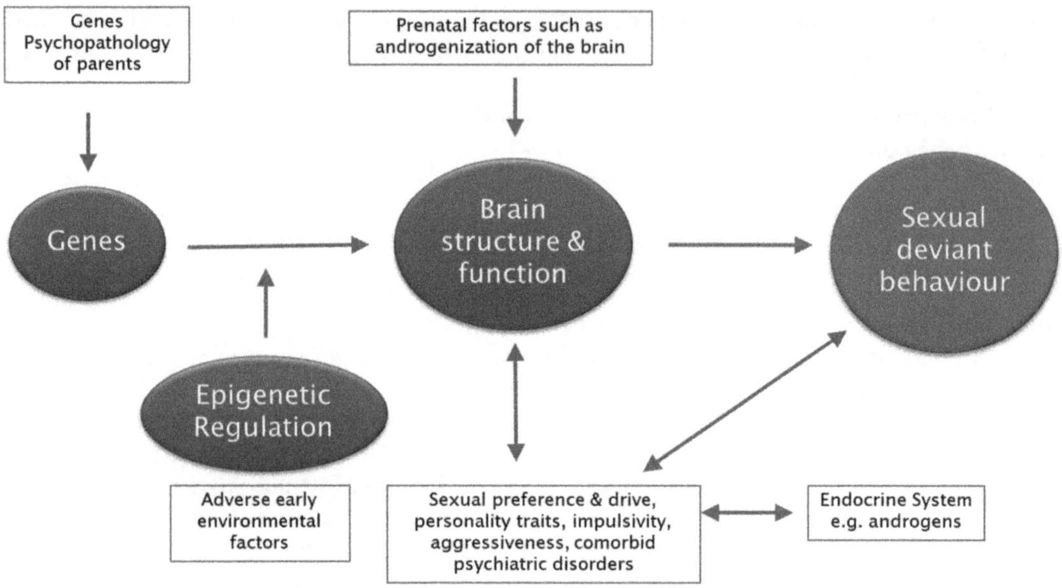

Figure 5.5 Neurobiological working model of trajectories on the road to sexual deviant behavior. Adapted from Kruger et al. (2019) with permission.

A recent study (Kruger et al., 2019) combined prenatal, genetic, epigenetic, and endocrine factors using the above mentioned NeMUP study group (2 × 2 factorial design). Independent of their sexual preference, CSOs showed signs of elevated prenatal androgen exposure, as assessed by the 2D:4D finger length ratio, compared to non-offending pedophiles and controls. The androgen receptor gene is more methylated in CSOs, indicating lower functionality of the testosterone system, as well as lower peripheral testosterone levels. Additionally, there was an interaction effect on methylation levels between offense status and androgen receptor functionality. Also, markers of prenatal androgenization and the methylation status of the androgen receptor gene were correlated with the total number of committed sexual offenses. Alterations in CAG repeat length were not found. Again, none of the findings are specific for pedophilia, but they are specific for child sexual offending. The authors suggested that these results may support theories of testosterone-linked abnormalities in early brain development in delinquent behavior and propose possible interactions of testosterone receptor gene methylation and plasma testosterone with environmental factors.

In conclusion, there is some evidence for a certain heritability and the involvement of androgenic factors on the road to sexual deviance. In the future, only combined multimodal approaches with large sample sizes will be able to further unravel the genetic, epigenetic, and hormonal underpinnings of sexual deviance. This endeavor will require substantial national and international research collaborations that may achieve the required numbers of clinically well-characterized subjects.

What Conclusions Can Be Drawn from the Current Findings?

Physiology

The previous sections demonstrated that we have quite a good understanding of the neuronal processing of sexual arousal in heterosexual men and women. The neuronal structures include limbic and paralimbic structures and known brain areas that are part of the salience network. Moreover, we know that homo- and heterosexual subjects show the same pattern of brain activation in response to visual sexual stimuli as long as their preferred stimulus is shown. A number of useful models and meta-analyses account for (neuro-)psychological as well as neurobiological components of sexual behavior.

Structure, Function, and Genes in Sexual Deviance

In contrast, the investigation of neurobiological factors that contribute to sexual deviance is still in its infancy. The majority of studies are conflicted by uncontrolled factors such as incarceration, delinquency, sexual preference and orientation, psychiatric comorbidities, and many others. Newer findings are challenging old assumptions and allow for a greater understanding of the differences between sexual preference and sexual delinquency. In summary, recent studies do not further support the theory of a sustained neurodevelopmental disorder for the case of (for example) pedophilia. fMRI research has revealed a similar activation pattern during the presentation of preferred sexual stimuli in pedophiles (and to some extent in sadists), indicating similar sexual stimuli processing in these individuals. Many previous results on functional and structural alterations in pedophiles (e.g., Schiffer et al., 2007; Walter et al., 2007) were not replicated by newer and better-controlled studies (Schiffer et al., 2017). These findings assume normal wiring in subjects with diverse sexual preference and orientation and/or may indicate a very subtle encoding (Poeppl et al., 2016). In the light of these considerations, sexual preference and orientation (as one part of sexual deviance) may reflect a physiological manifestation in a continuous and multidimensional concept of sexual behavior. On the other hand, delinquent behavior (e.g., rape, child sexual offending), as the other part of sexual deviance, is to be judged as criminal and more often depicts pathological signatures in psychological and biological studies. This delineation is consistent with the DSM-5 (American Psychiatric Association, 2013), where the mere presence of pedophilia is not seen as pathological unless it is accompanied by harm to oneself or others.

The Neurobiology of Sexual Deviance in a Nutshell

Using current neuroimaging techniques, the neurobiology of paraphilias (here pedophilia) indicates more normality compared to pathology, whereas delinquent behavior (here child sexual offending) and associated risk factors may have a neuronal signature.

References

Aigner, M., Eher, R., Fruehwald, S., Frottier, P., Gutierrez-Lobos, K., & Dwyer, S. M. (2000). Brain abnormalities and violent behavior. *Journal of Psychology & Human Sexuality, 11*(3), 57–64. https://doi.org/10.1300/J056v11n03_06

Alanko, K., Gunst, A., Mokros, A., & Santtila, P. (2016). Genetic variants associated with male pedophilic sexual interest. *The Journal of Sexual Medicine, 13*(5), 835–842. https://doi.org/10.1016/J.JSXM.2016.02.170

Alanko, K., Salo, B., Mokros, A., & Santtila, P. (2013). Evidence for heritability of adult men's sexual interest in youth under age 16 from a population-based extended twin design. *The Journal of Sexual Medicine, 10*(4), 1090–1099. https://doi.org/10.1111/JSM.12067

American Psychiatric Association. (2013). *Diagnostic and statistical manual of mental disorders* (5th ed.).

Bao, A. M., & Swaab, D. F. (2010). Sex differences in the brain, behavior, and neuropsychiatric disorders. *Neuroscientist, 16*(5), 550–565. https://doi.org/10.1177/1073858410377005

Bianchi-Demicheli, F., Cojan, Y., Waber, L., Recordon, N., Vuilleumier, P., & Ortigue, S. (2011). Neural bases of hypoactive sexual desire disorder in women: An event-related fMRI study. *The Journal of Sexual Medicine, 8*(9), 2546–2559. https://doi.org/10.1111/J.1743-6109.2011.02376.X

Blanchard, R. (2010). The DSM diagnostic criteria for pedophilia. *Archives of Sexual Behavior, 39*(2), 304–316. https://doi.org/10.1007/s10508-009-9536-0

Blanchard, R., Kolla, N. J., Cantor, J. M., Klassen, P. E., Dickey, R., Kuban, M. E., & Blak, T. (2007). IQ, handedness, and pedophilia in adult male patients stratified by referral source. *Sexual Abuse: A Journal of Research and Treatment, 19*(3), 285–309. https://doi.org/10.1177/107906320701900307

Bogaert, A. F. (2001). Handedness, criminality, and sexual offending. *Neuropsychologia, 39*(5), 465–469. https://doi.org/10.1016/S0028-3932(00)00134-2

Burns, J. M., & Swerdlow, R. H. (2003). Right orbitofrontal tumor with pedophilia symptom and constructional apraxia sign. *Archives of Neurology, 60*(3), 437. https://doi.org/10.1001/archneur.60.3.437

Cacioppo, S. (2017). Neuroimaging of female sexual desire and hypoactive sexual desire disorder. *Sexual Medicine Reviews, 5*(4), 434–444. https://doi.org/10.1016/j.sxmr.2017.07.006

Cantor, J. M., & Blanchard, R. (2012). White matter volumes in pedophiles, hebephiles, and teleiophiles. *Archives of Sexual Behavior, 41*(4), 749–752. https://doi.org/10.1007/s10508-012-9954-2

Cantor, J. M., Blanchard, R., Christensen, B. K., Dickey, R., Klassen, P. E., Beckstead, A. L., Blak, T., & Kuban, M. E. (2004). Intelligence, memory, and handedness in pedophilia. *Neuropsychology, 18*(1), 3–14. https://doi.org/10.1037/0894-4105.18.1.3

Cantor, J. M., Blanchard, R., Robichaud, L. K., & Christensen, B. K. (2005). Quantitative reanalysis of aggregate data on IQ in sexual offenders. *Psychological Bulletin, 131*(4), 555–568. https://doi.org/10.1037/0033-2909.131.4.555

Cantor, J. M., Kabani, N., Christensen, B. K., Zipursky, R. B., Barbaree, H. E., Dickey, R., Klassen, P. E., Mikulis, D. J., Kuban, M. E., Blak, T., & Blanchard, R. (2008). Cerebral white matter deficiencies in pedophilic men. *Journal of Psychiatric Research, 42*(3), 167–183. https://doi.org/10.1016/J.JPSYCHIRES.2007.10.013

Cantor, J. M., Lafaille, S. J., Hannah, J., Kucyi, A., Soh, D. W., Girard, T. A., & Mikulis, D. J. (2016). Independent component analysis of resting-state functional magnetic resonance imaging in pedophiles. *The Journal of Sexual Medicine, 13*(10), 1546–1554. https://doi.org/10.1016/j.jsxm.2016.08.004

Chamberlain, N. L., Driver, E. D., & Miesfeld, R. L. (1994). The length and location of CAG trinucleotide repeats in the androgen receptor N-terminal domain affect transactivation function. *Nucleic Acids Research, 22*(15), 3181–3186. https://doi.org/10.1093/nar/22.15.3181

Cheng, D., Hong, C.-J., Liao, D.-L., & Tsai, S.-J. (2006). Association study of androgen receptor CAG repeat polymorphism and male violent criminal activity. *Psychoneuroendocrinology, 31*(4), 548–552. https://doi.org/10.1016/J.PSYNEUEN.2005.11.004

Cohen, L. J., Nikiforov, K., Gans, S., Poznansky, O., McGeoch, P., Weaver, C., King, E. G., Cullen, K., & Galynker, I. (2002). Heterosexual male perpetrators of childhood sexual abuse: A preliminary neuropsychiatric model. *Psychiatric Quarterly, 73*(4), 313–336. https://doi.org/10.1023/A:1020416101092

Eastvold, A., Suchy, Y., & Strassberg, D. (2011). Executive function profiles of pedophilic and nonpedophilic child molesters. *Journal of the International Neuropsychological Society, 17*(2), 295–307. https://doi.org/10.1017/S1355617710001669

Eher, R., Aigner, M., Fruehwald, S., Frottier, P., & Gruenhut, C. (2000). Social information processed self-perceived aggression in relation to brain abnormalities in a sample of incarcerated sexual offenders. *Journal of Psychology & Human Sexuality, 11*(3), 37–47. https://doi.org/10.1300/J056v11n03_04

Eher, R., Aigner, M., Wagner, E., & Gutierrez, K. (1996). Magnetic resonance tomography of the brain in 21 sex offenders. *European Psychiatry, 11*(4). https://doi.org/10.1016/0924-9338(96)88861-4

Eisenegger, C., Naef, M., Snozzi, R., Heinrichs, M., & Fehr, E. (2010). Prejudice and truth about the effect of testosterone on human bargaining behaviour. *Nature, 463*(7279), 356–359. https://doi.org/10.1038/nature08711

Engel, J., Kessler, A., Veit, M., Sinke, C., Heitland, I., Kneer, J., Hartmann, U., & Kruger, T. H. C. (2019). Hypersexual behavior in a large online sample : Individual characteristics and signs of coercive sexual behavior. *Journal of Behavioral Addictions, 8*(2), 213–222. https://doi.org/10.1556/2006.8.2019.16

Engel, J., Veit, M., Sinke, C., Heitland, I., Kneer, J., Hillemacher, T., Hartmann, U., & Kruger, T. (2019). Same same but different: A clinical characterization of men with Hypersexual Disorder in the Sex@Brain study. *Journal of Clinical Medicine, 8*(2), 157. https://doi.org/10.3390/jcm8020157

Fabian, J. M. (2012). Neuropsychology, neuroscience, volitional impairment and sexually violent predators: A review of the literature and the law and their application to civil commitment proceedings. *Aggression and Violent Behavior, 17*(1), 1–15. https://doi.org/10.1016/j.avb.2011.07.002

Fazio, R. L. (2018). Toward a neurodevelopmental understanding of pedophilia. *The Journal of Sexual Medicine, 15*(9), 1205–1207. https://doi.org/10.1016/j.jsxm.2018.04.631

Fonteille, V., Redouté, J., Lamothe, P., Straub, D., Lavenne, F., Le Bars, D., Moulier, V., Marchand, J. J., Vittoz, A., Leriche, C., & Stoléru, S. (2019). Brain processing of pictures of children in men with pedophilic disorder: A positron emission tomography study. *NeuroImage: Clinical, 21*, 101647. https://doi.org/10.1016/j.nicl.2018.101647

Gaffney, G. R., Lurie, S. F., & Berlin, F. S. (1984). Is there familial transmission of Pedophilia? *Journal of Nervous and Mental Disease, 172*(9), 546–548. https://doi.org/10.1097/00005053-198409000-00006

Ganna, A., Verweij, K. J. H., Nivard, M. G., Maier, R., Wedow, R., Busch, A. S., Abdellaoui, A., Guo, S., Sathirapongsasuti, J. F., Lichtenstein, P., & Zietsch, B. P. (2019). Large-scale GWAS reveals insights into the genetic architecture of same-sex sexual behaviour. *Science, 365*(6456), eaat7693. https://doi.org/10.1126/science.aat7693

Georgiadis, J. R., & Kringelbach, M. L. (2012). The human sexual response cycle: Brain imaging evidence linking sex to other pleasures. *Progress in Neurobiology, 98*(1), 49–81. https://doi.org/10.1016/J.PNEUROBIO.2012.05.004

Gerwinn, H., Pohl, A., Granert, O., van Eimeren, T., Wolff, S., Jansen, O., Deuschl, G., Huchzermeier, C., Stirn, A., Siebner, H. R., & Ponseti, J. (2015). The (in)consistency of changes in brain macrostructure in male paedophiles: A combined T1-weighted and diffusion tensor imaging study. *Journal of Psychiatric Research, 68*, 246–253. https://doi.org/10.1016/j.jpsychires.2015.07.002

Graber, B., Hartmann, K., Coffman, J. A., Huey, C. J., & Golden, C. J. (1982). Brain damage among mentally disordered sex offenders. *Journal of Forensic Sciences, 27*(1), 11457J. https://doi.org/10.1520/jfs11457j

Habermeyer, B., Esposito, F., Händel, N., Lemoine, P., Klarhöfer, M., Mager, R., Dittmann, V., Seifritz, E., & Graf, M. (2013). Immediate processing of erotic stimuli in paedophilia and controls: A case control study. *BMC Psychiatry, 13*(1), 88. https://doi.org/10.1186/1471-244X-13-88

Hamann, S., Herman, R. A., Nolan, C. L., & Wallen, K. (2004). Men and women differ in amygdala response to visual sexual stimuli. *Nature Neuroscience, 7*(4), 411–416. https://doi.org/10.1038/nn1208

Harenski, C. L., Thornton, D. M., Harenski, K. A., Decety, J., & Kiehl, K. A. (2012). Increased frontotemporal activation during pain observation in sexual sadism. *Archives of General Psychiatry, 69*(3), 283. https://doi.org/10.1001/archgenpsychiatry.2011.1566

Hendricks, S. E., Fitzpatrick, D. F., Hartmann, K., Quaife, M. A., Stratbucker, R. A., & Graber, B. (1988). Brain structure and function in sexual molesters of children and adolescents. *The Journal of Clinical Psychiatry, 49*(3), 108–112. https://www.safetylit.org/citations/index.php?fuseaction=citations.viewdetails&citationIds[]=citjournalarticle_136122_38

Hucker, S., Langevin, R., Dickey, R., Handy, L., Chambers, J., Wright, S., Bain, J., & Wortzman, G. (1988). Cerebral damage and dysfunction in sexually aggressive men. *Annals of Sex Research, 1*(1), 33–47. https://doi.org/10.1007/BF00852881

Huettel, S. A., Song, A. W., & McCarthy, G. (2014). *Functional magnetic resonance imaging* (3rd ed.). Sinauer Associates.

Jakubczyk, A., Krasowska, A., Bugaj, M., Kopera, M., Klimkiewicz, A., Łoczewska, A., Michalska, A., Majewska, A., Szejko, N., Podgórska, A., Sołowiej, M., & Wojnar, M. (2017). Paraphilic sexual offenders do not differ from control subjects with respect to dopamine- and serotonin-related genetic polymorphisms. *Journal of Sexual Medicine, 14*(1), 125–133. https://doi.org/10.1016/j.jsxm.2016.11.309

Jordan, K., Fromberger, P., Stolpmann, G., & Müller, J. L. (2011a). The role of testosterone in sexuality and paraphilia: A neurobiological approach. Part I: Testosterone and sexuality. *The Journal of Sexual Medicine, 8*(11), 2993–3007. https://doi.org/10.1111/J.1743-6109.2011.02394.X

Jordan, K., Fromberger, P., Stolpmann, G., & Müller, J. L. (2011b). The role of testosterone in sexuality and paraphilia: A neurobiological approach. Part II: Testosterone and paraphilia. *The Journal of Sexual Medicine, 8*(11), 3008–3029. https://doi.org/10.1111/J.1743-6109.2011.02393.X

Joyal, C. C., Kärgel, C., Kneer, J., Amelung, T., Mohnke, S., Tenbergen, G., … Walter, H. (2019). The neurobiological origins of pedophilia: Not that simple. *Journal of Sexual Medicine, 16*(1), 153–154. https://doi.org/10.1016/j.jsxm.2018.10.015

Kärgel, C., Massau, C., Weiß, S., Walter, M., Borchardt, V., Krueger, T. H. C., Tenbergen, G., Kneer, J., Wittfoth, M., Pohl, A., Gerwinn, H., & Schiffer, B. (2017). Evidence for superior neurobiological and behavioral inhibitory control abilities in non-offending as compared to offending pedophiles. *Human Brain Mapping, 38*(2), 1092–1104. https://doi.org/10.1002/hbm.23443

Kärgel, C., Massau, C., Weiß, S., Walter, M., Kruger, T. H. C., & Schiffer, B. (2015). Diminished functional connectivity on the road to child sexual abuse in pedophilia. *The Journal of Sexual Medicine, 12*(3), 783–795. https://doi.org/10.1111/JSM.12819

Kazemi-Esfarjani, P., Trifiro, M. A., & Pinsky, L. (1995). Evidence for a repressive function of the long polyglutamine tract in the human androgen receptor: Possible pathogenetic relevance for the (CAG)n-expanded neuronopathies. *Human Molecular Genetics, 4*(4), 523–527. https://doi.org/10.1093/hmg/4.4.523

Kingston, D. A., Seto, M. C., Ahmed, A. G., Fedoroff, P., Firestone, P., & Bradford, J. M. (2012). The role of central and peripheral hormones in sexual and violent recidivism in sex offenders. *Journal of the American Academy of Psychiatry and the Law, 40*(4), 476–485.

Kneer, J., Borchardt, V., Kärgel, C., Sinke, C., Massau, C., Tenbergen, G., Ponseti, J., Walter, H., Beier, K. M., Schiffer, B., Schiltz, K., Walter, M., & Kruger, T. H. C. (2019). Diminished fronto-limbic functional connectivity in child sexual offenders. *Journal of Psychiatric Research, 108*, 48–56. https://doi.org/10.1016/j.jpsychires.2018.01.012

Kruger, T. H. C., & Schiffer, B. (2011). Neurocognitive and personality factors in homo- and heterosexual pedophiles and controls. *Journal of Sexual Medicine, 8*(6), 1650–1659. https://doi.org/10.1111/j.1743-6109.2009.01564.x

Kruger, T. H. C., Sinke, C., Kneer, J., Tenbergen, G., Khan, A. Q., Burkert, A., Müller-Engling, L., Engler, H., Gerwinn, H., von Wurmb-schwark, N., Pohl, A., Weiß, S., Amelung, T., Mohnke, S., Massau, C., Kärgel, C., Walter, M., Schiltz, K., Beier, K. M., & Frieling, H. (2019). Child sexual offenders show prenatal and epigenetic alterations of the androgen system. *Translational Psychiatry, 9*(1), 28. https://doi.org/10.1038/s41398-018-0326-0

Langevin, R., Wortzman, G., Dickey, R., Wright, P., & Handy, L. (1988). Neuropsychological impairment in incest offenders. *Sexual Abuse: A Journal of Research and Treatment, 1*(3), 401–415. https://doi.org/10.1177/107906328800100304

Langevin, R., Wortzman, G., Wright, P., & Handy, L. (1989). Studies of brain damage and dysfunction in sex offenders. *Sexual Abuse: A Journal of Research and Treatment, 2(2)*, 163–179. https://doi.org/10.1177/107906328900200204

Lenz, B., Müller, C. P., Stoessel, C., Sperling, W., Biermann, T., Hillemacher, T., Bleich, S., & Kornhuber, J. (2012). Sex hormone activity in alcohol addiction: Integrating organizational and activational effects. *Progress in Neurobiology, 96*(1), 136–163. https://doi.org/10.1016/J.PNEUROBIO.2011.11.001

Lesniak, R., Szymusik, A., & Chrzanowski, R. (1972). Multidirectional disorders of sexual drive in a case of brain tumour. *Forensic Science, 1*(3), 333–338. https://doi.org/10.1016/0300-9432(72)90031-3

Lett, T. A., Mohnke, S., Amelung, T., Brandl, E. J., Schiltz, K., Pohl, A., Gerwinn, H., Kärgel, C., Massau, C., Tenbergen, G., & Walter, H. (2018). Multimodal neuroimaging measures and intelligence influence pedophile child sexual offense behavior. *European Neuropsychopharmacology, 28*(7), 818–827. https://doi.org/10.1016/j.euroneuro.2018.05.002

Massau, C., Tenbergen, G., Kärgel, C., Weiß, S., Gerwinn, H., Pohl, A., Amelung, T., Mohnke, S., Kneer, J., Wittfoth, M., Ristow, I., Schiltz, K., Beier, K. M., Ponseti, J., Walter, M., Kruger, T. H. C., Walter, H., Schiffer, B. (2017). Executive functioning in pedophilia and child sexual offending. *Journal of the International Neuropsychological Society, 23*(6), 460–470. https://doi.org/10.1017/S1355617717000315

Masters, W. H., & Johnson, V. E. (1966). *Human sexual response.* Little, Brown and Company.

Mazur, A., & Booth, A. (1998). Testosterone and dominance in men. *Behavioral and Brain Sciences, 21*(3), 353–363. https://doi.org/10.1017/S0140525X98001228

Mendez, M. F., Chow, T., Ringman, J., Twitchell, G., & Hinkin, C. H. (2000). Pedophilia and temporal lobe disturbances. *The Journal of Neuropsychiatry and Clinical Neurosciences, 12*(1), 71–76. https://doi.org/10.1176/jnp.12.1.71

Mendez, M. F., & Shapira, J. S. (2011). Pedophilic behavior from brain disease. *The Journal of Sexual Medicine, 8*(4), 1092–1100. https://doi.org/10.1111/J.1743-6109.2010.02172.X

Miller, B. L., Cummings, J. L., McIntyre, H., Ebers, G., & Grode, M. (1986). Hypersexuality or altered sexual preference following brain injury. *Journal of Neurology, Neurosurgery, and Psychiatry, 49*(8), 867–873. https://doi.org/10.1136/jnnp.49.8.867

Mills, S., & Raine, A. (1994). Neuroimaging and aggression. *Journal of Offender Rehabilitation, 21*(3–4), 145–158. https://doi.org/10.1300/J076v21n03_09

Mohnke, S., Müller, S., Amelung, T., Krüger, T. H. C., Ponseti, J., Schiffer, B., Walter, M., Beier, K.M., & Walter, H. (2014). Brain alterations in paedophilia: A critical review. *Progress in Neurobiology*, *122*, 1–23. https://doi.org/10.1016/J.PNEUROBIO.2014.07.005

O'Donohue, W. (2010). A critique of the proposed DSM-V diagnosis of pedophilia. *Archives of Sexual Behavior*, *39*(3), 587–590. https://doi.org/10.1007/s10508-010-9604-5

Paul, T., Schiffer, B., Zwarg, T., Krüger, T. H. C., Karama, S., Schedlowski, M., Forsting, M., & Gizewski, E. R. (2008). Brain response to visual sexual stimuli in heterosexual and homosexual males. *Human Brain Mapping*, *29*(6), 726–735. https://doi.org/10.1002/hbm.20435

Phoenix, C. H., Goy, R. W., Gerall, A. A., & Young, W. C. (1959). Organizing action of prenatally administered testosterone propionate on the tissues mediating mating behavior in the female guinea pig. *Endocrinology*, *65*(3), 369–382. https://doi.org/10.1210/endo-65-3-369

Poeppl, T. B., Langguth, B., Laird, A. R., & Eickhoff, S. B. (2014). The functional neuroanatomy of male psychosexual and physiosexual arousal: A quantitative meta-analysis. *Human Brain Mapping*, *35*(4), 1404–1421. https://doi.org/10.1002/hbm.22262

Poeppl, T. B., Langguth, B., Rupprecht, R., Laird, A. R., & Eickhoff, S. B. (2016). A neural circuit encoding sexual preference in humans. *Neuroscience & Biobehavioral Reviews*, *68*, 530–536. https://doi.org/10.1016/J.NEUBIOREV.2016.06.025

Poeppl, T. B., Nitschke, J., Santtila, P., Schecklmann, M., Langguth, B., Greenlee, M. W., Osterheider, M., & Mokros, A. (2013). Association between brain structure and phenotypic characteristics in pedophilia. *Journal of Psychiatric Research*, *47*(5), 678–685. https://doi.org/10.1016/J.JPSYCHIRES.2013.01.003

Ponseti, J., Bruhn, D., Nolting, J., Gerwinn, H., Pohl, A., Stirn, A., Granert, O., Laufs, H., Deuschl, G., Wolff, S., & Kruger, T. H. C. (2018). Decoding pedophilia: Increased anterior insula response to infant animal pictures. *Frontiers in Human Neuroscience*, *11*, 645. https://doi.org/10.3389/fnhum.2017.00645

Ponseti, J., Granert, O., Jansen, O., Wolff, S., Beier, K., Neutze, J., Deuschl, G., Mehdorn, H., Siebner, H., & Bosinski, H. (2012). Assessment of pedophilia using hemodynamic brain response to sexual stimuli. *Archives of General Psychiatry*, *69*(2), 187–194. https://doi.org/10.1001/archgenpsychiatry.2011.130

Rahman, Q. (2005). The neurodevelopment of human sexual orientation. *Neuroscience & Biobehavioral Reviews*, *29*(7), 1057–1066. https://doi.org/10.1016/J.NEUBIOREV.2005.03.002

Rahman, Q., & Symeonides, D. J. (2008). Neurodevelopmental correlates of paraphilic sexual interests in men. *Archives of Sexual Behavior*, *37*(1), 166–172. https://doi.org/10.1007/s10508-007-9255-3

Rajender, S., Pandu, G., Sharma, J. D., Gandhi, K. P. C., Singh, L., & Thangaraj, K. (2008). Reduced CAG repeats length in androgen receptor gene is associated with violent criminal behavior. *International Journal of Legal Medicine*, *122*(5), 367–372. https://doi.org/10.1007/s00414-008-0225-7

Redouté, J., Stoléru, S., Grégoire, M.-C., Costes, N., Cinotti, L., Lavenne, F., Le Bars, D., Forest, M.G., & Pujol, J.-F. (2000). Brain processing of visual sexual stimuli in human males. *Human Brain Mapping*, *11*(3), 162–177. https://doi.org/10.1002/1097-0193(200011)11:3<62::aid-hbm30>3.0.CO;2-A

Schiffer, B., Amelung, T., Pohl, A., Kaergel, C., Tenbergen, G., Gerwinn, H., Mohnke, S., Massau, C., Matthias, W., Weiß, S., & Walter, H. (2017). Gray matter anomalies in pedophiles with and without a history of child sexual offending. *Translational Psychiatry*, *7*(5), e1129. https://doi.org/10.1038/tp.2017.96

Schiffer, B., Peschel, T., Paul, T., Gizewski, E., Forsting, M., Leygraf, N., Schedlowski, M., & Krueger, T. H. C. (2007). Structural brain abnormalities in the frontostriatal system and

cerebellum in pedophilia. *Journal of Psychiatric Research, 41*(9), 753–762. https://doi.org/10.1016/j.jpsychires.2006.06.003
Schiffer, B., & Vonlaufen, C. (2011). Executive dysfunctions in pedophilic and nonpedophilic child molesters. *The Journal of Sexual Medicine, 8*(7), 1975–1984. https://doi.org/10.1111/j.1743-6109.2010.02140.x
Schiltz, K., Witzel, J., Northoff, G., Zierhut, K., Gubka, U., Fellmann, H., Kaufmann, J., Tempelmann, C., Wiebking, C., & Bogerts, B. (2007). Brain pathology in pedophilic offenders. *Archives of General Psychiatry, 64*(6), 737. https://doi.org/10.1001/archpsyc.64.6.737
Schulz, K. M., Molenda-Figueira, H. A., & Sisk, C. L. (2009). Back to the future: The organizational–activational hypothesis adapted to puberty and adolescence. *Hormones and Behavior, 55*(5), 597–604. https://doi.org/10.1016/J.YHBEH.2009.03.010
Schulz, K. M., Zehr, J. L., Salas-Ramirez, K. Y., & Sisk, C. L. (2009). Testosterone programs adult social behavior before and during, but not after, Adolescence. *Endocrinology, 150*(8), 3690–3698. https://doi.org/10.1210/en.2008-1708
Seto, M. C. (2008). *Pedophilia and sexual offending against children: Theory, assessment, and intervention.* American Psychological Association.
Seto, M. C. (2012). Is pedophilia a sexual orientation? *Archives of Sexual Behavior, 41*(1), 231–236. https://doi.org/10.1007/s10508-011-9882-6
Siever, L. J. (2008). Neurobiology of aggression and violence. *American Journal of Psychiatry, 165*(4), 429–442. https://doi.org/10.1176/appi.ajp.2008.07111774
Stoléru, S., Fonteille, V., Cornélis, C., Joyal, C., & Moulier, V. (2012). Functional neuroimaging studies of sexual arousal and orgasm in healthy men and women: A review and meta-analysis. *Neuroscience and Biobehavioral Reviews, 36*(6), 1481–1509. https://doi.org/10.1016/j.neubiorev.2012.03.006
Stoleru, S., Gregoire, M.-C., Gerard, D., Decety, J., Lafarge, E., Cinotti, L., Lavenne, F., Le Bars, D., Vernet-Maury, E., Rada, H., Collet, C., Mazoyer, B., Forest, M. G., Magnin, F., Spira, A., & Comar, D. (1999). Neuroanatomical correlates of visually evoked sexual arousal in human males. *Archives of Sexual Behavior, 28*(1), 1–21. https://doi.org/10.1023/A:1018733420467
Studer, L. H., Aylwin, A. S., & Reddon, J. R. (2005). Testosterone, sexual offense recidivism, and treatment effect among adult male sex offenders. *Sexual Abuse: A Journal of Research and Treatment, 17*(2), 171–181. https://doi.org/10.1007/s11194-005-4603-0
Suchy, Y., Eastvold, A. D., Strassberg, D. S., & Franchow, E. I. (2014). Understanding processing speed weaknesses among pedophilic child molesters: Response style vs. Neuropathology. *Journal of Abnormal Psychology, 123*(1), 273–285. https://doi.org/10.1037/a0035812
Suchy, Y., Whittaker, J. W., Strassberg, D. S., & Eastvold, A. (2009). Neurocognitive differences between pedophilic and nonpedophilic child molesters. *Journal of the International Neuropsychological Society, 15*(2), 248–257. https://doi.org/10.1017/S1355617709090353
Tenbergen, G., Wittfoth, M., Frieling, H., Ponseti, J., Walter, M., Walter, H., Beier, K.M., Schiffer, B., & Kruger, T. H. C. (2015). The neurobiology and psychology of pedophilia: Recent advances and challenges. *Frontiers in Human Neuroscience, 9*, 344. https://doi.org/10.3389/fnhum.2015.00344
van Anders, S. M. (2013). Beyond masculinity: Testosterone, gender/sex, and human social behavior in a comparative context. *Frontiers in Neuroendocrinology, 34*(3), 198–210. https://doi.org/10.1016/J.YFRNE.2013.07.001
Walter, M., Witzel, J., Wiebking, C., Gubka, U., Rotte, M., Schiltz, K., Bermpohl, F., Tempelmann, C., Bogerts, B., Heinze, H. J., & Northoff, G. (2007). Pedophilia is linked to reduced activation in hypothalamus and lateral prefrontal cortex during visual erotic stimulation. *Biological Psychiatry, 62*(6), 698–701. https://doi.org/10.1016/J.BIOPSYCH.2006.10.018

Woodard, T. L., Nowak, N. T., Balon, R., Tancer, M., & Diamond, M. P. (2013). Brain activation patterns in women with acquired hypoactive sexual desire disorder and women with normal sexual function: A cross-sectional pilot study. *Fertility and Sterility, 100*(4), 1068–1076.e5. https://doi.org/10.1016/j.fertnstert.2013.05.041

World Health Organization. (2018). *International classification of diseases for mortality and morbidity statistics (11th Revision).* https://icd.who.int/browse11/l-m/en

Wright, P., Nobrega, J., Langevin, R., & Wortzman, G. (1990). Brain density and symmetry in pedophilic and sexually aggressive offenders. *Annals of Sex Research, 3*(3), 319–328. https://doi.org/10.1007/BF00849186

Part III

Assessing and Diagnosing Sexual Deviance

6

Problems and Controversies with Psychiatric Diagnoses of Paraphilia

Christian C. Joyal

Department of Psychology, University of Quebec at Trois-Rivières, Qc, Canada, International Center of Comparative Criminology, Trois-Rivières site, Canada, Groupe de Recherche sur les Agresseurs Sexuels, University of Montreal, Canada

> Often eroticism is just a manifestation of illness, emerging as a more or less severe symptom in a syndrome of manic exaltation
>
> -Joseph Guislain (1852)

> As a rule, [anomalies of the sexual instinct] are certainly only symptoms of a constitutional malady, or of a weakened state of the brain, which manifest themselves in the various forms of sexual perversions
>
> -Freiher Albert von Schrenck-Notzing (1892)

Introduction

Being influenced by social, cultural, moral, religious, political and legal factors, attempts to define pathological sexual interests have always been controversial (see Gert & Culver, 2009; Milner et al., 2008 for reviews). The term paraphilia (from the Greek *para*, "beside, aside," and *philia*, "love") is used in psychiatry to define "anomalous" or "atypical" sexual interests. Currently, definitions of mental disorders, paraphilia, and paraphilic disorders derive from two main psychiatry manuals used worldwide, the *Diagnostic and Statistical Manual of Mental Disorders*, 5th edition (DSM-5, APA, 2013), and the *International Classification of Diseases*, 11th revision (ICD-11, WHO, 2018). Each reference and problems related with their diagnostic criteria of paraphilias will be considered separately.

The DSM-5

In the DSM-5

> A mental disorder is a syndrome characterized by clinically significant disturbance in an individual's cognition, emotion regulation, or behavior that *reflects a dysfunction in the psychological, biological, or developmental processes underlying mental functioning.*

Sexual Deviance: Understanding and Managing Deviant Sexual Interests and Paraphilic Disorders,
First Edition. Edited by Leam A. Craig and Ross M. Bartels.
© 2021 John Wiley & Sons, Ltd. Published 2021 by John Wiley & Sons, Ltd.

> Mental disorders are usually associated with significant distress or disability in social, occupational, or other important activities. An expectable or culturally approved response to a common stressor or loss, such as the death of a loved one, is not a mental disorder. Socially deviant behavior (e.g., political, religious, or sexual) and conflicts that are primarily between the individual and society are not mental disorders unless the deviance or conflict results from a dysfunction in the individual. (p. 20, emphasis added)

Thus, signs and symptoms are measurable manifestations (cognitive, emotional or behavioral) of an underlying, deduced, psychopathology (a defective psychological, biological or developmental process). As described below, the main problem with the paraphilic disorder definitions is that signs (e.g., the behavioral manifestation of looking an unsuspecting stranger disrobing) and the supposed underlying defective process (voyeurism) are the same. Another important problem is that a growing number of studies fail to find signs (cognitive, emotional or behavioral disturbances) or evidence (dysfunctions in the psychological, biological, or developmental processes) of psychopathology in persons with certain paraphilias.

In the DMS-5, the term paraphilia refers to "non-normophilic" interest, i.e., "any intense and persistent sexual interest other than sexual interest in genital stimulation or preparatory fondling with phenotypically normal, physically mature, consenting human partners." Paraphilias become pathological (a paraphilic disorder) when they are illegal and acted upon or associated with clinically significant distress or impairment in social, occupational, or other areas of functioning (APA, 2013). The DSM-5 definitions of sexual normality ("normophilia") and "anomalous" sexual interests (paraphilia) have already been widely criticized (Balon, 2013; Downing, 2015; Fedoroff, 2011; Fedoroff et al., 2013; First, 2014; Hinderliter, 2010, 2011; Joyal, 2015, 2018; Moser, 2001, 2016, 2019; O'Donohue, 2010, 2016; Shindel & Moser, 2011; Singy, 2010; Wakefield, 2011). The goal of this chapter is not to reiterate all these critics, but to review and comment on the more important problems. Possible solutions to these problems will also be addressed.

Procreation or perversion: The bases of paraphilic definitions. In the DSM-5, the following sexual interests (fantasies, urges or behaviors) are listed as "anomalous": voyeurism, exhibitionism, frotteurism, sexual masochism, sexual sadism, pedophilia, fetishism, transvestism (main diagnoses), as well as telephone scatologia, necrophilia, zoophilia, coprophilia, klismaphilia, and urophilia (other specified paraphilic disorders). A first question concerning this list of "anomalous" sexual interests is: On which bases were they defined? A first hint is that none of them implies, by itself, a penile-vagina intercourse. Historically in Western cultures, early Christians (especially Saint Augustine, 354–430 AD) put great emphasis on procreation due, among other reasons, to a marked decrease in the birth rate of Italians following the fall of Rome (Kiefer, 1934/2009). The Doctors of the Church (especially Thomas Aquinas, 1224/1225–1274) also viewed sexuality negatively, a threat to the progress of moral and civilization, believing that open sexuality led to social chaos (Milhaven, 1977). According to Judeo-Christian ethic, coital relations should be used with parsimony, as a biological function (transmission of life), only under certain circumstances (e.g., within marriage), and within strict rules (restricted to coital intercourse; no masturbatory, oral, anal or homosexual behaviors; Bullough, 1976). As clearly stressed in the Catechism of the Catholic Church, "Sexual pleasure is morally disordered when sought for itself" (offenses against chastity, under the Sixth Commandment). In contrast, Eastern cultures traditionally had a positive view on sexuality, prompting classic books such as the ancient Indian Hindu *Kama Sutra* (Vatsyayana, 1883, original c. 400), medieval Indian *Koka Shastra* (Kokkoka, 1965, original c. 1150), and Arabic *The Perfumed Garden* (al-Nafzawi, 1886, original c. 1400) to recommend foreplays and non-coital behaviors to enhance sexual arousal (e.g., oral sex, biting, scratching, spanking, and hair pulling). Similarly, in Ancient China, fellatio, cunnilingus and anal intercourse were approved and practiced, as long as no semen was lost (the man yang essence; Tannahill, 1980). Therefore, definitions of paraphilic behaviors in Western culture are primarily based on historical, religious, and moral grounds. This is why homosexuality was listed in the DSM-II (APA, 1968). This is also why sadomasochism, fetishism, and fetishistic transvestism will be removed from the ICD-11 (discussed later).

In the West, psychiatry and forensic psychiatry were emerging during the 19th century, the first medical classifications of sexual perversions were established, and they were highly influenced by religious, societal and evolutionary factors. For instance, Krafft-Ebing (1886), a devoted Christian, defined sexual perversions as manifestations of the sexual instinct that "fails to reach the goal of nature," i.e., the perpetuation of the race ("perversion of the sexual instinct"). Similarly, Freud (1905/1920) defined sexual perversions as "substitutions of the normal sexual aim" (coital relation). It is worth noting, however, that Freud (1905/1920) underlined that the sole nature of a "sexual transgression" (i.e., oral sex, anal sex, fetishism, sadism, masochism, and voyeurism) should not be used to define perversions, as they were common: "Everyday experience has shown that most of these transgressions, at least the milder ones, are seldom wanting as components in the sexual life of normals who look upon them as upon other intimacies. [...] In no normal person does the normal sexual aim lack *some designable perverse element*, and this universality suffices in itself to prove the inexpediency of an opprobrious application of the name perversion" (p. 27, emphasis added). Thus, traditionally, it was not the non-coital sexual behavior, *per se*, that was problematic, but its exclusivity. As stressed by Hinderliter (2011), "Under a restrictive interpretation, [the DSM-5 definition of normophilia] means that if a certain instance of fondling is preparatory for genital stimulation, intense and persistent interest in it is not paraphilic; but if the same behavior is not preparatory for genital stimulation in another context, it might be" (p. 21). This dichotomy is highly reminiscent of Freud's perspective.

In the following section, the main issues with the DSM-5 diagnoses of paraphilia will be briefly reviewed. Pedophilia, which represents a particular, distinct (and the most studied) paraphilia, will be discussed afterward, in a separate section.

Paraphilic interests are rare, or are they? One basic criterion to define a paraphilic interest in psychiatric manuals is the unusual nature of the arousal source. According to the DSM-5 (APA, 2013) and the ICD-11 (WHO, 2018), paraphilic interests are anomalous or atypical, respectively, which means rare or uncommon. However, it is clear that many sexual fantasies or arousal based on paraphilic themes are not atypical in non-clinical/non-forensic samples of persons (Baur et al., 2016; Castellini et al., 2018; Dawson et al., 2016; Lodi-Smith et al., 2014; Mundy & Cioe, 2019; Renaud & Byers, 1999; Robinson & Parks, 2004; Roche & Staunton, 2018; Templeman & Stinnett, 1991; Watts et al., 2019; Williams et al., 2009). Therefore, the very basic criterion of atypicity (let alone anomalous) is not met for many paraphilic interests.

Based on objective statistical criteria, only two sexual fantasies out of 53 were found to be rare (having sex with a child under 12 and having sex with an animal) and nine were found to be atypical (urinating on partner; being urinated on; wearing clothes of the opposite gender; forcing someone to have sex; abusing a person who is drunk, asleep, or unconscious; having sex with a prostitute; and having sex with a women who has very small breasts, among women and urinating on partner; being urinated on; having sex with two other men; having sex with more than three other men among men) in a relatively large sample of adult participants recruited in the general population (Joyal et al., 2015). More than half of that sample (57%) actually met the DSM-5 criteria for paraphilic sexual interest (fantasies with intensity "greater than or equal to" normophilic fantasies; Joyal, 2015). Interestingly, two chief editors of the DSM-IV-TR (APA, 2000) acknowledged that a mistake was made in the DSM-IV revision of paraphilia diagnoses criteria: the word "and" was replaced by "or" in "sexually arousing fantasy, sexual urge *or* behaviors" (First & Frances, 2008). The authors warned (unsuccessfully) the DSM-5 subworkgroup that the word change left the door open to the interpretation that behaviors were now sufficient (e.g., repetitive child sexual abuse) to receive a diagnosis of mental disorder (e.g., pedophilia). However, another pernicious consequence of that use of the disjunction for the definition of paraphilia was that the sole presence of a fantasy was now sufficient to meet its criteria (Hinderliter, 2011).

As for paraphilic behaviors, earlier studies tended to report low prevalence among the general population. For instance, in a representative sample of 2,450 randomly selected adults, only 76 (3.1%) reported at least one incident of being sexually aroused by exposing their genitals to a stranger and only 191 (7.7%) reported at least one incident of being sexually aroused by spying on others having sex in Sweden (Langström & Seto, 2006). That study is often cited (including in the DSM-5) because it is based on state of the art person-to-person interviews. However, while questions related with sexuality were filled in without research assistants being able to see the answers, participants still had to eventually give the questionnaire to that person. This procedure might have led to an underestimate of the true prevalence of exhibitionistic and voyeuristic behaviors. In another study based on a representative sample of the population, 30% of women and 12% of men in the U.S. reported having faced unwanted genital flashing in their lifetime (UC San Diego Center on Gender Equity and Health, 2019). In the same study, 49% of women and 18% of men reported having been sexually touched in an unwelcome way at least once in their life. Indeed, a growing number of studies clearly demonstrate that many paraphilic behaviors are not atypical in non-clinical samples of participants (Ahlers et al., 2011; Androvicova et al., 2018; Castellini et al., 2018; Dawson et al., 2016; Eagan, 2017; Herbenick et al., 2017; Joyal & Carpentier, 2017; Jozifkova, 2018; Lodi-Smith et al., 2014; Mundy & Cioe, 2019; Noorishad et al., 2019). Approximately half of men recruited in non-clinical populations report having done a paraphilic behavior at least once in their lifetime (especially voyeurism and domination-submission themes; Apostolou & Khalil, 2019; Castellini et al., 2018; Dawson et al., 2016; Holvoet et al., 2017; Joyal & Carpentier, 2017; Noorishad et al., 2019). Rates of paraphilic behaviors might be lower in non-Western, non-Asian cultures (Abdullahi et al., 2015; Makanjuola et al., 2008), although many confounding factors might explain these differences (e.g., shyness, shame, fear, and/or religious beliefs restraining participants from divulging their sex life for research purposes).

Still, certain sexual interests are indeed rare or atypical among the general population, such as those involving prepubertal children, corpses, animals or excrements (Dawson et al., 2016; Dombert et al., 2016; Joyal & Carpentier, 2017; Rinehart & McCabe, 1998; Wurtele et al., 2014). These sexual interests are candidates for paraphilias (i.e., possible signs of mental disorder), which can only be assessed with developmental, neurological and psychological investigations. Future taxonomic studies should also include these rarer sexual interests in their analyses as they might represent distinct, categorical (and, perhaps, pathological) entities, contrarily to more common paraphilic interests, better conceptualized as dimensional variables (Thompson, 2016).

Paraphilias, sexual diversity and sexual drive. Another erroneous assumption is that most persons with paraphilic behaviors limit their sexual activities to these behaviors. As stressed by Moser (2016), most individuals with paraphilic interests also include genital stimulation and/or coital intercourse in their sexual behaviors. For example, the majority of BDSM (Bondage-Discipline-Domination/Submission-Sadism/Masochism) practitioners frequently engage (Botta et al., 2019; Connelly, 2006; Gosselin et al., 1991; Moser & Levitt, 1987; Sandnabba et al., 1999) and show interest (Chivers, Roy, Grimbos, Cantor, & Seto, 2014) in non-BDSM and more typical sexual behaviors. A similar diversity of sexual repertoire have been associated in such paraphilias as exhibitionism (Langevin et al., 1979), fetishism (Hawkinson & Zamboni, 2014;

Rees & Garcia, 2017), zoophilia (Williams & Weinberg, 2003), and necrophilia (Rosman & Resnick, 1989). Again, the nature of a sexual interest is usually not a category (an on/off function); it is often part of a larger continuum, as already stressed by Freud (1905/1962). Many adults in the general population have fantasies about, and/or experience with, sexual behaviors that are considered anomalous or atypical by current psychiatric nosology (Joyal & Carpentier, 2017; Joyal et al., 2015). However, such sexual behaviors as exhibitionism, voyeurism, masochism (including submission), sadism (including domination), and fetishism are dimensions, not categories (Hanson, 2010). Hair pulling, bondage, and spanking, for instance, can be placed near the center of a domination continuum running from absent (e.g., constant sexual mutuality) to problematic (coercive sexual sadism). Therefore, the place that a sexual interest takes on a continuum (e.g., necessity for satisfaction or exclusivity), could be more important to define sexual health than its nature.

In addition, persons who report paraphilic behaviors report having, on average, a higher sexual drive than persons who do not, whether they are recruited in clinical (e.g., Kafka, 1997), correctional (e.g., Abel et al., 1988) or non-clinical settings (Ahlers et al., 2011; Bouchard et al., 2017; Castellini et al., 2018; Långström & Hanson, 2006; Långström & Zucker, 2005; Shulman & Horne, 2006). This higher sexual drive might be associated with higher sexual diversity. Higher sexual drive should not be confounded with hypersexuality, however. Although hypersexuality necessarily involves a higher sexual drive, it is not necessarily true the other way around. While hypersexuality is problematic (involving sexual compulsions, lack of control and negative outcomes; Kafka, 2010), higher sexual drive and higher frequency of intercourse can simply be associated with higher sexual satisfaction (Långström & Hanson, 2006). Thus, the mere presence of a "non-normophilic" sexual interest equal or superior to that of a "normophilic" interest is not necessarily indicative of unhealthy sexuality. Therefore, the presence of sexual interest for a paraphilia might simply represent the sign of a higher sex drive and wider sexual interests. These results confirm the importance of exclusivity or necessity as criteria for unhealthy sexual behaviors. Sexual satisfaction that depend entirely on a single, precise behavior (e.g., being whipped, penile-vaginal intercourse) is not optimal.

Exclusivity of paraphilic interests: A lost notion. The crucial criteria of exclusivity, necessity and rigidity of paraphilic interests were gradually abandoned across editions of the DSM. Sexual deviations first appeared as a separate category in the second edition (APA, 1968). It described individuals whose sexual interests were "directed primarily toward objects other than people of the opposite sex, toward sexual acts not usually associated with coitus, or toward coitus performed under bizarre circumstances [...]" (p. 44). Notwithstanding the undefined adjective "bizarre," a deviant sexual behavior was seen as primary, in that the individual was not able to substitute typical sexual behavior for it. This notion was of utmost importance in the definition of paraphilia. In the third edition of the DSM (APA, 1980), the term paraphilia was introduced and defined as "Unusual or bizarre imagery or acts [that] are necessary for sexual excitement. Such imagery or acts tend to be insistently and involuntarily repetitive [...]" (p. 266). Again, the notions of necessity and loss of control were at the heart of the definition. Similarly, in 1984 Money, who popularized the term paraphilia, defined it as "An erotosexual condition of being recurrently responsive to, and *obsessively dependent on*, an unusual or unacceptable stimulus, perceptual or in fantasy, *in order to have a state of erotic arousal initiated or maintained, and in order to achieve or facilitate orgasm*" (p. 165, emphasis added). For Money (1984), an unacceptable stimulus was defined as a situation of behavior in which love and sex drive (lust) were mutually exclusive (distortion of the "Lovemap"). Therefore, not only the presence of obsessional components was required to meet the criteria of a paraphilia, but also the absence of love. In 1988, Money refined his definition of paraphilia as follows:

> A condition occurring in men and women of being *compulsively responsive to and obligatorily dependent* on an unusual and personally or socially unacceptable stimulus, perceived or in the ideation and imagery of fantasy, for optimal initiation and maintenance of sexuoerotic arousal and the facilitation or attainment of orgasm. Paraphilic imagery may be replayed in fantasy during solo masturbation or intercourse with a partner. In legal terminology, a paraphilia is a perversion or deviancy; and in the vernacular it is kinky or bizarre sex. Its antonym is normophilia. (p. 133, emphasis added)

Others also put emphasis on the criterion of necessity to define paraphilia using such terms as "consistently needed for sexual gratification" (Seto & Barbaree, 2000).

Intriguingly, these notions of exclusivity, necessity and rigidity to define paraphilia gradually faded over time. In the DSM-III-TR (APA, 1987), the condition of necessity was abandoned and the notion of "normative sexual arousal" was introduced. Today, a sexual interest simply has to be "greater than or equal to" a normophilic interest to be labelled as paraphilic and a repeated (over six months) illegal behavior (e.g., voyeurism) is sufficient to meet the criteria of a mental disorder (APA, 2013). As stressed by Wakefield (2011), paraphilias should not be merely optional preferences for maximizing pleasure when an activity is available or expressions of generally high and polymorphous sexual motivation.

> A paraphilia is a clear dysfunction for the same reasons that, say, impotence is a clear dysfunction, namely, there is an inability (*not mere preference* or circumstantial limitation) to have or enjoy normative sex. [...] One problem with using intensity as a criterion is that one risks pathologizing intensely sexual individuals who have a generally higher level of libido. This is why it is important, especially if exclusivity is lacking, to demand some evidence that a deviant desire is fixedly peremptory or compulsive. (p. 200, emphasis added)

Reliability of the diagnosis or lack thereof. During the development of the DSM-5, field trials were conducted for 33 separate diagnoses on 2,246 patients interviewed by 279 clinicians (Clarke et al., 2013). None of these field trials included a paraphilic disorder. Therefore, no data were collected about the reliability and validity of these diagnoses and it shows on the field. For instance, there is a lack of operationalization (and measurement) to assess crucial qualifiers such as "intense" and "persistent," jeopardizing reliability. In a landmark study, Levenson (2004) examined this issue within the context of Sexually Violent Predator commitments in the U.S. She found that none of the paraphilic diagnoses met acceptable standards, including the general category of "any paraphilia" with a coefficient clearly lower than expected (k = 0.47). Coefficients for specific disorders were also too low (pedophilia, k = 0.65; exhibitionism, k = 0.47; sexual sadism, k = 0.30; and paraphilia NOS, k = 0.36).

Validity of the diagnoses and the elusive underlying mental disorder. As can be seen with the two quotes in epigraph, nascent psychiatry in the 19th century began to consider perversions as symptoms of an underlying illness or mental disorder. If paraphilic behaviors are signs of a mental disorder they should, by definition, be associated with dysfunctions in psychological, biological or developmental processes underlying mental functioning. As repeatedly stressed (Joyal, 2018; Moser, 2001), however, signs (e.g., showing genitals to an unsuspected stranger) and syndromes (e.g., exhibitionism) are the same in the diagnoses of paraphilic disorders. Usually, diagnoses of underlying mental disorders (e.g., compulsive obsessional disorder, major depression, generalized anxiety) are based on distinct behaviors known to be signs or symptoms of the disorder (e.g., handwashing, weight loss, insomnia). Equating symptoms to syndrome would lead to such diagnosis as handwashing disorder and elevator-taking disorder. In their DSM-5 field trial for the proposed inclusion of a Hypersexuality Disorder (HD, eventually rejected), Reid and colleagues (Reid et al., 2012) correctly stressed that:

> the HD *criteria require more than simple manifestations of excessive sexual behavior* including an expansive range of associated features such as whether sexual thoughts, urges, and behaviors arise from stress or dysphoric mood states, create difficulties leading to dysfunctional consequences, and lead to a perceived diminished of sense of control. (Emphasis added, p. 2869)

In addition, complementary assessments are commonly available to confirm several diagnoses of mental disorders such as psychological (e.g., personality traits; Chioqueta & Stiles, 2005), neurological (e.g., cortico-limbic activation; Wang et al., 2012), neuropsychological (e.g., attentional deficits; Shenal et al., 2003), psychophysiological (e.g., higher P2 wave amplitude), and genetic (e.g., Brain-derived neurotrophic factor; Kemp et al., 2008) correlates of major depression, for instance. As discussed below, studies using these measures are either lacking or they generated negative results in the field of paraphilias (with the notable exception of child sexual abuse, to be discussed later).

The traditional view in psychiatry is that paraphilias are indeed associated with psychopathologies such as mood disorders, anxiety disorders, and substance abuse (e.g., Krueger & Kaplan, 2001). However, these classical associations are typically found among persons recruited in correctional, psychiatric or forensic settings (e.g., Bader et al., 2008; Drury et al., 2017; Dunsieth Jr. et al., 2004; Grant, 2005; Kafka & Hennen, 2002; Lee et al., 2001; Leue et al., 2004; Stinson et al., 2008; Taktak et al., 2016). These settings and participants include several possible confounding factors (e.g., depressive effects of incarceration; side effects of psychotropic medication). Although psychopathology and paraphilia commonly co-occur in sexual offenders (e.g., Marshall, 2007), the link between psychological imbalance and a sexual preference (vs. a sexual offense) is not well established. A member of the paraphilia workgroups for both the DSM-5 and ICD-11, Dr Krueger, even stated that "it is well known that there are few, if any, psychopathological or other variables that differentiate individuals with pedophilia or paraphilias from those without, and any such distinction would support the consideration of such individuals as constituting a separate group" (Krueger & Kaplan, 2002, p. 487). Even for such a diagnosis as conduct disorder (CD), entirely based on behaviors, it used to be clear that the disorder should not be diagnosed if the behaviors were not caused by an underlying dysfunction (Wakefield et al., 2006). The DSM-IV-TR, for instance, stated that "Consistent with the DSM-IV definition of mental disorder, the CD diagnosis should be applied only when the behavior in question is symptomatic of an underlying dysfunction within the individual [...]" (APA, 2000, p. 88). If paraphilic behaviors are not associated with any sign of psychopathology, on what ground can they be classified as manifestations of an underlying mental disorder? Again, this is achieved with evidence that a behavior (e.g., systematic avoidance of a particular situation such as crowded places) is due to a disorder (excessive anticipation of future threat), assessed with a validated measure of the disorder (anxiety). Attempts to do so with non-clinical/non-forensic persons with paraphilic interests are reviewed below.

The classic type of evidence that paraphilias emerge from cerebral dysfunction are neurological cases. Such neurological disorders as epilepsy, traumatic brain injury, brain tumor, sclerosis, neoplasm, and dementia can (infrequently) provoke paraphilic behaviors, including child molesting, exhibitionism, voyeurism, and bestiality (see Joyal et al., 2007 for a review). These cases are traditionally cited as evidence that neurological anomalies underlie paraphilias (e.g., Kolářský et al., 1967; Langevin, 1992). However, these signs of neurological disorders are generally not genuine paraphilias, being more closely related with a behavioral desinhibitory syndrome than a true modification of sexual preference (e.g., Sartori et al., 2016). Neurological anomalies were also reported in older brain imaging studies of persons with a diagnosis of paraphilia (e.g., exhibitionism; Langevin, Lang et al., 1989). These studies, however, were based on participants recruited in clinical or correctional settings and examined with crude methods (e.g., visual inspection of computerized tomography). Investigations with more recent technology (e.g., magnetic resonance imaging) and participants with paraphilic interests recruited in the general population are warranted.

Another approach to link paraphilias with mental disorders is the assessment of personality traits. A classic study from Wilson and Gosselin (1980) led to the conclusion that adepts of fetishism, sadomasochism or transvestism tended to be introvert, shy, anxious, and depressed, but "not to an extant that could be regarded as clinically significant" (p. 294). In addition, it was not clear if these results were genuine or due to the high social stigma of the time. More recently, among university students, voyeurism, exhibitionism, fetishism, frotteurism, bondage, sadism, child sexual abuse and sexual coercion all failed to be significantly associated with any of the Big Five factors of personality (Williams et al., 2009). When personality traits are associated with paraphilic behaviors, the most significant trait is openness (Lodi-Smith et al., 2014). Openness, in turn, is significantly associated with a liberal attitude toward sex (Allen & Walter, 2018), so we have a full circle. Paraphilic interests are generally not associated with intellectual quotient, handedness, susceptibility to illness, psychological functioning, general life satisfaction, and sex life satisfaction among adults recruited in the general population (Ahlers et al., 2011; Dawson et al., 2016; Robinson & Parks, 2004; Rogak & Connor, 2018). When correlations between paraphilic interests and signs of psychopathology are found in non-clinical samples, most lost significance after controlling for hypersexuality (Castellini et al., 2018). That is, hypersexuality is more closely associated with psychopathology than paraphilic interests are.

Interestingly, a growing number of studies suggest that individuals in non-clinical, non-forensic settings (typically university students) who engage in paraphilic behaviors have more "psychopathic" and "narcissistic" traits than persons who do not (Dawson et al., 2016; Lodi-Smith et al., 2014; Watts et al., 2019; Williams et al., 2009). It is important to note, however, that these associations are not indicative of psychopathology (i.e., these students are not necessarily psychopaths). They might simply indicate that persons engaging in paraphilic behaviors are more disinhibited, extravert, thrill-seekers, and self-centered than those who do not. In fact, an interesting correlate of paraphilic behaviors among persons recruited in non-clinical settings is sensation-seeking (Dawson et al., 2016; Turley & Butt, 2015). Given that many persons with paraphilic fantasies do not act upon these fantasies (Joyal & Carpentier, 2017), sensation-seeking and more impulsive traits might explain a significant part of paraphilic behaviors, as observed in sex offenders (Stinson et al., 2008). Because all these variables are dimensional, they would not necessarily be associated with pathology in the general population. Clearly, dimensional assessments of paraphilia are needed.

For instance, interests for either exhibitionism, fetishism, sexual sadism, transvestic fetishism or voyeurism were all found to be significantly associated with the disinhibition and meanness factors of the Triarchic Psychopathy Measure, the entitlement/exploitativeness factor of the Narcissistic Personality Inventory, and both antisocial and borderline personality traits among university students (Watts et al., 2019). These interesting results are not necessarily indicative of an underlying pathological process, as both personality traits and sexual interests are dimensional factors; their shared expression might simply reflect similar or related underlying constructs (e.g., empathy, self-esteem).

To date, most non-forensic, non-clinical studies assessing psychopathological signs in persons with paraphilic behaviors focused on behaviors related with BDSM. These studies strongly suggest that psychological health of BDSM practitioners is similar to (if not better than) that of non-practitioners (Brown et al., 2020; De Neef et al., 2019; Sandnabba et al., 1999; Wismeijer & Van Assen, 2013). Similar studies concerning interests for illegal paraphilic acts (e.g., voyeurism, exhibitionism, frotteurism) are still lacking.

Still, there are a few intriguing positive relationships between paraphilic interests and possible signs of psychopathology. Langström and Seto (2006) reported that being sexually aroused by exposing ones own genitals to a stranger or by spying on others having sex were associated with psychological problems and lower satisfaction with life in a representative sample of adults. However, both variables (psychological status and satisfaction in life) were based on a single self-reported Likert-type scale in that study (from very unsatisfying to very satisfying). Therefore, it remains possible that persons aroused by an exhibitionistic or voyeuristic behavior were simply less satisfied in general or less satisfied with themselves than others. Validated measures of psychological and sexual health are needed to assess their link with paraphilic interests. For instance, Ahlers and colleagues (Ahlers et al., 2011) found a strong association (odd ratio of 11.9) between interest for any paraphilic behavior and symptoms of psychopathology as assessed with the well-known Symptom Checklist-90 (SCL-90; Derogatis, 1975). However, the confidence intervals were extremely large for this odd (2.6-54.5), suggesting significant differences between the types of paraphilia. Therefore, different types of paraphilia should be considered separately. Exhibitionism is a good example. Although Langevin and colleagues (Langevin et al., 1978) first concluded that exhibitionists "appear normal with little evidence of a significant pathology," a more recent study concluded that exhibitionism was one of the few paraphilias (with transvestism and masochism) to retain its significant association with the SCL-90 after adjustment for hypersexuality among men (Castellini et al., 2018). More studies of this type are needed to conclude determine if paraphilia such as exhibitionism is (or is not) a sign of an underlying mental disorder.

The ICD-11

The ICD-11 definition of paraphilia and its implication. The International Classification of Diseases is published by the World Health Organization (World Health Organization, 2018). Although the 11th version (ICD-11) will officially come into effect on 1 January 2022, it is currently available (World Health Organization, 2018). In this edition, the definition of paraphilia changed significantly. First, it led to the removal of sadomasochism, fetishism, and fetishistic transvestism from the list of mental disorders because they are not associated with non-consent or dysfunction in psychological, biological, or developmental processes. That decision, reminiscent of a similar one made more than 40 years ago by the APA for the diagnosis of homosexuality (DSM-II), is an important step in the right direction. As stressed by the the Working Group on Sexual Disorders and Sexual Health (WGSDSH) for the ICD-11, "The regulation of private behaviour without health consequences to the individual or to others may be considered in different societies to be a matter for criminal laws, religious proscription, or public morality, but is not a legitimate focus of public health or of health classification" (Reed et al., 2016, p. 212). Second, however, because inter-personal criminality has public health implications, the definition of paraphilia could be entirely based on illegality. Apparently, the presence of an underlying mental disorder is no longer required. Implications of these modifications are discussed below.

As in the DSM-5, mental disorders are defined in the ICD-11 as follows:

> Mental, behavioural and neurodevelopmental disorders are syndromes characterized by clinically significant *disturbance* in an individual's cognition, emotional regulation, or behaviour that *reflects* a dysfunction in the psychological, biological, or developmental processes that *underlie* mental and behavioural functioning. These disturbances are usually associated with distress or impairment in personal, family, social, educational, occupational, or other important areas of functioning. (WHO, 2018)

In the ICD-11, only paraphilic disorders are defined (not paraphilias), as "persistent and intense patterns of atypical sexual arousal, manifested by sexual thoughts, fantasies, urges, or behaviours, with a focus on others whose age or status renders them unwilling or unable to consent and on which the person has acted or by which he or she is markedly distressed" (WHO, 2018). In the ICD-11, voyeurism, exhibitionism, frotteurism, pedophilia, coercive sexual sadism are listed, as well as an "other paraphilic disorder involving non-consenting individuals" category (only necrophilia and zoophilia are cited) and a "paraphilic disorder involving solitary behaviour or consenting individuals" category (i.e., involving significant risk of injury or death; only asphyxophilia is listed here).

More than 10 years ago, First and Halon (2008) suggested going back to the DSM-III-R criteria for paraphilic disorders, i.e., the requirement of both sexually arousing fantasies *and* urge, not mere behaviors. As they stressed, "Diagnostically, one error that can result in a false positive diagnosis (i.e., opining that a paraphilia is present in the respondent when it is not) is to *base the diagnosis solely on the presence of the criminal sexual behavior* without evidence causally connecting that behavior to the paraphilic arousal pattern" (p. 446, emphasis added). Other authors have also stressed that a criminal behavior is not necessarily the symptom of a mental disorder (Moser, 2016; O'Donohue, 2016). As stated by Halpern (2011), "Sexual assault is not a disorder—it is a crime; DSM [and ICD] is a classification of mental disorders, not a classification of criminal conduct" (p. 488). Hinderliter (2010) correctly stressed that certain paraphilias are in the list of psychiatric disorders simply because the act is illegal. "With this type of reasoning, perhaps 'Embezzlement Disorder' and 'Insider Trading Disorder' should be added to the DSM?" (p. 1236). Indeed, one can wonder why sex crimes are treated differently from other crimes in psychiatric manuals (Moser, 2016).

The category called "Other paraphilic disorder involving non-consenting individuals" is defined as:

> a persistent and intense pattern of atypical sexual arousal—manifested by sexual thoughts, fantasies, urges, or behaviours—in which the focus of the arousal pattern involves others who are unwilling or unable to consent but that is not specifically described in any of the other named Paraphilic Disorders categories (e.g., arousal patterns involving corpses or animals). The individual must have acted on these thoughts, fantasies or urges or be markedly distressed by them. The disorder specifically excludes sexual behaviours that occur with the consent of the person or persons involved, provided that they are considered able to provide such consent.

Notwithstanding that important terms such as "atypical," "persistent," and "intense" are still not defined, this new category seems to include rape. It is worth noting that the proposition to add a paraphilic coercive disorder was rejected for both DSM-IV and DSM-5, because it was based on criminal behavior alone (Zonana, 2011) and it had high potential for legal misuse (Knight, 2010). As stressed by Wakefield (2011):

> harm to self or others is not sufficient to warrant attribution of disorder—and many harmful but nondisordered conditions, from birth pain to body odor, confirm this view. The question that must be asked is whether the condition in question is a dysfunction. If a paraphilia is attributed when the dysfunction requirement is not satisfied, then that constitutes the pathologization of the individual's deviance and conflict with society. (p. 207)

Understandably, one important mandate of the ICD is to report behaviors that are relevant to public health, including sexual criminal acts (Reed et al., 2016). However, unless evidence-based data demonstrate that illegal sexual behaviors are truly symptoms of an underlying mental disorder, they could be reported without psychiatric implication in the International Classification of Functioning, Disability, and Health (ICF; WHO, 2001) instead of the ICD-11 (WHO, 2018).

The Special Case of Pedophilia (or More Precisely, Child Sexual Abuse)

As stressed so far, most consenting paraphilias do not seem to be associated with mental disorders and evidence-based data are still lacking concerning illegal paraphilias. One notable exception is child sexual abuse, with or without pedophilia. First, sexual interest for children (usually defined as aged 12 years or under) is statistically rare or atypical (less than 10%) among adults recruited in non-forensic/non-clinical populations (Ahlers et al., 2011; Dawson et al., 2016; Dombert et al., 2016; Joyal & Carpentier, 2017; Santtila et al., 2015; Wurtele et al., 2014). Second, in opposition to the dimensional aspect of more common paraphilic behaviors (i.e., voyeurism, sadomasochism, fetishism, frotteurism, exhibitionism; Thompson, 2016), child sexual molesting has distinct, categorical properties; it is either present or absent (Hanson, 2010; McPhail et al., 2018). Third, contrarily to adult sexual offending (19%) and non acted-out sexual interest in youth aged 15 or less (14.6%), genetic factors explain nearly half (46%) of variance for child sexual offending (Alanko et al., 2013; Långström et al., 2015). Fourth, psychiatric comorbidity is particularly high among child sexual offenders (Bogaerts et al., 2005; Garofalo & Bogaerts, 2019; Raymond et al., 1999). Finally, child sexual abuse is associated with a panoply of signs of neurobiological abnormalities, including neuroimaging anomalies (Hendricks et al., 1988; Wright et al., 1990), neurological damage (Alnemari et al., 2016; Burns & Swerdlow, 2003; Mendez et al., 2000; Mendez & Shapira, 2011; Poeppl et al., 2015) and neuropsychological deficits (Hucker et al., 1986; Joyal et al., 2007; Langevin & Curnoe, 2008; Langevin, Wortzman et al., 1989; Scott et al., 1984), Traditionally, these neurobiological findings are interpreted as evidence for a neurological origin of pedophilia (e.g., Flor-Henry et al., 1991; Wright et al., 1990).

More recent studies tend to show, however, that it is child sexual abuse, not pedophilia per se, that is associated with neuroimaging and neuropsychological impairments (e.g., Kärgel et al., 2017; Massau et al., 2017; Schiffer et al., 2017). In fact, a growing number of studies distinguish child sexual abuse and pedophilia (i.e., non-offending pedophiles) and demonstrate that it is the former, not the latter, that is associated with neurological and neuropsychological defects (see Joyal et al., 2019; Mohnke et al., 2014; Tenbergen et al., 2015 for reviews). Therefore, the search for signs and symptoms of an underlying mental disorder in paraphilias is still open, even for pedophilia. It is worth noting, however, that psychomotor slowness (Suchy et al., 2014) and associated white matter anomalies (Cantor et al., 2008) might be associated with pedophilia, although this possibility remains to be demonstrated with non-offending pedophiles.

Other, more controversial, variables thought to reflect neurodevelopmental anomalies have also been causally associated with pedophilia, including "non-right-handedness," lower I.Q., lower fraternal birth order, higher index finger/ring finger length and leg/torso length ratios (e.g., Blanchard et al. 1999, 2007, 2008; Cantor et al., 2004, 2005; Fazio et al., 2017). But again, these correlates of intrauterine hormonal defects were found in child molesters, not non-offending pedophiles (Kruger et al., 2019). In addition, these correlates are not specific to child sexual abuse, being also associated with sexual offending in general, nonsexual delinquency, thrill-seeking proclivity, aggressive traits, and impulsivity (e.g., Bailey & Hurd, 2005; Bogaert, 2001; Brower & Price, 2001; Fink et al., 2006; Guay et al., 2005; MacCulloch et al., 2004; Moffitt et al., 1994; Ogunfowokan et al., 2016). Therefore, it is difficult to disentangle a sexual preference for children from these possible confounding factors in these correlational studies. Besides, contrarily to earlier results obtained in adjudicated child molesters (Bogaert et al., 1997; Lalumière et al., 1998), men convicted for possession of child pornography (a much better sign of pedophilic preference) have significantly fewer older brothers (not more) than matched controls without sexual or nonsexual violent convictions (Babchishin et al., 2019). In fact, pedophilic interests per se do not appear to be associated with fraternal birth order (Côté et al., 2002).

Possible Solutions to Current Problems with Paraphilia Diagnoses

In view of the aforementioned problems with paraphilia diagnoses, certain solutions have been proposed, as described in this section.

Moser's Alternative Propositions

Charles Moser (2001) first suggested using a more general "sexual interest disorder" diagnosis to include any problematic sexual interest (i.e., inducing distress or impairment to the person or others), whatever its nature. This larger diagnosis would allow avoiding stigmatization associated with a definition of anomalous or atypical sexual interests It would also allow any individuals distressed or impaired by their sexual interests to receive a diagnosis and appropriate treatment (see also Joyal, 2014). However, such a diagnosis would still generate problems because distress related to sexual interest is much more closely related with sociocultural norms, religious beliefs and/or personal morality than with the idiosyncratic sexual inclination (e.g., Ahlers et al., 2011; Mundy & Cioe, 2019). In cases where mutual consent or no harm is involved (e.g., diaper fetishism), receiving a psychiatric diagnosis based on the presence of distress might actually be interpreted as a confirmation that a person has a mental disorder, which would further stigmatize/distress them. Thereafter, Moser and Kleinplatz (2005) suggested simply eradicating all diagnoses of paraphilia from psychiatric manuals. However, this might be premature at this time because evidence-based data demonstrating that all paraphilic interests are not manifestations a mental disorder are still lacking.

The Harmful Dysfunction Definition

Jerome Wakefield (1992) proposed an influential definition of mental disorders requiring both a dysfunction ("a failure of some mechanism in the organism to perform its function") and harmfulness to the individual ("must cause significant harm to the person") and to society ("only dysfunctions that are socially disvalued are disorders"). Wakefield (2011) subsequently applied his definition to paraphilia, refining his descriptions of dysfunction ("a failure of a 'natural' biologically designed function", i.e., "leading to greater inclusive reproductive fitness") and harmfulness ("has a negative or undesirable or harmful effect on the individual or on society at large as judged by social values") to define paraphilias. From this perspective, pedophilia, exhibitionism, voyeurism, frotteurism, zoophilia, necrophilia, scatologia are all paraphilias because they fail to lead to procreation and cause harm both to the individual (e.g., legal consequences) and to society (non-consent and possible adverse effects). In opposition, rape and homosexuality are not considered paraphilic, the first because it involves a coital intercourse (a biologically designed function), the second because it is not harmful. This interesting definition of paraphilia has two main limits, however. First, it is still too dependent on historical-social-legal factors. Male homosexuality, for instance, is still illegal in many countries worldwide (e.g., Afghanistan, Iran, Iraq, Pakistan, Qatar, Saudi Arabia), so it could be considered as a mental disorder simply because it is harmful for the individual (leading to the death penalty in certain cases) and contrary to certain social values in these jurisprudences. This criterion should not suffice to define a mental disorder. Second, the argument can be made that not only reproduction, but also pleasure can be an evolutionary product of sexual behaviors (e.g., Abramson & Pinkerton, 1995). Any heritable trait that increases the frequency of reproductive sexual intercourse will increase in prevalence because such a trait increases reproductive fitness (i.e., number of viable offspring). Therefore, sex pleasure can also be seen as a natural biologically designed function, even if it does not facilitate reproduction. A more promising approach to evaluating sexual health is based on the dimensional properties of most sexual interests.

The Dimensional Aspect of Sexual Interests

One of the classic criteria to validate a psychiatric category (or a disorder) is having clear diagnostic boundaries (Robins & Guze, 1970). A survey conducted with 505 mental health professionals revealed that they have three main criteria to suggest the removal of a diagnostic category from psychiatric manuals, all three related with boundaries: (1) problematic boundaries between healthy and pathologic; (2) problematic boundaries between different mental disorders; and (3) problematic boundaries between mental and physical disorders (Robles et al., 2015). The three diagnostic categories most commonly recommended for removal by these clinicians were all related with sexuality: gender identity disorder, sexual dysfunction, and paraphilia. Boundaries and diagnostic criteria are problematic with sexual interests and behaviors because most of them are better conceptualized as gradations on a continuum than as separate categories (Hyde & DeLamater, 2017). As for most human traits, sexual interests, including paraphilias and hypersexuality (Thompson, 2016; Walters et al., 2011), usually have a dimensional latent structure, which is at odds with current categorical diagnostics (the exception being, so far, child sexual molesting; McPhail et al., 2018).

An excellent example of an attempt to categorize a dimensional sexual construct is provided by Cantor and Sutton (2015), who proposed labeling sexual preference according to Tanner stages of the target, i.e., pedophilia (stage 1 or less than 11 years old), hebephilia (stages 2–3 or 11–14 years old), ephebophilia (stage 4 or 15 years to physical maturity), teleiophilia (stage 5, from physical maturity to physical decline, defined as between 17 and 45 years old), and gerontophilia (elderly persons, presumably defined as over 45 years old). All preferences except ephebophilia and teleophilia are considered paraphilic (Cantor & Sutton, 2015). This categorization defines "normophilia" as a sexual attraction to persons aged from 15 to 45. If someone's spouse is about to be 46 years old, does that make the person paraphilic if the spouse is still the center of their powerful erotic interests? Similarly, is a person aged 70 years old paraphilic because they are mostly attracted sexually to other 70 year-old persons? Therefore, for most sexual interests (except, as mentioned above, child sexual abuse) boundaries are a matter of degrees rather than of type (Hanson, 2010).

Karl Hanson, an advisor to the paraphilias subworkgroup of the DSM-5, suggested using dimensions to diagnose paraphilias (Hanson, 2010). This suggestion is interesting because it fits with the dimensional latent structure of paraphilias (at least in males; Thompson, 2016). However, Hanson proposed using three dimensions, including one based on atypicity and diversity of sexual interests (ranging from "multiple paraphilias to exclusive interest in ('normal') sexual behavior with consenting adults"). Thus, the distinction between "normal" and "abnormal" sexual interests was still present, which is problematic. For instance, someone interested in fetishistic, masochistic, sadistic and "normal" sexual behavior might have been considered mentally ill. Besides, his place on that dimension would not have been clear (toward the multiple paraphilias end or the "normal" sexual behavior with consenting adults end?). The proposition was ultimately rejected by the DSM-5 paraphilia subworkgroup, but it is promising. As stressed by Hanson (2010), extreme expressions of continuous distributions could represent distinct clinical entities (psychopathy and sexual interest in prepubescent children are good examples; Guay et al., 2007; McPhail et al., 2018). The challenge is to define what is an extreme expression or the cutoff point on the dimension indicating the boundary of pathology. Future taxonomic studies should assess the possible categorical nature of sexual interests that are atypical, such as interests in prepubescent children, corpses, animals or excrements (Dawson et al., 2016; Dombert et al., 2016; Joyal & Carpentier, 2017; Rinehart & McCabe, 1998; Wurtele et al., 2014). Meanwhile, three dimensions of sexual interests might help to assess healthy sexuality, as described below.

(1) *The preference level.* An interesting approach to delineate healthy vs. unhealthy sexual behaviors is based on the strength of preference (or necessity) for a behavior, no matter what its nature (Hyde & DeLamater, 2017). This continuum runs as follows: no preference (e.g., for G-string panties) → mild preference → strong preference → necessity (obligatory for sexual arousal) → complete substitute for a human partner. Whereas no, mild, and strong preferences are considered healthy (leading to sexual arousal), necessity (rigidity and fixity) and complete substitution (no interpersonal relation) are considered unhealthy (Hyde & DeLamater, 2017). Necessity and rigidity refer to the obligation of repeatedly using an exclusive mean to reach the same state. The fact that one specific behavior is absolutely and exclusively necessary to reach an orgasm or to be satisfied is a sign of rigidity, which is not a sign of optimal mental or sexual health. A sexually rigid person might have found their perfect partner and be perfectly happy, but that happiness depends on the satisfaction of a rigid behavior and a specific partner, which fails to meet the criteria of sexual health. In this case, the absence of the behavior leads to psychological discomfort. As stressed by Fedoroff (2011), however, most persons with paraphilic interests are not distressed or impaired by their own interests (e.g., Ahlers et al., 2011) except, of course, when it is due to social stigmatization or possible legal consequences (Mundy & Cioe, 2019). Therefore, he suggested that higher distress or lower sexual functioning should be associated with the absence (not the presence) of the paraphilic fantasy or behavior to be indicative of a pathology.

(2) *The volitional level of sexual thoughts or behaviors.* Another important aspect of sexual health is volition (the power of choosing). Fleeting sexual fantasies or desires are common in the general population; it is the way they emerge and how they are dealt with that is important. This continuum runs as follow: sexual thoughts and desires, when present, are acknowledged, accepted and let go easily → conscious, deliberate but temporary thinking about sex with effortless change of focus → involuntary thinking about sex with effortless change of focus → conscious, deliberate thinking about sex with difficulties to change focus when needed → involuntary thinking about sex with difficulties to change focus when needed → obsessional thinking about sex (recurrent thoughts, fantasies, or images that are experienced as intrusive and unwanted) → constant (50% of the time or more) involuntary thinking about sex.

For behaviors, the volitional continuum could be based on levels of inhibition capacities. It is interesting to know that the term "paraphilia" first appeared in a book written by Wilhem Stekel (1924) about impulsive behaviors. Likewise, paraphilias were defined as "recurrent intense sexual urges *and* sexually arousing fantasies" in the DSM-III-R (p. 279, emphasis added). Not only both urges and fantasies were required, but the sole behavior was insufficient; it has to be the result of an urge. Therefore, the notion of will was crucial in initial definitions of paraphilia. A sudden emergence of a sexual fantasy or desire to act sexually is very common among adults and adolescents in the general population. Still, when these cognitive manifestations are inappropriate (i.e., bad timing or target, such as at work, toward a stranger or during a family dinner), they are generally refrained with deliberate inhibitory mechanisms. For certain persons, however, these inhibitory mechanisms are defective, leading to an acting out. Impulsivity is a paramount aspect of the neuropsychological profiles of sexual offenders, both in adults (Joyal et al., 2014) and in adolescents (Joyal et al., 2020). Importantly, this acting out is not necessarily atypical or illegal, it might also concern typical sexual behaviors (non-paraphilic hypersexuality; Kafka, 2010). These urges, beyond the control of the person, generally provoke negative feelings, regrets and shame, just like compulsions or intermittent explosive violence. Therefore, the notions of control, will, timing, and positive effects of the sexual behavior are, again, more important than its nature to evaluate sexual health. Wanted, consenting use of an object for sexual arousal, for instance (e.g., fetishism), is far more sexually healthy than uncontrolled normophilic behaviors (e.g., excessive spouse harassment), unless, of course, these urges are satisfying for all parties. A behavioral impulsivity continuum could be: sexual behaviors are constantly accomplished voluntarily → sexual behaviors sometimes result from an irresistible impulse (compulsive, low will level) → most sexual behaviors result from an irresistible impulse → all sexual behaviors result from an irresistible impulse.

(3) *The type of affect associated with sexual thoughts or behaviors.* Sexual fantasies, thoughts or behaviors are not necessarily associated with positive feelings; some of them generate negative affect such as repulsion, disgust, and anxiety (Renaud & Byers, 1999). When sexual fantasies or behaviors are in opposition with one's values, moral, legal or religious beliefs, they generate negative feelings (Gil, 1990). For instance, the rate of distress among non offender or non-judiciarized pedophiles is particularly high (Dombert et al., 2016; Konrad et al., 2017). This simple continuum runs as follow (for fantasies or behaviors): constantly associated with positive feeling → mostly associated with positive feelings → neutral → mostly associated with negative feelings → constantly associated with negative feelings.

Conclusion

According to the World Health Organisation, sexual health is:

> ... a state of physical, emotional, mental and social well-being in relation to sexuality; it is not merely the absence of disease, dysfunction or infirmity. Sexual health requires a positive and respectful approach TO sexuality and sexual relationships, as well as the possibility of having pleasurable and safe sexual experiences, free of coercion, discrimination and violence. For sexual health to be attained and maintained, the sexual rights of all persons must be respected, protected and fulfilled. (WHO, 2006, p. 5)

It seems that in the future, the best way to assess sexual health will be based on multi-dimensional, non-judgmental, evidence-based instruments.

References

Abdullahi, H., Jafojo, R. O., & Udofia, O. (2015). Paraphilia among undergraduates in a Nigerian University. *Sexual Addiction & Compulsivity*, *22*(3), 249–257. https://doi.org/10.1080/10720162.2015.1057662

Abel, G. G., Becker, J. V., Cunningham-Rathner, J., Mittelman, M., & Rouleau, J. L. (1988). Multiple paraphilic diagnoses among sex offenders. *Journal of the American Academy of Psychiatry and the Law*, *16*(2), 153–168.

Abramson, P. R., & Pinkerton, S. D. (1995). *With pleasure: Thoughts on the nature of human sexuality*. Oxford University Press.

Ahlers, C. J., Schaefer, G. A., Mundt, I. A., Roll, S., Englert, H., Willich, S. N., & Beier, K. M. (2011). How unusual are the contents of paraphilias? Paraphilia-associated sexual arousal patterns in a community-based sample of men. *The Journal of Sexual Medicine*, *8*(5), 1362–1370. https://doi.org/10.1111/j.1743-6109.2009.01597.x

Alanko, K., Salo, B., Mokros, A., & Santtila, P. (2013). Evidence for heritability of adult men's sexual interest in youth under age 16 from a population-based extended twin design. *The Journal of Sexual Medicine, 10*(4), 1090–1099. https://doi.org/10.1111/jsm.12067

Allen, M. S., & Walter, E. E. (2018). Linking big five personality traits to sexuality and sexual health: A meta-analytic review. *Psychological Bulletin, 144*(10), 1081–1110. https://doi.org/10.1037/bul0000157

Al-Nafzawi, S. (1886). The perfumed garden (~1400), translated by Sir Richard Burton). Benares.

Alnemari, A. M., Mansour, T. R., Buehler, M., & Gaudin, D. (2016). Neural basis of pedophilia: Altered sexual preference following traumatic brain injury. *International Journal of Surgery Case Reports, 25*, 221–224. http://dx.doi.org/10.1016/j.ijscr.2016.06.035

American Psychiatric Association (APA). (1968). *Diagnostic and statistical manual of mental disorders* (2nd ed.). American Psychiatric Association.

American Psychiatric Association (APA). (1980). *Diagnostic and statistical manual of mental disorders* (3rd ed.). American Psychiatric Association.

American Psychiatric Association (APA). (1987). *Diagnostic and statistical manual of mental disorders* (3rd ed., Revised). American Psychiatric Association.

American Psychiatric Association (APA). (2000). *Diagnostic and statistical manual of mental disorders* (4th ed., text revised). American Psychiatric Association.

American Psychiatric Association (APA). (2013). *Diagnostic and statistical manual of mental disorders* (5th ed.). American Psychiatric Association.

Androvicova, R., Krejcova, L., Bartova, K., Weiss, P., & Klapilova, K. (2018). No 305 (Proceedings of the 21st world meeting on sexual meeting). Preferences for non-consensual sexual activities in the general population of Czech males (a representative survey). *The Journal of Sexual Medicine, 15*(7), supplement 3, S246. https://doi.org/10.1016/j.jsxm.2018.04.268

Apostolou, M., & Khalil, M. (2019). Aggressive and humiliating sexual play: Occurrence rates and discordance between the sexes. *Archives of Sexual Behavior, 48*(7), 2187–2200. https://doi.org/10.1007/s10508-018-1266-8

Babchishin, K. M., Seto, M. C., Fazel, S., & Långström, N. (2019). Are there early risk markers for pedophilia? A nationwide case-control study of child sexual exploitation material offenders. *The Journal of Sex Research, 56*(2), 203–212. https://doi.org/10.1080/00224499.2018.1492694

Bader, S. M., Schoeneman-Morris, K. A., Scalora, M. J., & Casady, T. K. (2008). Exhibitionism: Findings from a Midwestern police contact sample. *International Journal of Offender Therapy and Comparative Criminology, 52*(3), 270–279. http://10.1177/0306624X07307122

Bailey, A. A., & Hurd, P. L. (2005). Finger length ratio (2D: 4D) correlates with physical aggression in men but not in women. *Biological Psychology, 68*(3), 215–222. https://doi.org/10.1016/j.biopsycho.2004.05.001

Balon, R. (2013). Controversies in the diagnosis and treatment of paraphilias. *Journal of Sex & Marital Therapy, 39*(1), 7–20. https://doi.org/10.1080/0092623X.2012.709219

Baur, E., Forsman, M., Santtila, P., Johansson, A., Sandnabba, K., & Långström, N. (2016). Paraphilic sexual interests and sexually coercive behavior: A population-based twin study. *Archives of Sexual Behavior, 45*(5), 1163–1172. https://doi.org/10.1007/s10508-015-0674-2

Blanchard, R., Cantor, J. M., & Robichaud, L. K. (2008). Biological factors in the development of sexual deviance and aggression in males. In H. E. Barbaree & W. L. Marshall (Eds.), *The juvenile sex offender* (pp. 77–104). Guilford Press.

Blanchard, R., Kolla, N. J., Cantor, J. M., Klassen, P. E., Dickey, R., Kuban, M. E., & Blak, T. (2007). IQ, handedness, and pedophilia in adult male patients stratified by referral source. *Sexual Abuse, 19*(3), 285–309. https://doi.org/10.1177/107906320701900307

Blanchard, R., Watson, M. S., Choy, A., Dickey, R., Klassen, P., & Ferren, D. J. (1999). Pedophiles: Mental retardation, maternal age, and sexual orientation. *Archives of Sexual Behavior, 28*(2), 111–127. https://doi.org/10.1023/A:1018754004962

Bogaert, A. F. (2001). Handedness, criminality, and sexual offending. *Neuropsychologia, 39*(5), 465–469. https://doi.org/10.1016/S0028-3932(00)00134-2

Bogaert, A. F., Bezeau, S., Kuban, M., & Blanchard, R. (1997). Pedophilia, sexual orientation, and birth order. *Journal of Abnormal Psychology, 106*(2), 331–335. https://doi.org/10.1037/0021-843X.106.2.331

Bogaerts, S., Declercq, F., Vanheule, S., & Palmans, V. (2005). Interpersonal factors and personality disorders as discriminators between intra-familial and extra-familial child molesters. *International Journal of Offender Therapy and Comparative Criminology, 49*(1), 48–62. https://doi.org/10.1177/0306624X04271233

Botta, D., Nimbi, F. M., Tripodi, F., Silvaggi, M., & Simonelli, C. (2019). Are role and gender related to sexual function and satisfaction in men and women practicing BDSM? *The Journal of Sexual Medicine, 16*(3), 463–473. https://doi.org/10.1016/j.jsxm.2019.01.001

Bouchard, K. N., Dawson, S. J., & Lalumière, M. L. (2017). The effects of sex drive and paraphilic interests on paraphilic behaviours in a nonclinical sample of men and women. *The Canadian Journal of Human Sexuality, 26*(2), 97–111. https://doi.org/10.3138/cjhs.262-a8

Brower, M. C., & Price, B. H. (2001). Neuropsychiatry of frontal lobe dysfunction in violent and criminal behaviour: A critical review. *Journal of Neurology, Neurosurgery & Psychiatry, 71*(6), 720–726. http://dx.doi.org/10.1136/jnnp.71.6.720

Brown, A., Barker, E. D., & Rahman, Q. (2020). A systematic scoping review of the prevalence, etiological, psychological, and interpersonal factors associated with BDSM. *The Journal of Sex Research, 57*(6), 781–811. https://doi.org/10.1080/00224499.2019.1665619

Bullough, V. L. (1976). *Sexual variance in society and history*. University of Chicago Press.

Burns, J. M., & Swerdlow, R. H. (2003). Right orbitofrontal tumor with pedophilia symptom and constructional apraxia sign. *Archives of Neurology, 60*(3), 437–440. https://doi.org/10.1001/archneur.60.3.437

Cantor, J.M., & Sutton, K.S. (2015). Paraphilia, gender dysphoria, and hypersexuality. In P.H. Blaney, R.F. Krueger, and T. Millon (Eds.), *Oxford textbook of psychopathology* (3rd ed., pp. 589–614).

Cantor, J. M., Blanchard, R., Christensen, B. K., Dickey, R., Klassen, P. E., & Kuban, M. E. (2004). Intelligence, memory, and handedness in pedophilia. *Neuropsychology, 18*(1), 3–14. http://doi.org/10.1037/0894-4105.18.1.3

Cantor, J. M., Blanchard, R., Robichaud, L. K., & Christensen, B. K. (2005). Quantitative reanalysis of aggregate data on IQ in sexual offenders. *Psychological Bulletin, 131*(4), 555–568. https://doi.org/10.1037/0033-2909.131.5.661

Cantor, J. M., Kabani, N., Christensen, B. K., Zipursky, R. B., Barbaree, H. E., Dickey, R., ... & Richards, B. A. (2008). Cerebral white matter deficiencies in pedophilic men. *Journal of Psychiatric Research, 42*(3), 167–183. https://doi.org/10.1016/j.jpsychires.2007.10.013

Castellini, G., Rellini, A. H., Appignanesi, C., Pinucci, I., Fattorini, M., Grano, E., Fisher, A. D., Cassioli, E., Lelli, L., Maggi, M., & Ricca, V. (2018). Deviance or Normalcy? The relationship among paraphilic thoughts and behaviors, hypersexuality, and psychopathology in a sample of university students. *The Journal of Sexual Medicine, 15*(9), 1322–1335. https://doi.org/10.1016/j.jsxm.2018.07.015

Chioqueta, A. P., & Stiles, T. C. (2005). Personality traits and the development of depression, hopelessness, and suicide ideation. *Personality and Individual Differences, 38*(6), 1283–1291. https://doi.org/10.1016/j.paid.2004.08.010

Chivers, M. L., Roy, C., Grimbos, T., Cantor, J. M., & Seto, M. C. (2014). Specificity of sexual arousal for sexual activities in men and women with conventional and masochistic sexual interests. *Archives of Sexual Behavior, 43*(5), 931–940. https://doi.org/10.1007/s10508-013-0174-1

Clarke, D. E., Narrow, W. E., Regier, D. A., Kuramoto, S. J., Kupfer, D. J., Kuhl, E. A., Greiner, L., & Kraemer, H. C. (2013). DSM-5 field trials in the United States and Canada, part I: Study design, sampling strategy, implementation, and analytic approaches. *American Journal of Psychiatry, 170*(1), 43–58. https://doi.org/10.1176/appi.ajp.2012.12070998

Connolly, P. H. (2006). Psychological functioning of bondage/domination/sado-masochism (BDSM) practitioners. *Journal of Psychology & Human Sexuality, 18*(1), 79–120. https://doi.org/10.1300/J056v18n01_05

Côté, K., Earls, C. M., & Lalumiere, M. L. (2002). Birth order, birth interval, and deviant sexual preferences among sex offenders. *Sexual Abuse, 14*(1), 67–81. https://doi.org/10.1023/A:1013081527837

Dawson, S. J., Bannerman, B. A., & Lalumière, M. L. (2016). Paraphilic interests: An examination of sex differences in a nonclinical sample. *Sexual Abuse, 28*(1), 20–45. https://doi.org/10.1177/1079063214525645

De Neef, N., Coppens, V., Huys, W., & Morrens, M. (2019). Bondage-discipline, dominance-submission and sadomasochism (BDSM) from an integrative biopsychosocial perspective: A systematic review. *Sexual Medicine, 7*(2), 129–144. https://doi.org/10.1016/j.esxm.2019.02.002

Derogatis, L. R. (1975). *The SCL-90-R.* Clinical Psychometric Research.

Dombert, B., Schmidt, A. F., Banse, R., Briken, P., Hoyer, J., Neutze, J., & Osterheider, M. (2016). How common is men's self-reported sexual interest in prepubescent children? *The Journal of Sex Research, 53*(2), 214–223. https://doi.org/10.1080/00224499.2015.1020108

Downing, L. (2015). Heteronormativity and repronormativity in sexological "perversion theory" and the DSM-5's "paraphilic disorder" diagnoses. *Archives of Sexual Behavior, 44*(5), 1139–1145. https://doi.org/10.1007/s10508-015-0536-y

Drury, A., Heinrichs, T., Elbert, M., Tahja, K., DeLisi, M., & Caropreso, D. (2017). Adverse childhood experiences, paraphilias, and serious criminal violence among federal sex offenders. *Journal of Criminal Psychology, 7*(2), 105–119. https://doi.org/10.1108/JCP-11-2016-0039

Dunsieth Jr, N. W., Nelson, E. B., Brusman-Lovins, L. A., Holcomb, J. L., Beckman, D., Welge, J. A., Roby, D., Taylor, P., Soutullo, C. A., & McElroy, S. L. (2004). Psychiatric and legal features of 113 men convicted of sexual offenses. *The Journal of Clinical Psychiatry, 65*(3), 293–300. https://doi.org/10.4088/JCP.v65n0302

Eagan, A. (2017). Foot obsessed but not necessarily depressed: The relationship between paraphilias and mental health outcomes. Murray State Theses and Dissertations.

Fazio, R. L., Dyshniku, F., Lykins, A. D., & Cantor, J. M. (2017). Leg length versus torso length in pedophilia: Further evidence of atypical physical development early in life. *Sexual Abuse, 29*(5), 500–514. https://doi.org/10.1177/1079063215609936

Fedoroff, J. P. (2011). Forensic and diagnostic concerns arising from the proposed DSM-5 criteria for sexual paraphilic disorder. *Journal of the American Academy of Psychiatry and the Law, 39*(2), 238–241.

Fedoroff, J. P., Di Gioacchino, L., & Murphy, L. (2013). Problems with paraphilias in the DSM-5. *Current Psychiatry Reports, 15*(8), 363. http://10.1007/s11920-013-0363-6

Fink, B., Neave, N., Laughton, K., & Manning, J. T. (2006). Second to fourth digit ratio and sensation seeking. *Personality and Individual Differences, 41*(7), 1253–1262. https://doi.org/10.1016/j.paid.2006.05.002

First, M. B. (2014). DSM-5 and paraphilic disorders. *Journal of the American Academy of Psychiatry and the Law, 42*(2), 191–201.
First, M. B., & Frances, A. (2008). Issues for DSM-V: Unintended consequences of small changes: The case of paraphilias. *American Journal of Psychiatry, 165*(10), 1240–1241. https://doi.org/10.1176/appi.ajp.2008.08030361
First, M. B., & Halon, R. L. (2008). Use of DSM paraphilia diagnoses in sexually violent predator commitment cases. *Journal of the American Academy of Psychiatry and the Law, 36*(4), 443–454.
Flor-Henry, P., Lang, R. A., Koles, Z. J., & Frenzel, R. R. (1991). Quantitative EEG studies of pedophilia. *International Journal of Psychophysiology, 10*(3), 253–258. https://doi.org/10.1016/0167-8760(91)90036-W
Freud, S. (1905/1962). *Three essays on the theory of sexuality* [English translation]. Basic Books.
Garofalo, C., & Bogaerts, S. (2019). Attachment and personality disorders among child molesters: The role of trust. *Sexual Abuse, 31*(1), 97–124. https://doi.org/10.1177/1079063217720928
Gert, B., & Culver, C. M. (2009). Sex, immorality, and mental disorders. *Journal of Medicine and Philosophy, 34*(5), 487–495. https://doi.org/10.1093/jmp/jhp037
Gil, V. E. (1990). Sexual fantasy experiences and guilt among conservative Christians: An exploratory study. *The Journal of Sex Research, 27*(4), 629–638. https://doi.org/10.1080/00224499009551584
Gosselin, C., & Wilson, G. (1980). *Sexual variations: Fetishism, sadomasochism, transvestism.* Simon and Schuster.
Gosselin, C. C., Wilson, G. D., & Barrett, P. T. (1991). The personality and sexual preferences of sadomasochistic women. *Personality and Individual Differences, 12*(1), 11–15. https://doi.org//10.1016/0191-8869(91)90126-V
Grant, J. E. (2005). Clinical characteristics and psychiatric comorbidity in males with exhibitionism. *The Journal of Clinical Psychiatry, 66*(11), 1367–1371. doi: https://doi.org/10.4088/JCP.v66n1104
Guay, J. P., Ouimet, M., & Proulx, J. (2005). On intelligence and crime: A comparison of incarcerated sex offenders and serious non-sexual violent criminals. *International Journal of Law and Psychiatry, 28*(4), 405–417. https://doi.org/10.1016/j.ijlp.2004.03.010
Guay, J. P., Ruscio, J., Knight, R. A., & Hare, R. D. (2007). A taxometric analysis of the latent structure of psychopathy: Evidence for dimensionality. *Journal of Abnormal Psychology, 116*(4), 701–716. https://doi.org/10.1037/0021-843X.116.4.701
Guislain, J. (1852). Leçons orales sur les phrénopathies ou traité théorique et pratique des maladies mentales [Oral lessons on phrenopathies or theoretical and practical treatise of mental disorders]. Hebbelynck.
Halpern, A. L. (2011). The proposed diagnosis of hypersexual disorder for inclusion in DSM-5: Unnecessary and harmful. *Archives of Sexual Behavior, 40*(3), 487–488. doi: https://doi.org/10.1007/s10508-011-9727-3
Hanson, R. K. (2010). Dimensional measurement of sexual deviance. *Archives of Sexual Behavior, 39*(2), 401–404. https://doi.org/10.1007/s10508-009-9575-6
Hawkinson, K., & Zamboni, B. D. (2014). Adult baby/diaper lovers: An exploratory study of an online community sample. *Archives of Sexual Behavior, 43*(5), 863–877. https://doi.org/10.1007/s10508-013-0241-7
Hendricks, S. E., Fitzpatrick, D. F., Hartmann, K., Quaife, M. A., Stratbucker, R. A., & Graber, B. (1988). Brain structure and function in sexual molesters of children and adolescents. *Journal of Clinical Psychiatry, 49*(3), 108–112.
Herbenick, D., Bowling, J., Fu, T. C. J., Dodge, B., Guerra-Reyes, L., & Sanders, S. (2017). Sexual diversity in the United States: Results from a nationally representative probability sample of

adult women and men. *PloS One, 12*(7), e0181198. https://doi.org/10.1371/journal.pone.0181198
Hinderliter, A. C. (2010). Disregarding science, clinical utility, and the DSM's definition of mental disorder: The case of exhibitionism, voyeurism, and frotteurism. *Archives of Sexual Behavior, 39*(6), 1235–1237. https://doi.org/10.1007/s10508-010-9654-8
Hinderliter, A. C. (2011). Defining paraphilia in DSM-5: Do not disregard grammar. *Journal of Sex & Marital Therapy, 37*(1), 17–31. https://doi.org/10.1080/0092623X.2011.533567
Holvoet, L., Huys, W., Coppens, V., Seeuws, J., Goethals, K., & Morrens, M. (2017). Fifty shades of Belgian gray: The prevalence of BDSM-related fantasies and activities in the general population. *The Journal of Sexual Medicine, 14*(9), 1152–1159. https://doi.org/10.1016/j.jsxm.2017.07.003
Hucker, S., Langevin, R., Wortzman, G., Bain, J., Handy, L., Chambers, J., & Wright, S. (1986). Neuropsychological impairment in pedophiles. *Canadian Journal of Behavioral Sciences, 18*(4), 440–448. https://doi.org/10.1037/h0079965
Hyde, J. S., & DeLamater, J. D. (2017). *Understanding human sexuality* (13th ed.). McGraw-Hill.
Joyal, C. C. (2014). How anomalous are paraphilic interests? *Archives of Sexual Behavior, 43*(7), 1241–1243. https://doi.org/10.1007/s10508-014-0325-z
Joyal, C. C. (2015). Defining "normophilic" and "paraphilic" sexual fantasies in a population-based sample: On the importance of considering subgroups. *Sexual Medicine, 3*(4), 321–330. https://doi.org/10.1002/sm2.96
Joyal, C. C. (2018). Controversies in the Definition of Paraphilia. *The Journal of Sexual Medicine, 15*(10), 1378–1380. https://doi.org/10.1016/j.jsxm.2018.08.005
Joyal, C. C., Beaulieu-Plante, J., & de Chantérac, A. (2014). The neuropsychology of sex offenders: A meta-analysis. *Sexual Abuse, 26*(2), 149–177. https://doi.org/10.1177/1079063213482842
Joyal, C. C., Black, D. N., & Dassylva, B. (2007). The neuropsychology and neurology of sexual deviance: A review and pilot study. *Sexual Abuse, 19*(2), 155–173. https://doi.org/10.1177/107906320701900206
Joyal, C. C., & Carpentier, J. (2017). The prevalence of paraphilic interests and behaviors in the general population: A provincial survey. *The Journal of Sex Research, 54*(2), 161–171. https://doi.org/10.1080/00224499.2016.1139034
Joyal, C. C., Cossette, A., & Lapierre, V. (2015). What exactly is an unusual sexual fantasy? *The Journal of Sexual Medicine, 12*(2), 328–340. https://doi.org/10.1111/jsm.12734
Joyal, C. C., Kärgel, C., Kneer, J., Amelung, T., Mohnke, S., Tenbergen, G., Walter, H, & Kruger, T. H.C. (2019). The neurobiological origins of pedophilia: Not that simple. *The Journal of Sexual Medicine, 16*(1), 153–154. http://10.1016/j.jsxm.2018.10.015
Joyal, C. C., Tardif, M., & Spearson-Goulet, J. A. (2020). Executive functions and social cognition in juveniles who have sexually offended. *Sexual Abuse, 32*(2), 179–202. https://doi.org/10.1177/1079063218807487
Jozifkova, E. (2018). Sexual arousal by dominance and submissiveness in the general population: How many, how strongly, and why? *Deviant Behavior, 39*(9), 1229–1236. https://doi.org/10.1080/01639625.2017.1410607
Kafka, M. P. (1997). Hypersexual desire in males: An operational definition and clinical implications for males with paraphilias and paraphilia-related disorders. *Archives of Sexual Behavior, 26*(5), 505–526. https://doi.org/10.1023/A:1024507922470
Kafka, M. P. (2010). Hypersexual disorder: A proposed diagnosis for DSM-V. *Archives of Sexual Behavior, 39*(2), 377–400. https://doi.org/10.1007/s10508-009-9574-7
Kafka, M. P., & Hennen, J. (2002). A DSM-IV Axis I comorbidity study of males (n= 120) with paraphilias and paraphilia-related disorders. *Sexual Abuse, 14*(4), 349–366. https://doi.org/10.1023/A:1020007004436

Kärgel, C., Massau, C., Weiß, S., Walter, M., Borchardt, V., Krueger, T. H. C., Tenbergen, G., Kneer, J., Wittfoth, M., Pohl, A., Gerwinn, H., Ponseti, J., Amelung, T., Beier, K. M., Mohnke, S., Walter, H., & Schiffer, B. (2017). Evidence for superior neurobiological and behavioral inhibitory control abilities in nonoffending as compared to offending pedophiles. *Human Brain Mapping, 38*(2), 1092–1104. https://doi.org/10.1002/hbm.23443

Kemp, A. H., Gordon, E., Rush, A. J., & Williams, L. M. (2008). Improving the prediction of treatment response in depression: Integration of clinical, cognitive, psychophysiological, neuroimaging, and genetic measures. *CNS Spectrums, 13*(12), 1066–1086. https://doi.org/10.1017/S1092852900017120

Kiefer, O. (1934/2009). *Sexual life in Ancient Rome.* Routledge.

Kokkoka. (1965). The koka shastra. (Original work published ca. 1150). A. Comfort, Trans., Stein and Day.

Knight, R. A. (2010). Is a diagnostic category for paraphilic coercive disorder defensible? *Archives of Sexual Behavior, 39*(2), 419–426. https://doi.org/10.1007/s10508-009-9571-x

Kolářský, A., Freund, K., Machek, J., & Polak, O. (1967). Male sexual deviation: Association with early temporal lobe damage. *Archives of General Psychiatry, 17*(6), 735–743. https://doi.org/10.1001/archpsyc.1967.01730300095012

Konrad, A., Haag, S., Scherner, G., Amelung, T., & Beier, K. M. (2017). Previous judicial detection and paedophilic sexual interest partially predict psychological distress in a non-forensic sample of help-seeking men feeling inclined to sexually offend against children. *Journal of Sexual Aggression, 23*(3), 266–277. https://doi.org/10.1080/13552600.2017.1351264

Krafft-Ebing, R. (1886). Sexual psychopathy: A clinical-forensic study [Psychopathia sexualis: eine klinisch-forensische studie]. Verlag von Ferdinand Enke.

Krueger, R. B., & Kaplan, M. S. (2001). The paraphilic and hypersexual disorders: An overview. *Journal of Psychiatric Practice, 7*(6), 391–403. http://10.1097/00131746-200111000-00005.

Krueger, R. B., & Kaplan, M. S. (2002). A favorable view of the DSM-IV diagnosis of the pedophilia and empathy for the pedophile. Commentary. *Archives of Sexual Behavior, 31*(6), 486–488. https://doi-org.biblioproxy.uqtr.ca/10.1023/A:1020603214218

Kruger, T. H., Sinke, C., Kneer, J., Tenbergen, G., Khan, A. Q., Burkert, A., Müller-Engling Engler, H, Gerwinn, H., von Wurmb-Schwark, N., Pohl, A., Weiß, S., Amelung, T., Mohnke, S., Massau, C., Kärgel, C., Walter, M., Schiltz, K., Beier, K. M, Ponseti, J., Schiffer, B., Walter, H., Jahn, K., & Frieling, H. (2019). Child sexual offenders show prenatal and epigenetic alterations of the androgen system. *Translational Psychiatry, 9*(1), 1–11. https://doi.org/10.1038/s41398-018-0326-0

Lalumière, M. L., Harris, G. T., Quinsey, V. L., & Rice, M. E. (1998). Sexual deviance and number of older brothers among sexual offenders. *Sexual Abuse, 10*(1), 5–15. https://doi.org/10.1023/A:1022198329907

Langevin, R. (1992). Biological factors contributing to paraphilic behavior. *Psychiatric Annals, 22*(6), 307–314. https://doi.org/10.3928/0048-5713-19920601-07

Langevin, R., & Curnoe, S. (2008). Assessing neuropsychological impairment among sex offenders and paraphilics. *Journal of Forensic Psychology Practice, 8*(2), 150–173. https://doi.org/10.1080/15228930801963960

Langevin, R., Lang, R. A., Wortzman, G., Frentzel, R. R., & Wright, P. (1989). An examination of brain damage and dysfunction in genital exhibitionists. *Annals of Sex Research, 2*(1), 77–87. https://doi.org/10.1007/BF00850681

Langevin, R., Paitich, D., Freeman, R., Mann, K., & Handy, L. (1978). Personality characteristics and sexual anomalies in males. *Canadian Journal of Behavioural Science, 10*(3), 222–238. https://doi.org/10.1037/h0081551

Langevin, R., Paitich, D., Ramsay, G., Anderson, C., Kamrad, J., Pope, S., Geller, G., Peral, L., & Newman, S. (1979). Experimental studies of the etiology of genital exhibitionism. *Archives of Sexual Behavior, 8*(4), 307–331. https://doi.org/10.1007/BF01541876

Langevin, R., Wortzman, G., Wright, P., & Handy, L. (1989). Studies of brain damage and dysfunction in sex offenders. *Annals of Sex Research, 2*(2), 163–179. https://doi.org/10.1007/BF00851321

Långström, N., & Hanson, R. K. (2006). High rates of sexual behavior in the general population: Correlates and predictors. *Archives of Sexual Behavior, 35*(1), 37–52. https://doi.org/10.1007/s10508-006-8993-y

Långström, N., & Seto, M. C. (2006). Exhibitionistic and voyeuristic behavior in a Swedish national population survey. *Archives of Sexual Behavior, 35*(4), 427–435. https://doi.org/10.1007/s10508-006-9042-6

Långström, N., & Zucker, K. J. (2005). Transvestic fetishism in the general population. *Journal of Sex & Marital Therapy, 31*(2), 87–95. https://doi.org/10.1080/00926230590477934

Långström, N., Babchishin, K. M., Fazel, S., Lichtenstein, P., & Frisell, T. (2015). Sexual offending runs in families: A 37-year nationwide study. *International Journal of Epidemiology, 44*(2), 713–720. https://doi.org/10.1093/ije/dyv029

Lee, J. K., Pattison, P., Jackson, H. J., & Ward, T. (2001). The general, common, and specific features of psychopathology for different types of paraphilias. *Criminal Justice and Behavior, 28*(2), 227–256. https://doi.org/10.1177/0093854801028002005

Leue, A., Borchard, B., & Hoyer, J. (2004). Mental disorders in a forensic sample of sexual offenders. *European Psychiatry, 19*(3), 123–130. https://doi.org/10.1016/j.eurpsy.2003.08.001

Levenson, J. S. (2004). Reliability of sexually violent predator civil commitment criteria in Florida. *Law and Human Behavior, 28*(4), 357–368. https://doi.org/10.1023/B:LAHU.0000039330.22347.ad

Lodi-Smith, J., Shepard, K., & Wagner, S. (2014). Personality and sexually deviant behavior. *Personality and Individual Differences, 70*, 39–44. https://doi.org/10.1016/j.paid.2014.06.012

MacCulloch, S. I., Gray, N. S., Philips, H. K., Taylor, J., & MacCulloch, M. J. (2004). Birth order in sex-offending and aggressive-offending men. *Archives of Sexual Behavior, 33*(5), 467–474. http://10.1023/B:ASEB.0000037427.18474.1e.

Makanjuola, A. B., Adegunloye, O. A., & Adelekan, M. L. (2008). Disorders of sexual preference among secondary school teachers in Ilorin, Nigeria. *Nigerian Journal of Psychiatry, 6*(1), 26–30. http://10.4314/njpsyc.v6i1.39907

Marshall, W. L. (2007). Diagnostic issues, multiple paraphilias, and comorbid disorders in sexual offenders: Their incidence and treatment. *Aggression and Violent Behavior, 12*(1), 16–35. https://doi.org/10.1016/j.avb.2006.03.001

Kärgel, C., Massau, C., Weiß, S., Walter, M., Borchardt, V., Krueger, T. H., ... & Gerwinn, H. (2017). Evidence for superior neurobiological and behavioral inhibitory control abilities in non-offending as compared to offending pedophiles. *Human Brain Mapping, 38*(2), 1092–1104. https://doi.org/10.1002/hbm.23443

McPhail, I. V., Olver, M. E., Brouillette-Alarie, S., & Looman, J. (2018). Taxometric analysis of the latent structure of pedophilic interest. *Archives of Sexual Behavior, 47*(8), 2223–2240. https://doi.org/10.1007/s10508-018-1225-4

Mendez, M., & Shapira, J. S. (2011). Pedophilic behavior from brain disease. *The Journal of Sexual Medicine, 8*(4), 1092–1100. https://doi.org/10.1111/j.1743-6109.2010.02172.x

Mendez, M. F., Chow, T., Ringman, J., Twitchell, G., & Hinkin, C. H. (2000). Pedophilia and temporal lobe disturbances. *Journal of Neuropsychiatry and Clinical Neuroscience, 12*(1), 71–76. https://doi.org/10.1176/jnp.12.1.71

Milhaven, J. G. (1977). Thomas Aquinas on sexual pleasure. *The Journal of Religious Ethics, 5*(2), 157–181. https://www.jstor.org/stable/40017725

Milner, J. S., Dopke, C. A., & Crouch, J. L. (2008). Paraphilia not otherwise specified. In D. R. Laws & W. T. O'Donohue (Eds.), *Sexual deviance: Theory, assessment, and treatment* (2nd ed.) (pp. 384–418). Guilford Press.

Moffitt, T. E., Lynam, D. R., & Silva, P. A. (1994). Neuropsychological tests predicting persistent male delinquency. *Criminology, 32*(2), 277–300. https://doi.org/10.1111/j.1745-9125.1994.tb01155.x

Mohnke, S., Muller, S., Amelung, T., Kruger, T. H., Ponseti, J., Schiffer, B., Walter, M., Beier, K. M., & Walter, H. (2014). Brain alterations in paedophilia: A critical review. *Progress in Neurobiology, 122*, 1–23. https://doi.org/10.1016/j.pneurobio.2014.07.005

Money, J. (1984). Paraphilias: Phenomenology and classification. *American Journal of Psychotherapy, 38*(2), 164–179. https://doi.org/10.1176/appi.psychotherapy.1984.38.2.164

Moser, C. (2001). Paraphilia: A critique of a confused concept. In P. Kleinplatz (Ed.), *New directions in sex therapy: Innovations and alternatives* (pp. 91–108). Routledge.

Moser, C. (2016). DSM-5 and the paraphilic disorders: Conceptual issues. *Archives of Sexual Behavior, 45*(8), 2181–2186. https://doi.org/10.1007/s10508-016-0861-9

Moser, C. (2019). DSM-5, paraphilias, and the paraphilic disorders: Confusion Reigns. *Archives of Sexual Behavior, 48*(3), 681–689. https://doi.org/10.1007/s10508-018-1356-7

Moser, C., & Kleinplatz, P. J. (2005). DSM-IV-TR and the paraphilias: An argument for removal. *Journal of Psychology & Human Sexuality, 17*(3–4), 91–109. https://doi.org/10.1300/J056v17n03_05

Moser, C., & Levitt, E. E. (1987). An exploratory-descriptive study of a sadomasochistically oriented sample. *Journal of Sex Research, 23*(3), 322–337. https://doi.org/10.1080/00224498709551370

Mundy, C. L., & Cioe, J. D. (2019). Exploring the relationship between paraphilic interests, sex, and sexual and life satisfaction in non-clinical samples. *The Canadian Journal of Human Sexuality, 28*(3), 304–316. https://doi.org/10.3138/cjhs.2018-0041

Noorishad, P. G., Levaque, E., Byers, E. S., & Shaughnessy, K. (2019). More than one flavour: University students' specific sexual fantasies, interests, and experiences. *The Canadian Journal of Human Sexuality, 28*(2), 143–158. https://doi.org/10.3138/cjhs.2019-0024

O'Donohue, W. (2010). A critique of the proposed DSM-V diagnosis of pedophilia. *Archives of Sexual Behavior, 39*(3), 587–590. http://doi.org/10.1007/s10508-010-9604-5

O'Donohue, W. (2016). Problems in the classification and diagnosis of the paraphilias: What is the evidence that the DSM warrants use? In D. R. Laws & W. T. O'Donohue (Eds.), *Treatment of sex offenders: Strengths and weaknesses in assessment and intervention* (pp. 1–17). Springer.

Ogunfowokan, A. A., Olagunju, O. E., Olajubu, A. O., Faremi, F. A., Oloyede, A. S., & Sharps, P. W. (2016). Correlates of self-report of rape among male school adolescents in Ile-Ife, Nigeria. *Journal of Interpersonal Violence, 31*(4), 555–571. https://doi.org/10.1177/0886260514556104

Poeppl, T. B., Peytard, J., & Langguth, B. (2015). A temporal link between epileptiform brain activity, schizotypy, and pedophilia. *The Journal of Neuropsychiatry and Clinical Neurosciences, 27*(3), e204–e205. http://doi.org/10.1176/appi.neuropsych.14110305

Raymond, N. C., Coleman, E., Ohlerking, F., Christenson, G. A., & Miner, M. (1999). Psychiatric comorbidity in pedophilic sex offenders. *American Journal of Psychiatry, 156*(5), 786–788.

Reed, G. M., Drescher, J., Krueger, R. B., Atalla, E., Cochran, S. D., First, M. B., Cohen-Kettenis P. T, Arango-de Montis I., Parish S. J., Cottler S., Briken P., & Saxena, S. (2016). Disorders related to sexuality and gender identity in the ICD-11: Revising the ICD-10 classification based on current scientific evidence, best clinical practices, and human rights considerations. *World Psychiatry, 15*(3), 205–221. https://doi.org/10.1002/wps.20354

Rees, G., & Garcia, J. R. (2017). All I need is shoe: An investigation into the obligatory aspect of sexual object fetishism. *International Journal of Sexual Health, 29*(4), 303–312. https://doi.org/10.1080/19317611.2017.1309483

Reid, R. C., Carpenter, B. N., Hook, J. N., Garos, S., Manning, J. C., Gilliland, R., Cooper, E. B., McKittrick, H., Davtian, M., & Fong, T. (2012). Report of findings in a DSM-5 field trial for hypersexual disorder. *The Journal of Sexual Medicine, 9*(11), 2868–2877. https://doi.org/10.1111/j.1743-6109.2012.02936.x

Renaud, C. A., & Byers, E. S. (1999). Exploring the frequency, diversity, and content of university students' positive and negative sexual cognitions. *The Canadian Journal of Human Sexuality, 8*(1), 17–30.

Rinehart, N. J., & McCabe, M. P. (1998). An empirical investigation of hypersexuality. *Sexual and Marital Therapy, 13*(4), 369–384. https://doi.org/10.1080/02674659808404255

Robins, E., & Guze, S. B. (1970). Establishment of diagnostic validity in psychiatric illness: Its application to schizophrenia. *American Journal of Psychiatry, 126*(7), 983–987. https://doi.org/10.1176/ajp.126.7.983

Robinson, J. D., & Parks, C. W. (2004). Lesbian and bisexual women's sexual fantasies, psychological adjustment, and close relationship functioning. *Journal of Psychology & Human Sexuality, 15*(4), 185–203. https://doi.org/10.1300/J056v15n04_03

Robles, R., Fresán, A., Medina-Mora, M. E., Sharan, P., Roberts, M. C., de Jesus Mari, J., Matsumoto, C., Maruta, T., Gureje, O., Ayuso-Mateos, J. L., Xiao, Z., & Reed, G. M. (2015). Categories that should be removed from mental disorders classifications: Perspectives and rationales of clinicians from eight countries. *Journal of Clinical Psychology, 71*(3), 267–281. https://doi.org/10.1002/jclp.22145

Roche, E., & Staunton, C. (2018). An exploration of sexual fantasies among an Irish sample: Implications for forensic populations. *The Open Journal of Criminology and Sociology, 1,* 71–86.

Rogak, H. M., & Connor, J. J. (2018). Practice of consensual BDSM and relationship satisfaction. *Sexual and Relationship Therapy, 33*(4), 454–469. https://doi.org/10.1080/14681994.2017.1419560

Rosman, J. P., & Resnick, P. J. (1989). Sexual attraction to corpses: A psychiatric review of necrophilia. *Bulletin of the American Academy of Psychiatry and the Law, 17*(2), 153–163.

Sandnabba, N. K., Santtila, P., & Nordling, N. (1999). Sexual behavior and social adaptation among sadomasochistically-oriented males. *Journal of Sex Research, 36*(3), 273–282. https://doi.org/10.1080/00224499909551997

Santtila, P., Antfolk, J., Räfså, A., Hartwig, M., Sariola, H., Sandnabba, N. K., & Mokros, A. (2015). Men's sexual interest in children: One-year incidence and correlates in a population-based sample of Finnish male twins. *Journal of Child Sexual Abuse, 24*(2), 115–134. https://doi.org/10.1080/10538712.2015.997410

Sartori, G., Scarpazza, C., Codognotto, S., & Pietrini, P. (2016). An unusual case of acquired pedophilic behavior following compression of orbitofrontal cortex 10.1007/s00415-016-8143-y and hypothalamus by a Clivus Chordoma. *Journal of Neurology, 263*(7), 1454–1455. https://doi.org/10.1007/s00415-016-8143-y

Schiffer, B., Amelung, T., Pohl, A., Kaergel, C., Tenbergen, G., Gerwinn, H., Mohnke, S., Massau, C., Matthias, W., Weiß, S., Marr, V., Beier, K.M., Walter, M., Ponseti, J., Krüger, T.H.C., Schiltz, K., & Walter, H. (2017). Gray matter anomalies in pedophiles with and without a history of child sexual offending. *Translational Psychiatry, 7,* e1129. https://doi.org/10.1038/tp.2017.96

Schrenck-Notzing, F. A. (1892). *Die suggestions-therapie bei krankhaften erscheinungen des geschlechts sinnes mit besonderer berucksichtigung des contraren sexualempfindung [The suggestion therapy in cases of morbid phenomena of the sex sense with special consideration for the contrarian sexual sensation].* F. Enke.

Scott, M. L., Cole, J. K., McKay, S. E., Golden, C. J., & Liggett, K. R. (1984). Neuropsychological performance of sexual assaulters and pedophiles. *Journal of Forensic Science, 29*(4), 1114–1118.

Seto, M. C., & Barbaree, H. E. (2000). Paraphilia. In V. B. Van Hasselt & M. Hersen (Eds.), *Aggression and violence: An introductory text* (pp. 198-213). Allyn and Bacon.

Shenal, B. V., Harrison, D. W., & Demaree, H. A. (2003). The neuropsychology of depression: A literature review and preliminary model. *Neuropsychology Review, 13*(1), 33–42. https://doi.org/10.1023/A:1022300622902

Shindel, A. W., & Moser, C. A. (2011). Why are the paraphilias mental disorders? *The Journal of Sexual Medicine, 8*(3), 927–929. https://doi.org/10.1111/j.1743-6109.2010.02087.x

Shulman, J. L., & Horne, S. G. (2006). Guilty or not? A path model of women's forceful sexual fantasies. *Journal of Sex Research, 43*(4), 368–377. https://doi.org/10.1080/00224490609552336

Singy, P. (2010). What's wrong with sex? *Archives of Sexual Behavior, 39*(6), 1231–1233. https://doi.org/10.1007/s10508-010-9650-z

Stekel, W. (1924). Peculiarities of behavior: Wandering mania, dipsomania, cleptomania, pyromania and allied impulsive acts [English translation]. Boni and Liveright.

Stinson, J. D., Becker, J. V., & Sales, B. D. (2008). Self-regulation and the etiology of sexual deviance: Evaluating causal theory. *Violence and Victims, 23*(1), 35–51. https://doi.org/10.1891/0886-6708.23.1.35

Suchy, Y., Eastvold, A. D., Strassberg, D. S., & Franchow, E. I. (2014). Understanding processing speed weaknesses among pedophilic child molesters: Response style vs. Neuropathology. *Journal of Abnormal Psychology, 123*(1), 273–285. https://doi.org/10.1037/a0035812

Taktak, Ş., Yılmaz, E., Karamustafalıoglu, O., & Ünsal, A. (2016). Characteristics of paraphilics in Turkey: A retrospective study–20 years. *International Journal of Law and Psychiatry, 49*(Pt A), 22–30. https://doi.org/10.1016/j.ijlp.2016.05.004

Tannahill, R. (1980). *Sex in history*. Stein and Day Publishers.

Templeman, T. L., & Stinnett, R. D. (1991). Patterns of sexual arousal and history in a "normal" sample of young men. *Archives of Sexual Behavior, 20*(2), 137–150. https://doi.org/10.1007/BF01541940

Tenbergen, G., Wittfoth, M., Frieling, H., Ponseti, J., Walter, M., Beier, K. M., Schiffer, B., & Krueger, T. H. C. (2015). The neurobiology and psychology of pedophilia: Recent advances and challenges. *Frontiers in Human Neuroscience, 9*, Article 344, 1–21. https://doi.org/10.3389/fnhum.2015.00344

Thompson, L. (2016). *Latent structure of paraphilic disorders in male and female college-aged samples* Master's thesis. Brandeis University, MA.

Turley, E. L., & Butt, T. (2015). Bdsm–bondage and discipline; dominance and submission; sadism and masochism. In C. Richards & M. J. Barker (Eds.), *The Palgrave handbook of the psychology of sexuality and gender* (pp. 24–41). Palgrave Macmillan.

UC San Diego Center on Gender Equity and Health (2019). Measuring #MeToo: *A national study on sexual harassment and assault.* UCSD Center on Gender Equity and Health. Document retrieved 13 December 2019 http://geh.ucsd.edu/wp-content/uploads/2019/05/2019-metoo-national-sexual-harassment-and-assault-report.pdf

Vatsyayana, M., (c. 300 A.D.). (1883). The kama sutra of Vatsyayana. Retrieved March 2020, from www.gutenberg.org/ebooks/27827

Wakefield, J. C. (1992). The concept of mental disorder: On the boundary between biological facts and social values. *American Psychologist, 47*(3), 373–388. https://doi.org/10.1037/0003-066X.47.3.373

Wakefield, J. C. (2011). DSM-5 proposed diagnostic criteria for sexual paraphilias: Tensions between diagnostic validity and forensic utility. *International Journal of Law and Psychiatry, 34*(3), 195–209. https://doi.org/10.1016/j.ijlp.2011.04.012

Wakefield, J. C., Kirk, S. A., Pottick, K. J., Hsieh, D. K., & Tian, X. (2006). The lay concept of conduct disorder: Do nonprofessionals use syndromal symptoms or internal dysfunction to distinguish disorder from delinquency? *The Canadian Journal of Psychiatry, 51*(4), 210–217. https://doi.org/10.1177/070674370605100402

Walters, G. D., Knight, R. A., & Långström, N. (2011). Is hypersexuality dimensional? Evidence for the DSM-5 from general population and clinical samples. *Archives of Sexual Behavior, 40*(6), 1309–1321. https://doi.org/10.1007/s10508-010-9719-8

Wang, L., Hermens, D. F., Hickie, I. B., & Lagopoulos, J. (2012). A systematic review of resting-state functional-MRI studies in major depression. *Journal of Affective Disorders, 142*(1–3), 6–12. https://doi.org/10.1016/j.jad.2012.04.013

Watts, A. L., Nagel, M. G., Latzman, R. D., & Lilienfeld, S. O. (2019). Personality disorder features and paraphilic interests among undergraduates: Differential relations and potential antecedents. *Journal of Personality Disorders, 33*(1), 22–48. https://doi.org/10.1521/pedi_2017_31_327

Williams, C. J., & Weinberg, M. S. (2003). Zoophilia in men: A study of sexual interest in animals. *Archives of Sexual Behavior, 32*(6), 523–535. https://doi.org/10.1023/A:1026085410617

Williams, K. M., Cooper, B. S., Howell, T. M., Yuille, J. C., & Paulhus, D. L. (2009). Inferring sexually deviant behavior from corresponding fantasies: The role of personality and pornography consumption. *Criminal Justice and Behavior, 36*(2), 198–222. https://doi.org/10.1177/0093854808327277

Wismeijer, A. A., & Van Assen, M. A. (2013). Psychological characteristics of BDSM practitioners. *The Journal of Sexual Medicine, 10*(8), 1943–1952. https://doi.org/10.1111/jsm.12192

World Health Organization (WHO). (2001). International classification of functioning, disability, and health (ICF). WHO. https://www.who.int/classifications/icf/en

World Health Organization (WHO). (2006). Defining sexual health: Report of a technical consultation on sexual health. WHO. Retrived February 2019, from www.who.int/reproductivehealth/publications/sexual_health/defining_sexual_health.pdf

World Health Organization (WHO). (2018). *Classifications.* WHO. Retrieved December 22, 2019, from http://www.who.int/classifications/en.

Wright, P., Nobrega, J., Langevin, R., & Wortzman, G. (1990). Brain density and symmetry in pedophilic and sexually aggressive offenders. *Annals of Sex Research, 3*(3), 319–328. https://doi.org/10.1007/BF00849186

Wurtele, S. K., Simons, D. A., & Moreno, T. (2014). Sexual interest in children among an online sample of men and women: Prevalence and correlates. *Sexual Abuse, 26*(6), 546–568. https://doi.org/10.1177/1079063213503688

Zonana, H. (2011). Sexual disorders: New and expanded proposals for the DSM-5–do we need them? *Journal of the American Academy of Psychiatry and the Law, 39*(2), 245–249.

7

Diagnosing Sexual Sadism and Other Paraphilic Disorders on the Agonistic Continuum

Deirdre M. D'Orazio[1] *and Charles A. Flinton*[2]

[1] *Central Coast Clinical and Forensic Psychological Services, USA*
[2] *San Francisco Forensic Institute, USA*

Introduction

Sexual abuse prevention starts with proper identification of those at risk of acting on sexually abusive interests. Sexual abuse is associated with numerous psychological and physical problems to victims and perpetrators (Dong et al., 2003; Levenson et al., 2016). Sexual abuse prevention is a matter of public health impacting the safety, wellbeing, and fiscal budget of communities. Nearly one in three women and one in four men experience violent sexual contact at some point in their lives (Centers for Disease Control and Prevention (CDC), 2020). In the European Union, the cost of sexual assault is about 2% of the Gross Domestic Product (Perryer, 2018). In the U.S., preventing one rape saves about $164,000 (Miller et al., 2018).

Agonistic paraphilic disorders are a subcategory of mental disorders involving persistent, atypical, algolagnic sexual interests. The use of the term "deviant sexual interests" is not used in this chapter because it may discourage treatment engagement and cause other unintended negative impacts. However, the paraphilic focus goes beyond that implied by the term "atypical sexual interests," for example, consensual bondage or kink, and beyond that implied by "problematic sexual behaviors," for example, excessive pornography consumption. Agonistic paraphilic disorders are mental disorders involving sexual gratification by the infliction of agony which, when acted upon, result in serious harm, distress, or impairment.

Mental disorders are dysfunctions in the psychological, biological, or developmental processes underlying mental functioning (APA, 2013). Paraphilic disorders are a category of mental disorders. They manifest in persistent, atypical, problematic sexual activity or sexual target preferences in a variety of ways.

The purpose of diagnostic systems is to facilitate the identification, categorization, and communication of disorders (APA, 2013; Mezzich, 2002). Thus, diagnosis often serves as a gateway to access medical and mental health services. Accurate diagnosis of paraphilic disorders has many benefits, including potential reductions in the prevalence of sexual abuse. Accurate information about mental disorders is foundational to community education and prevention of mental illness. In more recent years, reduced stigma about mental illness along with increased sexual abuse prevention and education efforts have contributed to increased self-initiated help-seeking behaviors among those with problematic sexual interests. This help-seeking behavior typically occurs either when sexual offending has not yet occurred or when it has occurred but has not been officially detected. Secondary prevention efforts targeting outreach to those showing symptoms of paraphilic disorders potentiates significant enhancements in wellbeing and reductions in sexual abuse.

Accurate diagnosis increases the likelihood that individuals who sexually offend will receive interventions necessary to refrain from further sexual abuse. Roughly 5% to 15% of those

Sexual Deviance: Understanding and Managing Deviant Sexual Interests and Paraphilic Disorders, First Edition. Edited by Leam A. Craig and Ross M. Bartels.
© 2021 John Wiley & Sons, Ltd. Published 2021 by John Wiley & Sons, Ltd.

arrested for a sex crime get re-arrested for a sexual offense within five years (Phenix et al., 2017). However, these statistics include the subgroup that prolifically reoffend and those that never reoffend. Despite an increase of individuals seeking self-initiated treatment for paraphilic interests, most treatment occurs through criminal justice mandates or in response to civil commitment. Examples include sexual offense-specific treatment to achieve early release from incarceration sentences; as a condition of parole or probation community sentences; and to show readiness for release from civil commitment.

Forensic experts are often called upon to educate courts by responding to various psycholegal referral questions involving the diagnosis of mental disorders. For example:

- What are the individual's risk for sexual reoffending and treatment needs?
- Can the individual's risk be managed through community treatment and supervision or is incarceration necessary?
- Does the individual suffer from a mental disorder that makes the individual likely to sexually reoffend and in need of detainment and treatment?
- In a child custody case, does a parent with a history of sexual offending have a paraphilic disorder that compromises his ability to parent without putting the child at risk?
- Is the individual convicted of sexual offending safe to work with vulnerable others?
- Is the individual safe enough to be released from the institution?

A large number of paraphilias have been identified and described in the scientific literature (APA, 2013). These include more commonly discussed paraphilias such as pedophilia, exhibitionism, voyeurism, and sexual sadism, and those less commonly discussed such as coprophilia, somnophilia, and gerontophilia. The diagnoses of countless paraphilic disorders are possible, as long as they meet the general definition of a paraphilic disorder.

Paraphilic disorders that entail non-consensual acts with other humans are generally considered more dangerous than those that involve consenting others or do not involve others, for example, pedophilic disorder versus fetishistic disorder. Likewise, paraphilic disorders involving physical contact are generally considered more harmful than those exhibited through non-contact, for example, sexual sadism disorder versus voyeuristic disorder. Indeed, although non-contact sexual offenses, for example, exhibitionism, reoccur with more frequency (Hanson & Morton-Bourgon, 2004), the less frequent but more harm-inducing contact sexual offenses are the focus of intensive criminal justice interventions.

Detecting the subgroup of sexual offending individuals with paraphilic disorders is arguably the best first step in reducing reoffense rates; however, this is a challenging task. Sexual offending individuals with paraphilic disorders are more likely to sexually reoffend than those without paraphilic disorders (Hanson & Morton-Bourgon, 2005; Lalumiere et al., 2005). The risk of incorrectly detecting a paraphilic disorder when it is not present, a false positive, is elevated because the majority of detected sexual offenders are not driven by paraphilic disorders. Although all sexual criminals have perpetrated socially aberrant acts, less than one out of five have paraphilic sexual preferences (Hanson et al., 2007). Most sexual offending individuals are adult men (Greenfeld, 1997) with consensual sexual preferences, not paraphilic sexual preferences (e.g., Kingston et al., 2010). On the other hand, it is common for paraphilic individuals, especially those within the criminal justice system, to conceal paraphilic interests, which may inflate the likelihood of false negative diagnoses.

It is incumbent on those providing expertise and intervention with sexual offending individuals to correctly discern those with agonistic paraphilic disorders from the larger portion of non-paraphilic sexual offending individuals. The smaller portion of sexual offending individuals persistently and intensely driven to perpetrate agonistic sexual acts presents significant risk for sexual reoffense, dangerousness by way of victim impact, and need for intensive treatment. Accurate identification of agonistic paraphilic disorders is essential to prevent first acts of sexual offending, to identify the smaller portion of sexual offenders most likely to reoffend, and identify targets for treatment to reduce sexual offense likelihood.

This chapter offers a deep examination of the agonistic continuum of paraphilic disorders, which range from lower levels of coercion to extreme brutality. The goal is to facilitate and enhance accurate diagnosis and communication about paraphilic disorders on the agonistic continuum. Lacking abundant and definitive quantitative research, along with the unfortunate prejudicial impact of paraphilic disorder diagnoses, agonistic paraphilic disorders are rarely discussed without acknowledgment of the controversies that surround them. As the evolving field of study works toward formalizing operational definitions, it is crucial to proceed in a manner that combines available research, theory, and clinical experience and that reflects best practice.

The Role of Agonistic Paraphilic Disorders in Best Practice Standards for Interventions with Sexual Offending Individuals

Prior to the 21st century, the question of whether sexual offending individuals could be successfully treated was seriously debated, as the available research was mixed (Barbaree, 1997; Furby et al., 1989; Gallagher et al., 1999; Hall, 1995; Hanson et al., 1991; Harris et al., 1998; Marques et al., 1994). Since the turn of the 21st century, the field of general offender research and its subspecialty, sexual offender research, have seen immense growth (Harris & Hanson, 2010). It is now widely accepted that general offender and sexual offender treatment can effectively reduce reoffense rates (Hanson et al., 2002; Schmucker & Losel, 2015), when applied according to best practice principles (Bonta & Andrews, 2017; Hanson et al., 2009).

Risk, Needs, Responsivity Principles

The Risk, Needs, Responsivity (RNR) model provides guiding principles for effective correctional interventions (Bonta & Andrews, 2017). Meta-analytic research shows that participants in sexual offense treatment programs where all three principles are followed are about five times more likely to refrain from further sexually offending than those receiving no treatment. In contrast, when none of the principles are followed, treatment participants are about 20% *more* likely to sexually reoffend than untreated individuals (Hanson et al., 2009). Given the robust empirical outcomes of RNR, it is not surprising that RNR is widely considered the best practice guidance for sexual offender treatment (Thornton & D'Orazio, 2013).

The vast body of research underlying RNR identifies the internal and external attributes of offending individuals and assists the evaluator in differentiating those that reoffend from those that desist (Bonta & Andrews, 2017). RNR is a distillation of these research findings into principles that guides any correctional intervention whose goal is to maximally reduce reoffending while balancing community safety and offender rehabilitation.

The Place for Agonistic Paraphilic Disorders in RNR

Below is a description of each principle followed by a description of its application to the subpopulation of sexually abusive individuals with agonistic paraphilic disorders.

Risk Principle

The intensity and dosage of interventions should be proportionate to the risk for recidivism. For example, higher-risk offending individuals should receive more treatment and risk management services than lower-risk offending individuals.

Applying the Risk Principle to those with agonistic paraphilic disorders means conducting a comprehensive risk assessment; assigning the dose and intensity of interventions according to risk level and titrating them as risk is reduced. Tools and methods aid in discerning higher- from lower-risk individuals. Appropriately identifying higher-risk individuals enhances outcomes, allows use of resources, and prevents iatrogenic effects caused by excessive or unnecessary treatment (e.g., Lovins et al., 2009).

Common indicators of paraphilic disorders, and specifically the agonistic type, are empirically associated with sexual reoffense risk. This is exemplified by their inclusion in the most researched and used actuarial risk assessment tool for sexual offenders in the world, the Static99R (Helmus et al., 2012). Half of the Static99R items include indicators of agonistic paraphilic disorders: non-sexual violence at the time of the index sex offense and prior; persistent sexual offending; stranger and unrelated victim selection (i.e. items 3, 4, 5, 8, 9, and 10). Research has additionally shown phallometrically assessed sexual arousal to sexual and non-sexual violence; violent sexual offending; and intrusive sexual offending as predictive of sexual recidivism (Kingston et al., 2010). Meta-analytic research further shows the dangerous combination of elevated psychopathy plus sexual deviance as predictive of sexual reoffense, although notably "sexual deviance" includes both agonistic and child focus preferences (Hawes et al., 2013).

Need Principle

Interventions should target empirically supported criminogenic needs. Criminogenic needs are psychologically meaningful factors that predispose an individual to offending. As such, an assessment of criminogenic needs explains the sources of risk (Thornton & D'Orazio, 2016). Reduced risk occurs when there is change in the underlying criminogenic needs.

Applying the Need Principle to those with agonistic paraphilic disorders means strategically applying interventions to target the internal and external features that predispose the individual to sexual offending behavior. Ample research indicates sexual deviance is a criminogenic need that must be addressed in order to mitigate the likelihood of sexual offending. Table 7.1 lists several empirically supported tools that aid the detection of agonistic sexual preferences. These include objective measures of sexual response (i.e., penile plethysmograph, PPG), behavior indicator checklists, and items from comprehensive need assessment tools.

Responsivity Principle

The responsivity principle means that only evidence-based interventions should be utilized and that they are adapted and delivered to maximize participants' response, for example, by attending to individual learning style, motivation, abilities, and culture.

Applying the Responsivity Principle to individuals with agonistic sexual preferences means finding ways to motivate and engage them in treatment. The sexual attraction to pain and suffering in others is often associated with any number of other co-occurring conditions including psychopathy, antisociality, attachment disorders, and adverse early life experiences including childhood abuse and neglect. Because the very nature of the change requires disruption of conditioned arousal to distress in others, interventions that focus on empathy, compassion, and victim awareness may be unhelpful. Further, paraphilic sexual preferences tend to be persistent and intense, requiring multiple arousal reconditioning strategies such as cognitive interventions and behavioral interventions (such as aversion therapy, e.g., olfactory, taste and masturbatory reconditioning).

Table 7.1 Tools that aid diagnosing agonistic paraphilic disorders

Tool	Description	Item(s)	Validated Population Use	Citation
Violence Risk Scale Sex Offender Version	Comprehensive risk, need, and progress assessment tool	Sexually deviant lifestyle Sexual compulsivity Offense planning Sexual offending cycle Deviant sexual preference	Adult males with sexual offenses	VRSSO, Olver et al. (2007)
Structured Risk Assessment-Forensic Version	Comprehensive need assessment tool	Sexualized violence Sexual preoccupation	Adult males with sexual offenses	SRA-FV, Thornton and Knight (2015)
Stable-2007	Comprehensive need assessment tool	Sex drive/preoccupation Sex as coping Deviant sexual preference	Adult males with sexual offenses	Hanson et al., (2007)
Sexual Sadism Scale	Eleven-item offense behavior checklist plus three additional indicators	Items assess crime scene behaviors including arousal, power, control, domination, torture, humiliation, mutilation, excessive violence, object insertion, ritual, confinement, trophies, planning and fantasies	Adult males and females	SeSaS, Mokros et al. (2014)
Multi-Dimensional Inventory of Development Sex and Aggression	Computerized self-report inventory that provides a clinical report to support therapeutic interventions	Scales assessing: Sadism Paraphilias Sexualization	Adult and juvenile males with sexual offenses; non-offending adult and juvenile males	MIDSA clinical manual (2011)
Penile Plethysmograph	Audio and visual stimuli depicting various sexual and non-sexual violent acts	Measures penile circumference responses to presented stimuli	Adult males with sexual offenses	Freund (1958)
Multiphasic Sexual Inventory-II	A 560-question self-report inventory	Measures cognitive distortions, denial and accountability, scheming, sexual development, and sexual interest and experiences	Offending and non-offending adult and juvenile males, and females	Nichols and Molinder (2000)

The Agonistic Continuum

> *... scientific evidence now places many, if not most, disorders on a spectrum with closely related disorders that have shared symptoms.* (DSM-5, APA, 2013, p. 6)

Diagnostic systems, such as the Diagnostic and Statistical Manual (DSM) of Mental Disorders, assign underlying mental conditions to categories based on prototypical outward manifestations, called symptoms. Diagnostic symptoms included are those most commonly shown by available research, but not the entire range of symptoms. The categorical approach to mental disorders is fundamentally faulty because the underlying mental conditions are not discrete entities. Boundaries between disorders are often fluid. The same symptoms cut across numerous disorders, and individual manifestation of the same disorder often vastly differs.

In the Preface and Introduction, DSM-5 acknowledges its diagnostic system is flawed due to its premise that narrow diagnostic categories could capture clinical reality, and it suggests future improvement will occur through a dimensional approach. DSM-5 currently takes a categorical approach to paraphilic disorders, assuming the same structural problems. DSM-5 includes several paraphilic disorders but allows the diagnosis of innumerable other specified and unspecified paraphilic disorders, which shows an understanding that discrete finite categories do not exist. Diagnosis occurs by assigning the individual case to the category that best fits the individual's symptom presentation.

Salient aspects of sexual preferences are more accurately understood as occurring on continuums rather than as discrete categorical entities. This means there is a progression in values from one end to the other, and that adjacent points on the continuum are very similar, whereas distant points are distinct. The agonistic continuum model acknowledges that what is commonly referred to as sexual sadism occurs along a continuum much like any other disorder. As a medical analogy, it is not uncommon to have a mild cold on one end of a severity spectrum and pneumonia on the other.

The agonistic continuum is an evidence-supported conceptual model referring to the individual's sexual preference regarding the degree of agony of the sexual partner. As Figure 7.1 indicates, mutual consenting preference is at one end of the continuum, depicting an absence

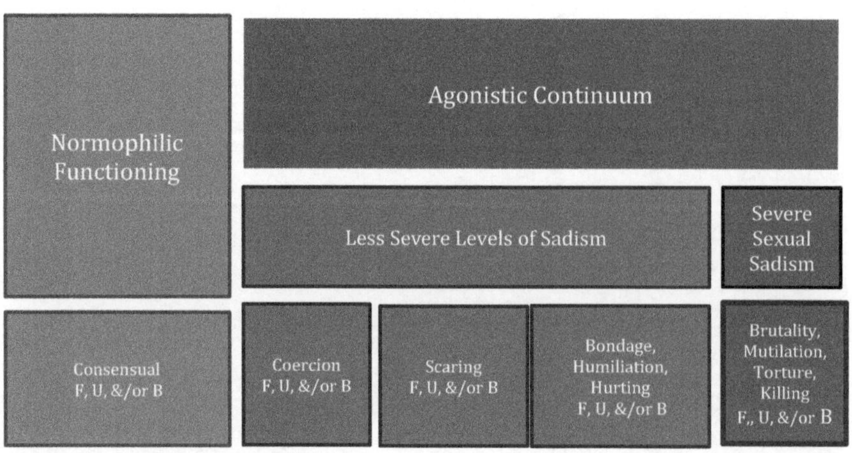

Figure 7.1 Agonistic Continuum Model.
F = Fantasies; U = Urges; B = Behaviors

of agonistic preference. In the middle is a preference for sex acts that are coercive but do not involve gratuitous brutality. At the other end of the continuum are forms of extreme sexual sadism involving high levels of physical brutality. There are many gradations on the continuum between these points, resulting in precise communication of individual preferences. The range of sexual target agony preferences includes persuasion, obedience, humiliation/mental anguish, coercion, subjugation, fear, threatening physical harm, physical pain, torture, injury, mutilation, up to and including and death.

Empirical support for this continuum comes mostly from Knight and colleagues (e.g., Longpré et al., 2019). Whereas some authors find it worthwhile to distinguish excitatory from inhibitory causes (e.g., Knight et al., 2013), disorders on the agonistic continuum can be diagnosed for individuals abnormally excited by agony cues or abnormally uninhibited by agony cues because both result in abnormal sexual arousal.

Diagnosing on the Agonistic Continuum

Evolution of Paraphilic Disorders in the Diagnostic Manual of Mental Disorders

When the first DSM (APA, 1952) was released, it included just one diagnosis for problematic sexual behavior, "sexual deviation," a personality disorder, defined on page 38 as:

> … deviant sexuality which is not symptomatic of more extensive syndromes, such as schizophrenic and obsessional reactions. The term includes most of the cases formally classed as "psychopathic personality with pathologic sexuality." The diagnosis will specify the type of pathologic behavior, such as homosexuality, transvestism, pedophilia, fetishism and sexual sadism (including rape, sexual assault, mutilation).

On pages 41 and 42 of the original DSM, "sexual offenses" were listed under "conduct disturbances":

> When the transient reaction manifests itself primarily as a disturbance in social conduct or behavior, it will be classified here […] for example, truancy, stealing, destructiveness, cruelty, sexual offenses, use of alcohol, etc.

Over the years, treatment providers and criminal justice system stakeholders helped propel research advances and DSM revisions by demanding more understanding and specificity regarding coercive and violent sexual behaviors and the motivating forces behind them. The DSM-III (APA, 1980, p. 266) first introduced the category *paraphilias* indicating that this term is preferable over the term *sexual deviations*. This change emphasized that paraphilic behavior is motivated by individual sexual interests and arousal patterns, and not simply a disregard for social mores. DSM-III emphasized that paraphilias are a pattern of sexual arousal that "may interfere with the capacity for reciprocal affectionate sexual activity" (DSM-III-R; APA, 1987, p. 292). The DSM-IV (APA, 1994) became more specific, indicating the essential features of paraphilias are "recurrent, intense sexually arousing fantasies, sexual urges, or behaviors" (p. 566).

Instead of describing what a paraphilia *is*, DSM-5 (APA, 2013) indicates that a paraphilia is any intense and persistent sexual interest that is *not* normophilic. The DSM-5 initiates the distinction between a paraphilia and a paraphilic disorder. This is a bold step toward non-pathologizing atypical but non problematic sexual interests. Whereas for both, sexual fantasies, urges, or behaviors signal the underlying paraphilia, it becomes a disorder when they cause clinically significant negative effects, including harm, to the person or others. Within the DSM-5 paraphilic disorders section, there are eight paraphilic disorders, each distinguished by the target focus or activity focus plus an "other specified" paraphilic disorder to utilize when diagnosing specific paraphilic disorders other than the eight provided. DSM-5 adds a disclaimer that many dozens exist and thus may be diagnosed. The changes from DSM-IV to DSM-5 that add "other specified" eliminate "not otherwise specified," and the disclaimer greatly expands the potential to diagnose paraphilic disorders using DSM-5.

Making Accurate and Reliable Agonistic Disorder Diagnoses

Diagnosing paraphilic disorders on the agonistic continuum is challenging and requires thorough training, not merely on diagnostic tools and interview techniques, but also on the myriad clinical presentations of paraphilic disorders. Accurate diagnosis flows from a thorough clinical case formulation and requires richly detailed sources of information. The dimensions quantifiable in research manifest in a wide range of ways across individuals. Rendering diagnoses always involves integrating multiple data points. Diagnosing individuals along the agonistic continuum is a developing application. Like all diagnoses, agonistic diagnoses are continually evolving alongside the evidence base.

Mental Disorder

Diagnosis of a paraphilic disorder means a *mental disorder* is present. Mental disorders are not abnormal behaviors, but rather are the underlying dysfunctional processes that motivate, or explain, abnormal behavior. Mental disorders are expressed as syndromes, of "clinically significant disturbance in cognition, emotion regulation, or behavior" (DSM-5, p. 20). The symptoms are signals of the underlying dysfunctional psychological, biological, or developmental processes.

Paraphilic Disorder

Diagnosis of a specific disorder, notably including other Specified Paraphilic Disorder, on the agonistic continuum means a *paraphilic disorder* is present. Proper assessment focuses on the underlying motivation for the behavior. Any specific paraphilic disorder diagnosis should meet the criterion for paraphilia and disorder, which is currently defined by DSM-5 in criterion A (paraphilia) and B (disorder).

DSM-5 Paraphilia, Criterion A: Any intense and persistent (i.e., generally at least six months) sexual interest other than "normophilic" sexual interest. Not without criticism, DSM-5 defines "normophilic" as "genital stimulation or preparatory fondling with phenotypically normal, physically mature, consenting human partners" (DSM-5, p. 685).

DSM-5, Disorder, Criterion B: The paraphilia causes significant distress, impairment, harm, or risk of harm.

Diagnostic Indicators

Diagnostic reliability and validity are enhanced by conscientious application of knowledge and skills. Frequently, individuals undergoing assessment are resistant to honest disclosure for fear of legal or social consequences. Accurate diagnosis includes a thorough review of all available sources of information; a confluence of multiple data points; and clear communication of diagnostic rationale. Sources of information include self-report, collateral interviews, information from psychological tests or tools, police reports, crime scene reports/photographs, prison and community supervision records, victim statements, medical reports, previous psychological evaluations, and school records. Keen diagnosticians assess for salient indicators of paraphilic disorders across multiple domains of functioning:

(1) *Sexual thoughts* associated with a paraphilic disorder are the general attitudes, core beliefs, and specific cognitions and affects that precede, coexist, or follow the sexual fantasy, urge, or behavior. This includes the content, frequency, and intensity of sexual thoughts, and those associated with the sexual target, sexual script, and associated triggers. In addition to direct verbalizations, thoughts can be assessed through plans, motives, and ruminations.
(2) *Sexual fantasies* are internal mental imagery, wish-states, or imaginary scenarios played, and are intentional or automatic (e.g., intrusive). Sexual fantasy, in combination with masturbation, sometimes acts as rehearsal and conditioning for behavior.
(3) *Sexual urges* are often associated with a physiological genital arousal response, or physical craving. Information about sexual urges helps determine the strength and direction of sex excitatory and inhibitory processes, that influence sexual self-regulation.
(4) *Sexual behaviors* are the physical actions that relate to, or include, sexual activity. In the absence of self-disclosure or evidence of fantasies or thoughts, patterns of behavior are essential to assessing coercive paraphilic disorders. Nonetheless, diagnosing paraphilic disorders based solely on observed, reported, or documented behavior, e.g., victim statements, crime scene evidence, police reports, court documents, is controversial. Making inferences about underlying mental processes based on observed behavior may lead to erroneous diagnosis, especially if the behavior is equated with the diagnosis instead of as an indicator of the underlying sexual interest. However, as pointed out by First and Tasman (2004), "Paraphilias are recognized by unusual eroticism and often socially destructive behaviors such as sex with children, rape, exhibitionism, voyeurism, masochism, obscene phone calling, or sexually touching strangers" (p. 1085). Inferences from behaviors are regularly used in the assessment of medical and psychological syndromes, for example, such as schizophrenia and depression.
(5) *Minimum Victim Count*: DSM-5 explicitly allows diagnosis of sexual sadism disorder despite negative self-report when there are multiple victims, defined as "three or more victims on separate occasions, or fewer than three, if there are multiple instances of infliction of pain and suffering to the same victim, or if there is evidence of strong or preferential interest in pain and suffering involving multiple victims" (p. 696). Further, preliminarily research supports the use of a minimum victim count to indicate coercive preference on the agonistic continuum (Thornton & D'Orazio, 2012).
(6) *Scripts*: In diagnosing agonistic disorders, it is necessary not only to identify manifest symptoms, but also their underlying motivation in the overall pattern of agonistic arousal. The pattern is referred to as a "sexual script," a concept first coined in 1973 by sociologists Gagnon and Simon. Analysis of the script facilitates understanding of the relationship between behavior and its motivation, allowing a window into the underlying sexual arousal pattern. All sexual humans have scripts for sexual behavior ranging from normative non-paraphilic to sexually sadistic (Table 7.2). Scripts help answer questions about the sources of arousal for example: Was the individual aroused by the experience of dominating the victim? What was the desired response from the sexual target? What is satisfying about the behavior?

Table 7.2 Examples of sexual scripts

Sexual Scripts Examples
Script 1 (normophilic: non-paraphilic): adult male seeks out and finds adult women with specific physical and personality characteristics; sexual thoughts, fantasies, and arousal begins (1); flirts and engages in conversation (2); buys flowers, offers to pay for dinner (3); has a drink and dinner (4); seeks out approval/validation (5); prefers oral sex before intercourse (6); intercourse commences in missionary position (7); moves to a different position (8); cuddles (9); smokes a cigarette (10).
Script 2: (coercion preference: paraphilic): adult male seeks out middle-aged married women for sexual contacts; sexual thoughts, fantasies, arousal begins (1); flirts and engages in conversation (2); uses deceit to induce them into an affair (3); increases demands for frequent sex, planned for them to resist (4); when they resist, he threatens to expose the affair (5); their fear is sexually arousing (6); the more the sexual target resists, the more sexually arousing the interaction (7); repeats the sequence with multiple women.
Script 3: (sexual sadism preference: paraphilic): adult male identifies houses where single women live; mental rehearsal and begins (1); enters the house while the woman sleeps, walks around the house, then departs (2); similarly returns on another occasion, puts a hand over the woman's mouth and wakes her (3); makes efforts to scare her with threats- until he perceives fear (4); calms her and reassures her (5); invokes her fear again then rapes her (6); flees stating he will be back (7).

Sexual Sadism Disorder

Unfortunately, DSM-5 includes only two paraphilia diagnoses on the agonistic continuum, Sexual Sadism Disorder and Other Specified Paraphilic Disorder. Sexual Sadism Disorder includes a significant portion of the agonistic continuum. To diagnose this, the criteria for a paraphilic disorder are met, plus a qualitative specification of the type of paraphilia (i.e. Criteria A and B plus type specifier), "recurrent and intense sexual arousal from the physical or psychological suffering of another person" (DSM-5: APA, p. 695). Notably, sexual sadism disorder diagnosis here does not require the person diagnosed to cause the other's suffering. Further, contrary to the image conjured by lay people, sexual sadism does not always include overt physical brutality; it may comprise arousal to lesser agony for example psychological distress. The prevalence of sexual sadism disorder in forensic populations varies from 2% to 30%, and the population prevalence is unknown (APA, 2013).

Lower Preferences on the Agonistic Continuum

The only available DSM-5 diagnosis other than Sexual Sadism Disorder to capture agonistic clinical realities is Other Specified Paraphilic Disorder. This means agonistic preferences lower than Sexual Sadism on the continuum should be diagnosed through "Other Specified Paraphilic Disorder," which applies when the full criteria for a paraphilic disorder are present but the type is other than the eight DSM-5 specifies (APA, p. 705). Diagnoses of Other Specified Paraphilic Disorder require the full criteria for paraphilic disorder to be met.

Paraphilic Arousal to Coercion

When the paraphilic disorder focus is on coercion, where there is sexual interest to coercing sexual targets without overt brutality, but not overt brutality, two different DSM-5 paraphilic disorder diagnoses are applicable. Review of the text changes from DSM-IV to DSM-5 clearly provides support for diagnosing Sexual Sadism Disorder in these circumstances. However, some choose to utilize the diagnosis of "other specified paraphilic disorder" with a descriptive qualifier that best reflects the individual's preferences, e.g., coercion, non-consent, resistance, biastophilia, etc. Money (1999) introduced the term "biastophilic rapism" to refer to paraphilic interest in rape, underscoring that the target is “terror stricken and resistant.” Notably, during the DSM-5 development process, “Paraphilic Coercive Disorder” was proposed for inclusion but it was ultimately rejected by the DSM-5 Board of Trustees. Nonetheless, research illustrates the existence of paraphilic preference for coercive acts, e.g., Thornton (2010). Further, preliminary research showed that adding the diagnosis would significantly reduce the number of cases formerly diagnosed with Paraphilia, Not Otherwise Specified, and would not significantly increase the total number diagnosed with a paraphilic disorder (D’Orazio et al., 2011).

Penile Plethysmography

A useful tool in the assessment of agonistic disorders is the penile plethysmograph (PPG). The PPG is a physiological instrument that measures a male’s erectile responses to stimuli depicting various “sexual targets” involved in various sexual activities. These targets are males, females, adults, and children engage in a variety of behaviors including consensual sexual activity, oral sex, intercourse, the use of coercion, rape, manipulation, sexual sadism, and non-sexual physical violence. As with any assessment tool, the PPG should be utilized in combination with other data points. Any result from the PPG should be matched with actual behavior, and other information about the individual’s sexual preferences. Quantitative research on the PPG suggests it can be helpful in identifying paraphilic interest (Howes, 1998; Looman, 2000; Quinsey et al., 1984). More recently, Kingston et al. (2010) found that significant PPG arousal is significantly associated with violent (including sexual) recidivism. The PPG can be a useful tool when used alongside other data engaging in an identifying diagnoses on the agonistic continuum.

Challenges, and Controversies

Agonistic paraphilic disorders influence contribute to the risk, criminogenic needs, and responsivity of sexual offending individuals. A limitation of DSM-5 is its failure to include specifiers or diagnoses to capture the range of agonistic preferences. Specifically, DSM-5 users must select either sexual sadism disorder or other specified paraphilic disorder when rendering diagnoses on the agonistic continuum. This fuels problems with rater reliability and diagnostic utility. Improvements in DSM are crucial to enhancing diagnostic reliability and promoting future research on agonistic disorders.

The agonistic continuum is an evidence-supported conceptual model that responds to the need to evolve toward dimensional diagnostic models that better represent underlying mental conditions. Diagnoses can be made for any preference point on the agonistic continuum but must meet the general criteria for paraphilic disorder, i.e. intense, persistent, atypical sexual interest plus clinically significant negative consequences. Clinical case formulation, scripts, tools, and indicators facilitate diagnostic decision making. Sexual sadism disorder in DSM-5 includes “arousal from the physical or psychological suffering of another” and can be utilized to diagnose a significant portion of the agonistic range of preferences, including paraphilic arousal to coercion without gratuitous brutality. Sexual sadism disorder diagnosis is preferable over other specified paraphilic disorder for this purpose. Despite the unfortunate reality that the diagnosis can fit either label, diagnosticians should clear clinical justification and specify the paraphilic focus, e.g., torture, humiliation, psychological coercion, non-consent, unconscious sexual partners, etc.

A significant cause of unreliability across raters of the same case when agonistic preferences are present is the mixed application of sexual sadism and pedophilia diagnoses to individuals with agonistic preferences targeted exclusively toward children. In cases where sadistic or other agonistic activity preferences are targeted toward children, diagnosing pedophilic disorder plus an agonistic disorder are typically appropriate.

Rendering paraphilic disorder diagnoses requires inferences about underlying sexual arousal patterns and preferences. Manifest behaviors are not paraphilic disorders. Behaviors are helpful indicators of underlying conditions. It is not necessary to ascertain whether the person is sexually excited by the agonistic preference or failed to inhibit sexual arousal to agonistic cues in order to render diagnoses on the agonistic continuum.

When diagnostic criteria are met, sexual arousal patterns indicating problematic agonistic sexual interest, and not necessarily preference, may be diagnosed. It is not uncommon for some with agonistic paraphilic disorders to show sporadic or intermittent periods of intense agonistic interest that is greater than or equal to consensual sexual interest. Differential diagnosis is an important consideration when assessing for agonistic disorders. When agnostic behavior is subtle, rare, or at the low end of the continuum, the potential of competing diagnostic causes or no diagnosis is elevated. Sexual misconduct associated with entitlement, general difficulty adhering to socially acceptable boundaries, dispositional impulsivity, chronic rule-breaking, or perceived abandonment oftentimes derives from personality disorders, rather than agonistic sexual interests. Likewise, the role of substances (e.g., methamphetamine, alcohol, etc.) should be considered along with other temporary mental states and contexts in ruling out paraphilic disorders.

Further research on the agonistic continuum is recommended. Research is needed to test the validity and reliability of diagnoses on the agonistic continuum which will facilitate the refinement of diagnostic systems. Further research on the use of minimum victim counts and other behavioral indicators in absence of reliable self-report is suggested, along with population prevalence rates and information about change across the lifespan. The impact of race, socioeconomic level, culture, and ecological influences on both the expression of paraphilic interests and their diagnosis is an often overlooked research need.

Conclusions

Sexual abuse is a public health problem. Accurate diagnosis of paraphilic disorders is necessary for primary, secondary, and tertiary prevention. Diagnoses of paraphilic disorders often occur in the context of high-stakes forensic and clinical decision-making that significantly impacts the lives of many individuals. Evaluators must apply utmost professional ethics and objectivity. Communications about diagnoses must be free from pejorative or value-laden language and respect the dignity of all parties.

Most sexual offenders are perpetrated by non-paraphilic individuals. However, sexual offending individuals with paraphilic disorders are responsible for a disproportionately high number of sexual offenses, and offending is often chronic and persistent. Rendering diagnoses of agonistic paraphilic disorders in forensic matters a common but challenging task for forensic experts, requiring advanced skill and training, along with rich sources of case information.

References

American Psychiatric Association. (1952). *Diagnostic and statistical manual: Mental disorders.* Washington, D.C.: American Psychiatric Association Mental Hospital Service.

American Psychiatric Association. (1967). *Diagnostic and statistical manual of mental disorders* (2nd ed.). Washington, DC.: The Committee on Nomenclature and Statistics of the American Psychiatric Association.

American Psychiatric Association. (1980). *Diagnostic and statistical manual of mental disorders-III* (3rd ed.). Washington, D.C.:American Psychiatric Association.

American Psychiatric Association. (1987). *Diagnostic and statistical manual of mental disorders-III-R* (3rd ed. revised ed.). Washington, D.C.: American Psychiatric Association.

American Psychiatric Association. (1994). *Diagnostic and statistical manual of mental disorders-IV* (4th ed.). Washington, D.C.: American Psychiatric Association.

American Psychiatric Association. (2013). *Diagnostic and statistical manual of mental disorders-5* (5th ed.). American Psychiatric Publishing.

Barbaree, H. (1997). Evaluating treatment efficacy with sexual offenders: The insensitivity of recidivism studies to treatment effects. *Sexual Abuse: A Journal of Research and Treatment*, 9(2), 111–128. doi: https://doi.org/10.1007/BF02674862

Bonta, J., & Andrews, D. A. (2017). *The psychology of criminal conduct.* Taylor & Francis. doi: https://doi.org/10.4324/9781315677187

Centers for Disease Control and Prevention (CDC). (2020). Sexual violence is preventable. Retrieved May 1, 2020, from Center on Disease Control, Washington, DC, https://www.cdc.gov/features/sexualviolence/index.html.

D'Orazio, D., Wilson, R., & Thornton, D. (2011). *Prevalence of pedohebephilia, paraphilic coercive disorder, and sexual sadism diagnoses with the proposed DSM-5 criterion sets.* Paper presented at the Association for the Treatment of Sexual Abusers 30th Annual Research and Treatment Conference, Toronto Canada, November 4.

Dong, M., Anda, R. F., Dube, S. R., Giles, W. H., & Felitti, V. J. (2003). The relationship of exposure to childhood sexual abuse to other forms of abuse, neglect, and household dysfunction during childhood. *Child Abuse & Neglect*, 27(6), 625–639. doi: 10.1016/s0145-2134(03)00105-4

First, M. B., & Tasman, A. (2004). *DSM-IV-TR: Diagnosis, etiology, and treatment.* John Wiley & Sons, Ltd.

Freund, K., Diamant, J., & Pinkava, V. (1958). On the validity and reliability of the phalloplethysmographic diagnosis of some sexual deviations. *Review of Czechoslovak medicine*, 4(2), 145–151.

Furby, L., Weinrott, M. R., & Blackshaw, L. (1989). Sex offender recidivism: A review. *Psychological Bulletin*, 105(1), 3–30. doi: https://doi.org/10.1037/0033-2909.105.1.3

Gagnon, J., & Simon, W. (1974). *Sexual conduct: The social sources of human sexuality.* Aldine Press. doi: https://doi.org/10.1177/136346099002001006

Gallagher, C. A., Wilson, D. B., Hirschfield, P., Coggeshall, M. B., & MacKenzie, D. L. (1999). Quantitative review of the effects of sex offender treatment on sexual reoffending. *Corrections Management Quarterly*, 3(4), 11. doi: 10.1016/j.avb.2006.03.002

Greenfeld, L. (1997). *Sex offenses and offenders: An analysis of data on rape and sexual assault.* U.S. Department of Justice, Bureau of Justice Statistics. http://www.ncjrs.gov/App/publications/abstract.aspx?ID=163931

Hall, G. C. N. (1995). Sexual offender recidivism revisited: A meta-analysis of recent treatment studies. *Journal of Consulting and Clinical Psychology*, 63(5), 802. doi: 10.1037//0022-006x.63.5.802

Hanson, R. K., Bourgon, G., Helmus, L., & Hodgson, S. (2009). The principles of effective correctional treatment also apply to sexual offenders: A meta-analysis. *Criminal Justice and Behavior*, 36(9), 865–891. doi: https://doi.org/10.1177/0093854809338545

Hanson, R. K., Cox, B., & Woszczyna, C. (1991). Assessing treatment outcome for sexual offenders. *Annals of Sex Research*, 4(3), 177–208. doi: https://doi.org/10.1007/BF00850052

Hanson, R. K., Gordon, A., Harris, A. J., Marques, J. K., Murphy, W., Quinsey, V. L., & Seto, M. C. (2002). First report of the collaborative outcome data project on the effectiveness of psychological treatment for sex offenders. *Sexual Abuse: A Journal of Research and Treatment*, 14(2), 169–194. doi: 10.1177/107906320201400207

Hanson, R. K., Harris, A. J., Scott, T. L., & Helmus, L. (2007). *Assessing the risk of sexual offenders on community supervision: The dynamic supervision project* (Vol. 5, No. 6). Public Safety Canada.

Hanson, R. K., & Morton-Bourgon, K. (2004). *Predictors of sexual recidivism: An updated meta-analysis.* Public works and government services Canada. https://www.publicsafety.gc.ca/cnt/rsrcs/pblctns/2004-02-prdctrs-sxl-rcdvsm-pdtd/index-en.aspx

Hanson, R. K., & Morton-Bourgon, K. E. (2005). The characteristics of persistent sexual offenders: A meta-analysis of recidivism studies. *Journal of Consulting and Clinical Psychology*, 73(6), 1154. doi: https://doi.org/10.1037/0022-006X.73.6.1154

Harris, A. J. R., & Hanson, R. K. (2010). Clinical, actuarial and dynamic risk assessment of sexual offenders: Why do things keep changing? *Journal of Sexual Aggression*, 16(3), 296–310. doi: https://doi.org/10.1080/13552600.2010.494772

Harris, G. T., Rice, M. E., & Quinsey, V. L. (1998). Appraisal and management of risk in sexual aggressors: Implications for criminal justice policy. *Psychology, Public Policy, and Law*, 4(1–2), 73–115. doi: https://doi.org/10.1037/1076-8971.4.1-2.73

Hawes, S. W., Boccaccini, M. T., & Murrie, D. C. (2013). Psychopathy and the combination of psychopathy and sexual deviance as predictors of sexual recidivism: Meta-analytic findings using the psychopathy checklist—revised. *Psychological Assessment*, 25(1), 233. doi: https://doi.org/10.1037/a0030391

Helmus, L., Thornton, D., Hanson, R. K., & Babchishin, K. M. (2012). Improving the predictive accuracy of static-99 and static-2002 with older sex offenders: Revised age weights. *Sexual Abuse*, 24(1), 64–101. doi: https://doi.org/10.1177/1079063211409951

Howes, R. J. (1998). Plethysmographic assessment of incarcerated nonsexual offenders: A comparison with rapists. *Sexual Abuse*, 10(3), 183–194. doi: https://doi.org/10.1023/A:1021313820005

Kingston, D. A., Seto, M. C., Firestone, P., & Bradford, J. M. (2010). Comparing indicators of sexual sadism as predictors of recidivism among adult male sexual offenders. *Journal of Consulting and Clinical Psychology*, 78(4), 574. doi: https://doi.org/10.1037/a0019734

Knight, R. A., Sims-Knight, J., & Guay, J. P. (2013). Is a separate diagnostic category defensible for paraphilic coercion? *Journal of Criminal Justice*, 41(2), 90–99. doi: http://doi-org-443.webvpn.fjmu.edu.cn/10.1016/j.jcrimjus.2012.11.002

Lalumière, M.L., Harris, G., Quinsey, V., & Rice, M. (2005). *The causes of rape: Understanding individual differences in the male propensity for sexual aggression*. American Psychological Association.

Levenson, J. S., Willis, G. M., & Prescott, D. S. (2016). Adverse childhood experiences in the lives of male sex offenders: Implications for trauma-informed care. *Sexual Abuse*, 28(4), 340–359. doi: https://doi.org/10.1177/1079063214535819

Longpré, N., Guay, J. P., & Knight, R. A. (2019). MTC sadism scale: Toward a dimensional assessment of severe sexual sadism with behavioral markers. *Assessment*, 26(1), 70–84. doi: https://doi.org/10.1177/1073191117737377

Looman, J. (2000). Sexual arousal in rapists as measured by two stimulus sets. *Sexual Abuse: A Journal of Research and Treatment*, 12(4), 235–248. doi: https://doi.org/10.1023/A:1009590225937

Lovins, B., Lowenkamp, C. T., & Latessa, E. J. (2009). Applying the risk principle to sex offenders: Can treatment make some sex offenders worse? *The Prison Journal*, 89(3), 344–357. doi: https://doi.org/10.1177/0032885509339509

Marques, J. K., Day, D. M., Nelson, C., & West, M. A. (1994). Effects of cognitive-behavioral treatment on sex offender recidivism: Preliminary results of a longitudinal study. *Criminal Justice and Behavior*, 21(1), 28–54. doi: https://doi.org/10.1177/0093854894021001004

Mezzich, J. E. (2002). Comprehensive diagnosis: A conceptual basis for future diagnostic systems. *Psychopathology*, 35(2–3), 162–165. doi: https://doi.org/10.1159/000065138

MIDSA clinical manual. (2011). *Bend, OR*: Augur Enterprises, Inc. www.midsa.us.

Miller, T., Fulton, D., & Lee, D. (2018). *The cost and consequences of sexual violence in California.* California Coalition Against Sexual Assault (CALCASA). Downloaded, 05/09/2020 from https://www.calcasa.org/wp-content/uploads/2018/02/CALCASA_CCofSV_FINALSpreads_2018.pdf

Mokros, A., Schilling, F., Weiss, K., Nitschke, J., & Eher, R. (2014). Sadism in sexual offenders: Evidence for dimensionality. *Psychological Assessment*, 26(1), 138. doi: https://doi.org/10.1037/a0034861

Money, J. (1999). *The lovemap guidebook: A definitive statement.* Bloomsbury Continuum.

Nichols, H. R., & Molinder, I. (2000). *MSI II: Multiphasic sex inventory II handbook.* Nichols & Molinder.

Olver, M. E., Wong, S. C., Nicholaichuk, T., & Gordon, A. (2007). The validity and reliability of the violence risk scale-sexual offender version: Assessing sex offender risk and evaluating therapeutic change. *Psychological Assessment*, 19(3), 318. doi: 10.1037/1040-3590.19.3.318

Perryer, S. (2018). The cost of sexual assault, European CEO, 23 October 2018. National Institute of Justice, Washing to DC. Retrieved May 29, 2020, from https://www.europeanceo.com/business-and-management/the-cost-of-sexual-assault

Phenix, A., Fernandez, Y., Harris, A. J., Helmus, M., Hanson, R. K., & Thornton, D. (2017). *Static-99R coding rules, revised-2016.* Public Safety Canada. www.static99.org.

Quinsey, V. L., Chaplin, T. C., & Upfold, D. (1984). Sexual arousal to nonsexual violence and sadomasochistic themes among rapists and non-sex-offenders. *Journal of Consulting and Clinical Psychology*, 52(4), 651. doi: https://doi.org/10.1037/0022-006X.52.4.651

Schmucker, M., & Lösel, F. (2015). The effects of sexual offender treatment on recidivism: An international meta-analysis of sound quality evaluations. *Journal of Experimental Criminology*, 11(4), 597–630. doi: https://psycnet.apa.org/doi/10.1007/s11292-015-9241–z

Thornton, D. (2010). Evidence regarding the need for a diagnostic category for a coercive paraphilia. *Archives of Sexual Behavior*, 39(2), 411–418. doi: https://doi.org/10.1007/s10508-009-9583-6

Thornton, D., & D'Orazio, D. (2012). *Diagnosing paraphilia when facts are thin: The diagnostic significance of the minimum victim count.* Paper presented at the Association for the Treatment of Sexual Abusers 31th Annual Research and Treatment Conference, Denver Colorado, October 18.

Thornton, D., & D'Orazio, D. (2013). Best practice in SVP treatment programs. In L. A. Craig, L. Dixon, & T. Gannon (Eds.), *What works in offender rehabilitation: An evidenced based approach to assessment and treatment* (pp. 359–385). Wiley-Blackwell.

Thornton, D., & D'Orazio, D. M. (2016). Advancing the evolution of sexual offender risk assessment: The relevance of psychological risk factors. In L. A. Craig & M. Rettenberger (Eds.), *Volume 2: The Wiley handbook on the theories, assessment and treatment of sexual offending* (pp. 667–693). Wiley-Blackwell.

Thornton, D., & Knight, R. A. (2015). Construction and validation of SRA-FV need assessment. *Sexual Abuse*, 27(4), 360–375.) doi: 10.1177/1079063213511120

8

Understanding Minor Attraction

Rebecca Lievesley[1] and Craig Harper[2]

[1,2] *Department of Psychology, Nottingham Trent University, UK*

Introduction

Individuals who have a sexual attraction to minors face vast amounts of social stigma within the general population (Jahnke, Imhoff et al., 2015), and often come to internalize that stigma in relation to their self-perceptions (Lievesley et al., 2020). These experiences can lead to stigma-related stress and poor mental health (Jahnke, Imhoff et al., 2015). While the vast majority of research focuses on the narrower category of pedophilia (e.g., Cantor & McPhail, 2016; Harper et al., 2018; Jahnke, 2018a, 2018b), our focus here looks at "minor attraction" in a more general sense, encompassing a range of chronophilic attraction categories (Seto, 2017). In this chapter we explore the definition of minor attraction and explore when this becomes disordered, before setting out some recommendations for promoting the wellbeing of individuals with this sexual arousal pattern, and reducing their risk of sexual offending.

Understanding Minor Attraction

While "minor attraction" (as a specific label) is a relatively new label, the study of individuals having sexual attractions towards children has been a popular topic of forensic psychological research for some time. Under the umbrella of "minor attraction" there is a constellation of specific age attraction categories, called *chronophilias* by Seto (2017). His chronophilic continuum acts as an age- and developmentally-graded model for identifying the primary targets of sexual attraction and preference. The continuum begins with nepiophilia (a sexual attraction towards infants, typically between the ages of 0 to 2 years), through pedophilia (a sexual attraction to prepubescent children, typically 3–10 years), hebephilia (a sexual attraction to pubescent children between the ages of approximately 11 and 14 years), and ephebophilia (a sexual attraction to older children). The chronophilic model then works through attractions towards adults of reproductive age (teleiophilia), middle age (mesophilia), and old age (gerontophilia). Evidence for the distinctiveness of each chronophilic category typically comes from phallometric studies that measure genital arousal to a range of differently-aged visual stimuli. For example, the distinctiveness of hebephilia was supported by Blanchard et al. (2009), who found that men who self-report having a greater level of sexual arousal towards pubescent children than prepubescent children demonstrated this arousal pattern physiologically, with both groups differing in their genital responses to adult stimuli, as compared to teleiophilic participants. Nonetheless, there is an acknowledgment within the field that a majority of individuals with sexual attractions to children are not exclusively aroused by specific chronophilic age

Sexual Deviance: Understanding and Managing Deviant Sexual Interests and Paraphilic Disorders,
First Edition. Edited by Leam A. Craig and Ross M. Bartels.
© 2021 John Wiley & Sons, Ltd. Published 2021 by John Wiley & Sons, Ltd.

categories (Lievesley & Harper, 2019; Martijn et al., 2018; McPhail et al., 2018). As such, we adopt the phrase "minor-attracted persons" (MAPs) to describe individuals with attractions that fall into the nepiophilic, pedophilic, hebephilic, and ephebophilic chronophilia categories.

To contextualize minor attraction research, we root our discussion in the domain of sexual orientation, defining this as "a stable tendency to preferentially orient—in terms of attention, interest, attraction, and genital arousal—to particular classes of sexual stimuli" (Seto, 2017, p. 3). According to Seto (2012), a sexual orientation is something that has an early age of onset, is resistant to attempts to change it, and contributes to a congruence between the targets of sexual and romantic attractions. While there is limited evidence for other chronophilic categories, pedophilia appears to meet each of these criteria. For example, MAPs with pedophilic sexual attractions report first acknowledging these between the ages of 12 and 14, around the age of puberty (Grundmann et al., 2016). Similarly, attempts to alter pedophilic sexual attractions have been unsuccessful, with phallometric measures supporting the temporal stability of this arousal pattern (Mokros & Habermeyer, 2016). Until recently there was minimal evidence in relation to the correspondence between sexual and romantic attractions to children among MAPs. However, Martijn et al. (2018) reported data suggesting that there is a relationship between the exclusivity of minor attraction and the odds of only having ever fallen in love with children (vs. falling in love with adults, which was more prevalent among non-exclusive MAPs). As such, we conclude that, on the balance of evidence, minor attraction operates psychologically as a form of sexual orientation (for a fuller review of the available evidence, see Seto, 2012).

Prevalence of Minor Attraction

While the true rate of minor attraction within the general population is unknown due to limitations in data collection (i.e., large samples are difficult to obtain, and there are social desirability issues related to this topic), some data are available that act as a useful starting point. For example, when looking at pedophilia specifically (the most commonly studied chronophilic category), the estimated prevalence rate within the general (male) population is between < .1 and 5% (Dombert et al., 2016; Seto, 2018). However, when looking at community-based males' self-reported sexual attraction to "children" in a more general sense (i.e., not limiting oneself to the pedophilic age bracket), this estimate increases substantially. For example, Ahlers et al. (2011) reported how approximately 10% of German men admitted to using sexual fantasies involving children (broadly defined) when masturbating. Further, when Bergen et al. (2013) disclosed to adult men on a chat room that the person they were speaking to was a child, around 25% of those adults continued to sexualize their conversations. These statistics indicate that low-level sexual interests in children may be widespread within the general population.

When Does Attraction Become Disordered?

Diagnostic manuals for mental health problems list specific types of paraphilic interests and behaviors as having the potential for becoming disordered. For example, the Diagnostic and Statistical Manual (DSM), currently in its fifth edition (DSM-5; American Psychiatric Association, 2013), includes such conditions as:

1. Voyeuristic disorder (covertly watching others engaged in sexual activities)
2. Exhibitionistic disorder (non-consensual display of one's genitals)
3. Frotteuristic disorder (non-consensual touching or rubbing against another individual)

4. Fetishistic disorder (the use of inanimate objects or a focus on non-sexual body parts for sexual arousal or gratification)
5. Pedophilic disorder (having a sexual focus on prepubescent children)
6. Sexual masochism disorder (undergoing humiliation or experiencing suffering for sexual pleasure)
7. Sexual sadism disorder (inflicting humiliation or suffering for one's own sexual pleasure)
8. Transvestic disorder (engaging in cross-sex dressing for sexual arousal or gratification)

The only one of these diagnoses that relates specifically to minor attraction is pedophilic disorder. Table 8.1 presents the current DSM-5 criteria for this diagnosis.

There are substantial issues with some of the criteria used to diagnose pedophilic disorder. For example, the criteria referring to the targets of attraction being aged 13 years or younger is inconsistent with both Seto's (2017) proposed upper cutoff age of 11 years, and the research base where Tanner stages of physical development are used. That is, researchers tend to measure physiological (i.e., erectile) responses, reaction and viewing times, and self-reported attractiveness ratings of images purporting to present the Tanner stages of physical development (Marshall & Tanner, 1969) to classify individuals as "pedophiles" (e.g., Banse et al., 2010; Ristow et al., 2018; Schmidt et al., 2013). Further, a range of research evidence suggests that individuals recognize their minor-attraction between the ages of 12 and 14 years (Bailey et al., 2016; Lievesley & Harper, 2019; Tozdan & Briken, 2015). This potentially means that the lower age limit of 16 years in the diagnostic criteria excludes some individuals (who may be experiencing distress due to their sexual attractions) from accessing treatment.

While the paraphilic disorders listed each have their own specific diagnostic criteria, there is an acknowledgment by the American Psychiatric Association (2013) that the list is not exhaustive. This means that the experience of other paraphilic interests can be considered disordered if they are accompanied by the essential characteristics of other paraphilic diagnoses (i.e., causing harm to others, or the experience of distress or disturbed interpersonal functioning). This is particularly important in relation to minor attraction for two key reasons. First, we know that "pedophilia" is used as a synonym for a range of distinct age of attraction categories (Harper & Hogue, 2017) in spite of Seto's (2017) exploration of a range of chronophilic age preferences. Second, MAPs who have pedophilic attractions commonly experience these alongside an

Table 8.1 DSM-5 diagnostic criteria for pedophilic disorder

Criteria for Diagnosis	Specifications to Be Clarified
Criterion A Over a period of at least six months, the individual has recurrent, intense, sexually arousing fantasies, sexual urges, or behaviors involving sexual activity with a prepubescent child or children (generally aged 13 years or younger)	*Sex of attraction targets* • Male • Female • Both
Criterion B The fantasies, urges, or behaviors cause clinically significant distress or impairment in social, occupational, or other important areas of functioning	*Relationship to attraction targets* • Limited to incest • Not limited to incest
Criterion C The person is at least aged 16 years and at least five years older than the child or children in Criterion A	*Exclusivity of attraction targets* • Exclusive attractions to children • Non-exclusive attractions to children

attraction to other age categories, including those that span arbitrary legal and social distinctions between "children" and "adults" (Lievesley & Harper, 2019; Tozdan & Briken, 2015). Therefore, while the current diagnostic criteria do not explicitly exclude those with non-pedophilic chronophilic attraction patterns from seeking help, there may be some merit to moving away from explicit diagnostic criteria in relation to specific attraction targets, and instead focusing on disordered attraction patterns in a more general sense. The next sections of this chapter explore the aforementioned essential characteristics of "harm" and "distress" for the diagnosis of disordered attraction in more depth.

Minor Attraction and the Conflation with Offending Behavior

While sexual offending behavior is built into the DSM-5 criteria as an indicator of pedophilic disorder, a number of authors have identified issues with the conflation between minor attraction (or "pedophilia," as is typically the topic of investigation in such research) and the sexual abuse of children. These terms are used interchangeably in a number of contexts. For example, in recent analyses of press coverage related to sexual crime, Harper and Hogue (2015) and Harper and Harris (2017) reported how offenses against children are over-represented in news stories, and that these offenses and perpetrators are usually described as "pedophilia" and "pedophiles," respectively. This media conflation feeds into a social conversation where the public believes that "a pedophile" is somebody who sexually abuses children (Kitzinger, 2002; Silverman & Wilson, 2002). Not only this, academics working in the area of forensic psychology also fall prey to this conflation (Feelgood & Hoyer, 2008), with the vast majority of the available evidence stemming from samples of individuals convicted of sexual offenses. The academic conflation further translates into clinicians' attitudes towards MAPs too, with Stiels-Glenn (2010) reporting how slightly less than 5% of psychotherapists show some willingness to accept people with pedophilic sexual attractions into their treatment settings. This rate was equivalent to the proportion who were willing to accept individuals convicted of child sexual offenses, potentially indicating a conflation between these terms being made by psychotherapists.

In reality, though, while minor attraction (and other paraphilias) has been cited as an important risk factor for sexual (re-)offending (Hanson & Morton-Bourgon, 2004; Helmus et al., 2015; Seto, 2019), Schmidt et al. (2013) found that fewer than half of all individuals convicted of child abuse actually have a predominant sexual preference for children. They determined this using the Explicit and Implicit Sexual Interest Profile (EISIP; Banse et al., 2010)—an assessment procedure that combines self-report questionnaires with viewing time and reaction time measures to determine an individual's sexual interest and preference profile. Similarly, we also know that there is a large number of non-offending MAPs within the general population (Cantor & McPhail, 2016). Taken together, these findings suggest that minor attraction alone (specifically pedophilia in the aforementioned studies, though this arousal pattern is commonly not exclusive) is neither a necessary nor a sufficient condition for sexual offending behavior to take place.

This conclusion raises questions as to what the link between minor attraction and sexual offending actually is. Theoretical insights from Seto (2019) shed light on this link, with his Motivation-Facilitation Model of sexual offending separating risk factors into motivational and facilitating domains. Sexual attractions (along with sexual blockage) are motivating factors that orient an individual towards seeking out a sexually arousing stimulus, such as individuals that match their arousal patterns, sexually explicit materials, or sexual fantasy. While these attractions do motivate sexual activity, in the case of attractions that could involve illegal acts (e.g., attractions to minors, or coercive sexual practices), this is not always the case. These behaviors, according to Seto's (2019) model, will only be enacted if other facilitating factors are present, such as antisocial personality traits, or implicit theories (cognitions) that support offending behavior. These ideas correspond to Finkelhor's (1984) preconditions model of sexual offending. However, where Seto (2019) deviates from Finkelhor (1984) is in the temporality of the offense chain. While Finkelhor (1984) viewed sexual arousal as a precondition to sexual offending that is linear in nature (i.e., an initial motivation that leads an individual to subsequently try to overcome other inhibitors to sexual offending), Seto (2019) sees these motivators as interacting with facilitating factors simultaneously. This theoretical position is consistent with work suggesting a link between psychopathy and antisocial personality on the consumption of child sexual exploitation material (Williams et al., 2009) and sexual offending against children (Klein et al., 2015). These theoretical models suggest that minor attraction is not destined to lead to sexual offending, but instead is associated with this type of behavior through moderation by other relevant factors.

Minor Attraction and the Experience of Distress

Stigmatization relates to the negative evaluation of an individual or group that is based upon a specific or very limited set of characteristics, and is comprised of affective (emotional feelings about the target), cognitive (attributions made about the target), and behavioral (how one interacts with the target) domains (Corrigan et al., 2012). Within the context of minor attraction, stigmatization has tended to be studied in relation to individuals with pedophilic sexual attractions (Jahnke & Hoyer, 2013; Jahnke, Imhoff et al., 2015). However, given the pervasiveness of the "pedophile" label (Harper & Hogue, 2017), these findings likely apply to the stigmatization of MAPs across the chronophilic spectrum.

Emotionally, members of the general public tend to experience automatic negative feelings about MAPs when they encounter information about this group (Harper et al., 2018; Jahnke, 2018b). Emotional responses, including fear, anger, and disgust, make up a state of emotional arousal known as moral outrage (Bastian et al., 2013), with this being a common response to information about MAPs who both do and do not commit sexual offenses (King & Roberts, 2017). Behaviorally, there is widespread support for punitive policy positions in relation to MAPs, such as preventative incarcerated and castration (Jahnke, Imhoff et al., 2015). These responses may stem from cognitive evaluations of MAPs, such that people ascribe choice to MAPs' sexual attractions (Jahnke, 2018a), and a presumption of offending behavior (Cantor & McPhail, 2016; Feelgood & Hoyer, 2008).

The social roots of such beliefs may be found in news stories about sexual crime (which, as stated previously, use "pedophilia" as a synonym for child abuse), where the use of dehumanizing descriptions of the individuals convicted of such offenses (Harper & Hogue, 2017), such as "beasts," "fiends," and "monsters" is commonplace. Harper and Hogue (2017) suggested that this language use contributes to societal negativity about individuals convicted of sexual offenses. However, the same argument can also be made in relation to minor attraction due to the mass conflation of terms set out above. McCartan (2013) argued that the social construction of "the pedophile" portrays this group as a collective group of predatory individuals who commit sexual offenses against children, consistent with the arguments subsequently made by King and Roberts (2017). In doing so, these types of representations contribute to the strengthening of negative stereotypes and implicit theories about this group, which perpetuates the widespread social stigmatization of MAPs that we observe in contemporary society (Harper et al., 2018; Jahnke & Hoyer, 2013).

The psychological origins of the stigmatization of MAPs may ultimately be rooted in fundamental aspects of human moral psychology. Jahnke (2018a) reported how community members feel emotions such as anger and disgust towards non-offending MAPs, with these feelings being exaggerated when the motivations for not committing offending were presented as being extrinsic (i.e., a fear of incarceration or punishment) rather than intrinsic (i.e., knowing that offending would be wrong). This matches Harper and Harris's (2017) conceptual argument that an individual's moral foundations may guide their responses to themes related to sexual offending. That is, sexual relations between adults and children are seen by most of society as being impure and abusive from a moral and legal perspective. Those who engage in such behaviors (either in a non-offending way through sexual fantasy, or by committing acts of sexual abuse) trigger punitive responses in an intuitive way. That is, individuals feel that the behavior is wrong before putting together an argument as to why this is the case. These instinctual responses then lead to support for punitive policies directed towards MAPs.

It is important to note that such moral and emotional responses to MAPs do not merely come from the community, but MAPs also self-stigmatize for similar reasons. According to Jahnke et al. (2015), this process of self-stigmatization has been linked to a fear of discovery among the MAP community, as well as with lower levels of psychological wellbeing. These deficits are also associated with MAPs perceiving themselves to be different from the "normal" (teleiophilic) population, which further results in lower levels of self-esteem and a greater propensity for MAPs to isolate themselves (Jahnke, Imhoff et al., 2015). While these factors are important from a health and wellbeing perspective, they are also important risk factors for sexual offending (Gillespie et al., 2012). In recent work, Lievesley et al. (2020) reported how levels of thought suppression among MAPs was equivalent to or greater than those observed in other clinical populations, such as individuals with depression, eating disorders, and obsessive-compulsive disorder (OCD). Thought suppression was also associated with increased levels of shame and guilt about having attractions to minors, lower levels of hope for the future, and a desire for more support for their sexual attractions. Lievesley et al. (2020) suggested that thought suppression, therefore, represents a form of internalized stigma, and indicates a desire to distance oneself from the MAP identity. This is consistent with a self-concealment process that might be expected as a symptom of minority stress (Meyer, 2003), indicating a potential need to address mental health difficulties within the MAP community.

These psychosocial issues were all recently reported as being associated with sexual offending in a community sample of MAPs in a paper published by Cohen et al. (2018). Further, the social isolation of MAPs has also been linked to a lack of willingness to actively seek therapeutic support for these sexual interests (Jahnke & Hoyer, 2013), potentially compounding both low levels of wellbeing and further distancing this group from services aimed at both improving MAP wellbeing and preventing child sexual abuse (Lievesley et al., 2020). In addition to these findings, Grady et al. (2019) spoke with MAPs about their help-seeking behaviors and found that social stigma and a fear of discovery were the most important barriers to seeking professional support, with internalized stigma (i.e., seeing themselves as a "bad person" because of their unchosen sexual attractions; Grady et al., 2019, p. 400) and a fear of being reported to legal authorities also being prominent themes in participant narratives (see also Lievesley et al., 2020). As such, by not adequately addressing one of the diagnostic criteria for pedophilic disorder (distress), we may actually be increasing the risk that an individual will ultimately present in custodial settings with the other criteria (causing harm).

Future Directions and Recommendations

What is clear from the review provided in this chapter is that minor attraction is commonly misunderstood within society and, in spite of evidence to the contrary, is a relatively common experience among men (Ahlers et al., 2011; Bergen et al., 2013). In spite of this, those who are attracted to minors perceive themselves as being different to those around them, are on the receiving end of widespread and severe social stigma (Jahnke, 2018b; Jahnke & Hoyer, 2013), and experience stigma-related stress as a result of both their internal feelings about their attractions, and society's response to them as individuals (Jahnke, 2018b). It is our central premise that simply being attracted to minors is not problematic in and of itself, but rather becomes so when there is harm or distress being caused to oneself or others. This is in line with the current DSM-5 criteria for the diagnosis of a paraphilic disorder (American Psychiatric Association, 2013). As such, our recommendations for future directions in the treatment and management of minor attraction do not focus on the attraction patterns themselves, but on helping MAPs work through and manage their experiences of these attractions. In doing so, we advocate a health and wellbeing-based approach to the management of minor attraction, with sexual abuse prevention being a secondary aim within this paradigm. In the sections that follow, we consider two key areas of potential focus—social attitudes and the subsequent indirect effects that these have on MAP wellbeing, and the specific treatment of MAPs in a direct therapeutic context.

Beyond the "Beast" Paradigm—Humanizing Minor-Attracted People

As stated earlier in this chapter, we (as a society) respond to minor attraction in a particularly punitive manner. For example, our news media use chronophilic labels (i.e., "pedophile" and "pedophilia") as synonyms for the sexual abuse of children (Harper & Hogue, 2017; Harrison et al., 2010), leading to a social conflation of these terms whereby most members of the general public are unaware of the differences between these groups (Feelgood & Hoyer, 2008). This conflation leads to attributions of psychopathy being made about people with pedophilic sexual attractions (and, thus, those with a minor-attracted arousal pattern more generally), with some even calling for preventative incarceration or violence against these groups (Jahnke, Imhoff et al., 2015). The linguistic strategies employed by news outlets and high-profile campaigners about minor-attracted groups further lead to the dehumanization of MAPs (Harper et al., 2018)—a process that has been shown to predict punitive attitudes and negative automatic responses to numerous different target groups (Bastian et al., 2013; Kteily & Bruneau, 2017; Viki et al., 2012).

In recent years, research has examined attitudes towards people with pedophilic sexual attractions (and thus minor attraction more generally). Specifically, research has investigated whether presenting information in a way that rehumanizes MAPs can improve attitudes and reverse the media effects on stigmatization reported previously. This body of research has demonstrated how presenting information about pedophilia from the perspective of somebody with such sexual attraction patterns can contribute to significant improvements in participants' attitudes towards this group. Importantly, this effect has been found in a range of participant groups, including undergraduate and postgraduate psychology students (Harper et al., 2018), trainee psychotherapists (Jahnke, Philipp et al., 2015), and lay members of the general public (Harper et al., 2019). Moreover, this effect has been observed to still be present in follow-up testing (though to a lesser extent) up to four months following the initial presentation of the humanizing stimulus (Harper et al., 2019; Jahnke, Philipp et al., 2015). This suggests that these changes in attitudes and levels of stigmatization are relatively stable over time as a result of this type of presentation intervention. This long-term change in attitudes is particularly important in relation to encouraging a more dispassionate social conversation about minor attraction and may also play an important role in encouraging a higher rate of help-seeking behavior among MAPs. For example, we know that a large proportion of MAPs internalize social stigma (Lievesley et al., 2020), and that this decreases the likelihood that they will seek help if or when it is required (Grady et al., 2019).

Beyond the "Risk" Paradigm—Towards a Health-Based Approach to Treating Minor-Attracted People

Having created a social environment within which MAPs feel comfortable to seek help, it is important to ensure that the services available to them are appropriately marketed, staffed, and operated. This means that the central aims of MAP treatment (i.e., addressing psychological and social wellbeing) should be promoted as being at the forefront of such treatment provision. At present, high profile schemes in this area of clinical work are explicitly labeled as being designed to prevent or reduce the incidence of child sexual abuse (e.g., Germany's Dunkelfeld Prevention Project; Beier et al., 2009). While the aim of sexual abuse prevention is to be commended, the framing of these interventions makes an implicit assumption that MAPs need to be prevented from committing acts of child sexual abuse (Lievesley & Harper, 2019), rather than them requiring support though the management of their sexual attractions and the psychosocial effects that accompany these feelings (Grady et al., 2019; Jahnke, 2018b).

In addition to this philosophical point, while some evaluations of prevention schemes have reported reductions in risk-relevant outcomes (e.g., pro-criminal attitudes and beliefs; Beier et al., 2009, 2015), more robust re-analyses of the data have demonstrated that any positive effects of these schemes in relation to criminogenic factors are no greater than those observed in control groups (Mokros & Banse, 2019). Again this highlights a potential shortcoming in the focus of prevention schemes. While this lack of "treatment success" questions the necessity and utility of prevention programs, it may be that these schemes emerge as being much more successful if broader psychosocial constructs related to wellbeing and interpersonal functioning were also assessed. As identified in the early stages of this chapter, the literature suggests that a large proportion of MAPs will never commit sexual offenses (Cantor & McPhail, 2016), possibly due to them not possessing high levels of psychological or situational facilitators of abusive behavior (Seto, 2019). In having a narrow focus on evaluating offense-related outcomes but not those related to wellbeing, programs may not be finding a lack of treatment effect, but instead are simply examining factors that are not relevant to a substantial proportion of the population under investigation.

The focus on abuse prevention in existing treatment programs leads to a mismatch between MAP needs and treatment goals. This is a claim supported by self-reported experiences and expectations of MAPs when surveyed about what they believe therapist aims are (B4U-ACT, 2011). The implication of such an incongruence in treatment aims may be that those wishing to distance themselves from the assertion or suspicion of offending behavior simply do not seek out services that could lead to significant wellbeing improvements (Grady et al., 2019; Lievesley & Harper, 2019). Instead, taking a wellbeing approach to treatment could foster trust in professionals and encourage more MAPs to look for professional support and improve their mental health (Goodier & Lievesley, 2018). A secondary effect of this type of approach may be to reduce offense risk, as improving psychological wellbeing is associated with a lower risk of sexual offending within the broader forensic literature (Ward & Stewart, 2003).

One way to address these issues may be to adopt acceptance-based approaches to treatment programs aimed at MAPs. This was discussed by Lievesley et al. (2018), and is consistent with a positive psychological approach to sexual abuse prevention. This type of treatment paradigm is recognized as an alternative to traditional Cognitive Behavioral Therapy (CBT) models, and moves away from a therapeutic mindset that is focused on individual deficits (Walton & Hocken, 2019). Instead, acceptance-based models of treatment help service users to work through feelings that they typically would attempt to avoid or suppress (Hayes et al., 1999; Hayes & Wilson, 1994)—an issue that has recently been identified among the MAP community (Lievesley et al., 2020). Thus, we recommend that treatment approaches tackle the negative self-image experienced by many MAPs by encouraging them to view their sexual interests as a core part of their identities (acceptance), but also support them to live crime-free lives (commitment). Treatment may thus be aligned with established principles within the area of sexual crime desistance, such as those embedded within the Good Lives Model (GLM; Ward & Stewart, 2003) by encouraging therapists to assist service users in achieving primary human goods related to inner peace, rather than fixating on managing or changing their sexual attractions.

Conclusions

In this chapter, we have presented the argument that current research on "pedophilia" and "pedophilic disorder" is too narrow in focus, and advocate for the study of "minor attraction" as an alternative. There are issues with the diagnostic criteria for pedophilic disorder (as set out in the DSM-5; American Psychiatric Association, 2013), with individuals being medicalized for normal responses to an unchosen sexual arousal pattern. We advocate for a social and professional change in how we view minor attraction, with more services being made available for MAPs who experience distress, and a focus on their wellbeing as opposed to sexual abuse prevention.

References

Ahlers, C. J., Schaefer, G. A., Mundt, I. A., Roll, S., Englert, H., Willich, S. N., & Beier, K. M. (2011). How unusual are the contents of paraphilias? Paraphilia-associated sexual arousal patterns in a community-based sample of men. *The Journal of Sexual Medicine*, 8(5), 1362–1370. https://doi.org/10.1111/j.1743-6109.2009.01597.x

American Psychiatric Association. (2013). *Diagnostic and statistical manual of mental disorders* (5th ed.). Author.

B4U-ACT (2011). Mental health care & professional literature. https://www.b4uact.org/research/survey-results/spring-2011-survey.

Bailey, J. M., Hsu, K. J., & Bernhard, P. A. (2016). An internet study of men sexually attracted to children: Sexual attraction patterns. *Journal of Abnormal Psychology*, 125(7), 976–988. https://doi.org/10.1037/abn0000212

Banse, R., Schmidt, A. F., & Clarbour, J. (2010). Indirect measures of sexual interest in child sex offenders: A multi-method approach. *Criminal Justice and Behavior*, 37(3), 319–335. https://doi.org/10.1177/0093854809357598

Bastian, B., Denson, T. F., & Haslam, N. (2013). The roles of dehumanization and moral outrage in retributive justice. *PLoS ONE*, 8(e61842). https://doi.org/10.1371/journal.pone.0061842

Beier, K. M., Ahlers, C. J., Goecker, D., Neutze, J., Mundt, I. A., Hupp, E., & Schaefer, G. A. (2009). Can pedophiles be reached for primary prevention of child sexual abuse? First results of the Berlin Prevention Project Dunkelfeld (PPD). *The Journal of Forensic Psychiatry & Psychology*, 20(6), 851–867. https://doi.org/10.1080/14789940903174188

Beier, K. M., Grundmann, D., Kuhle, L. F., Scherner, G., Konrad, A., & Amelung, T. (2015). The German Dunkelfeld project: A pilot study to prevent child sexual abuse and the use of child abusive images. *The Journal of Sexual Medicine*, 12(2), 529–542. https://doi.org/10.1111/jsm.12785

Bergen, E., Antfolk, J., Jern, P., Alanko, K., & Santtila, P. (2013). Adults' sexual interest in children: A quasi-experimental study. *International Journal of Cyber Criminology*, 7(2), 94–111. http://www.cybercrimejournal.com/bergenetalijcc2013vol7issue2.pdf

Blanchard, R., Lykins, A. D., Wherrett, D., Kuban, M. E., Cantor, J. M., Blak, T., Dickey, R., & Klassen, P. E. (2009). Pedophilia, hebephilia, and the DSM-V. *Archives of Sexual Behavior*, 38(3), 335–350. https://doi.org/10.1007/s10508-008-9399-9

Cantor, J. M., & McPhail, I. V. (2016). Non-offending pedophiles. *Current Sexual Health Reports*, 8(3), 121–128. https://doi.org/10.1007/s11930-016-0076-z

Cohen, L., Ndukwe, N., Yaseen, Z., & Galynker, I. (2018). Comparison of self-identified minor-attracted persons who have and have not successfully refrained from sexual activity with children. *Journal of Sex & Marital Therapy*, 44(3), 217–230. https://doi.org/10.1080/0092623X.2017.1377129

Corrigan, P. W., Morris, S. B., Michaels, P. J., Rafacz, J. D., & Rusch, N. (2012). Challenging the public stigma of mental illness: A meta-analysis of outcome studies. *Psychiatric Services*, 63(10), 963–973. https://doi.org/10.1176/appi.ps.201100529

Dombert, B., Schmidt, A. F., Banse, R., Briken, P., Hoyer, J., Neutze, J., & Osterheider, M. (2016). How common is men's self-reported sexual interest in prepubescent children? *The Journal of Sex Research*, 53(2), 214–223. https://doi.org/10.1080/00224499.2015.1020108

Feelgood, S., & Hoyer, J. (2008). Child molester or paedophile? Sociolegal versus psychopathological classification of sexual offenders against children. *Journal of Sexual Aggression*, 14(1), 33–43. https://doi.org/10.1080/13552600802133860

Finkelhor, D. (1984). *Child sexual abuse: New theory and research*. The Free Press.

Gillespie, S. M., Mitchell, I. J., Fisher, D., & Beech, A. R. (2012). Treating disturbed emotional regulation in sexual offenders: The potential applications of mindful self-regulation and controlled breathing techniques. *Aggression and Violent Behavior*, 17(4), 333–343. https://doi.org/10.1016/j.avb.2012.03.005

Goodier, S., & Lievesley, R. (2018). Understanding the needs of individuals at risk of perpetrating child sexual abuse: A practitioner perspective. *Journal of Forensic Psychology Research and Practice*, 18(1), 77–98. https://doi.org/10.1080/24732850.2018.1432185

Grady, M. D., Levenson, J. S., Mesias, G., Kavanagh, S., & Charles, J. (2019). "I can't talk about that": Stigma and fear as barriers to preventive services for minor-attracted persons. *Stigma and Health, 4(4), 400–410.* https://doi.org/10.1037/sah0000154

Grundmann, D., Krupp, J., Scherner, G., Amelung, T., & Beier, K. M. (2016). Stability of self-reported arousal to sexual fantasies involving children in a clinical sample of pedophiles and hebephiles. *Archives of Sexual Behavior*, 45(5), 1153–1162. https://doi.org/10.1007/s10508-016-0729-z

Hanson, R. K., & Morton-Bourgon, K. (2004). *Predictors of sexual recidivism: An updated meta-analysis* (Corrections Research User Report No. 2004–02). Public Safety and Emergency Preparedness Canada.

Harper, C. A., Bartels, R. M., & Hogue, T. E. (2018). Reducing stigma and punitive attitudes towards pedophiles through narrative humanization. *Sexual Abuse*, 30(5), 533–555. https://doi.org/10.1177/1079063216681561

Harper, C. A., & Harris, A. J. (2017). Applying moral foundations theory to understanding public views of sexual offending. *Journal of Sexual Aggression*, 23(2), 111–123. https://doi.org/10.1080/13552600.2016.1217086

Harper, C. A., & Hogue, T. E. (2015). The emotional representation of sexual crime in the national British press. *Journal of Language and Social Psychology*, 34(1), 3–24. https://doi.org/10.1177/0261927X14544474

Harper, C. A., & Hogue, T. E. (2017). Press coverage as a heuristic guide for social decision-making about sexual offenders. *Psychology, Crime & Law*, 23(2), 118–134. https://doi.org/10.1080/1068316X.2016.1227816

Harper, C. A., Lievesley, R., Carpenter, T., Blagden, N., & Hocken, K. (2019). Using personal narratives to humanize people with pedophilic sexual interests. *PsyArXiv Preprints*. https://doi.org/10.31234/osf.io/9c3s2

Harrison, K., Manning, R., & McCartan, K. (2010). Multi-disciplinary definitions and understandings of "paedophilia". *Social & Legal Studies*, 19(4), 481–496. https://doi.org/10.1177/0964663910369054

Hayes, S. C., Strosahl, K. D., & Wilson, K. G. (1999). *Acceptance and commitment therapy. An experiential approach to behavior change*. Guilford.

Hayes, S. C., & Wilson, K. G. (1994). Acceptance and commitment therapy: Altering the verbal support for experiential avoidance. *The Behavior Analyst*, 17(2), 289–303. https://doi.org/10.1007/BF03392677

Helmus, L., Ó Ciardha, C., & Seto, M. C. (2015). The Screening Scale for Pedophilic Interests (SSPI): Construct, predictive, and incremental validity. *Law and Human Behavior*, 39(1), 35–43. https://doi.org/10.1037/lhb0000099

Jahnke, S. (2018a). Emotions and cognitions associated with stigma of non-offending pedophilia: A vignette experiment. *Archives of Sexual Behavior*, 47(2), 363–373. https://doi.org/10.1007/s10508-017-1073-7

Jahnke, S. (2018b). The stigma of pedophilia: Clinical and forensic implications. *European Psychologist*, 23(2), 144–153. https://doi.org/10.1027/1016-9040/a000325

Jahnke, S., & Hoyer, J. (2013). Stigmatization of people with pedophilia: A blind spot in stigma research. *International Journal of Sexual Health*, 25(3), 169–184. https://doi.org/10.1080/19317611.2013.795921

Jahnke, S., Imhoff, R., & Hoyer, J. (2015). Stigmatization of people with pedophilia: Two comparative surveys. *Archives of Sexual Behavior*, 44(1), 21–34. https://doi.org/10.1007/s10508-0140312-4

Jahnke, S., Philipp, K., & Hoyer, J. (2015). Stigmatizing attitudes towards people with pedophilia and their malleability among psychotherapists in training. *Child Abuse & Neglect*, 40, 93–102. https://doi.org/10.1016/j.chiabu.2014.07.008

King, L. L., & Roberts, J. J. (2017). The complexity of public attitudes toward sex crimes. *Victims and Offenders*, 12(1), 71–89. https://doi.org/10.1080/15564886.2015.1005266

Kitzinger, J. (2002). The ultimate neighbour from hell? Stranger danger and the media framing of paedophiles. In Y. Jewkes, & G. Letherby (Eds.), *Criminology: A reader* (pp. 145–158). Sage Publications.

Klein, V., Schmidt, A. F., Turner, D., & Briken, P. (2015). Are sex drive and hypersexuality associated with pedophilic interest and child sexual abuse in a male community sample? *PLoS ONE*, 10, e0129730. https://doi.org/10.1371/journal.pone.0129730

Kteily, N., & Bruneau, E. (2017). Backlash: The politics and real-world consequences of minority group dehumanization. *Personality and Social Psychology Bulletin*, 43(1), 87–104. https://doi.org/10.1177/0146167216675334

Lievesley, R., Eliiott, H., & Hocken, K. (2018). Future directions: Moving forward with sexual crime prevention. In R. Lievesley, K. Hocken, H. Elliott, B. Winder, N. Blagden, and P. BanyardKHocken, H. Elliott(Eds.), *Sexual crime and prevention* (pp. 181–200). Springer Nature.

Lievesley, R., & Harper, C. (2019, April). *Understanding the needs and experiences of people living with a sexual interest in children. Workshop presented at the NOTA (Scotland) Conference. Stirling*, Scotland. https://osf.io/cwvf9.

Lievesley, R., Harper, C. A., & Elliott, H. (2020). The internalization of social stigma among minor-attracted persons: Implications for treatment. *Archives of Sexual Behavior*, 49(4), 1291–1304. https://doi.org/10.1007/s10508-019-01569-x

Marshall, W. A., & Tanner, J. A. (1969). Variations in pattern of pubertal changes in girls. *Archives of Disease in Childhood*, 44(235), 291–303. https://doi.org/10.1136/adc.44.235.291

Martijn, F., Babchishin, K. M., Pullman, L., & Seto, M. C. (2018, August). *Experiences of sexual and romantic attraction to children and/or adults in persons with pedohebephilia. Paper presented at the 15th International Association for the Treatment of Sexual Offenders (IATSO) Conference.* Vilnius, Lithuania.

McCartan, K. (2013). Media constructions of, and reactions to, paedophilia in society. In K. Harrison (Ed.), *Managing high-risk sex offenders in the community: Risk management, treatment and social responsibility* (pp. 249–268). Routledge.

McPhail, I. V., Stephens, S., & Heasman, A. (2018). Legal and ethical issues in treating clients with pedohebephilic interests. *Canadian Psychology*, 59(4), 369–381. https://doi.org/10.1037/cap0000157

Meyer, I. H. (2003). Prejudice, social stress, and mental health in lesbian, gay, and bisexual populations: Conceptual issues and research evidence. *Psychological Bulletin*, 129(5), 674–697. https://doi.org/10.1037/0033-2909.129.5.674

Mokros, A., & Banse, R. (2019). The "Dunkelfeld" project for self-identified pedophiles: A reappraisal of its effectiveness. *The Journal of Sexual Medicine*, 16(5), 609–613. https://doi.org/10.1016/j.jsxm.2019.02.009

Mokros, A., & Habermeyer, E. (2016). Regression to the mean mimicking changes in sexual arousal to child stimuli in pedophiles. *Archives of Sexual Behavior*, 45(7), 1863–1867. https://doi.org/10.1007/s10508-015-0652-8

Ristow, I., Li, M., Colic, L., Marr, V., Födisch, C., von Düring, F., Schiltz, K., Drumkova, K., Witzel, J., Walter, H., Beier, K., Kruger, T. H. C., Ponseti, J., Schiffer, B., & Walter, M. (2018). Pedophilic sex offenders are characterised by reduced GABA concentration in dorsal anterior cingulate cortex. *NeuroImage: Clinical*, 18, 335–341. https://doi.org/10.1016/j.nicl.2018.01.018

Schmidt, A. F., Mokros, A., & Banse, R. (2013). Is pedophilic sexual preference continuous? A taxometric analysis based on direct and indirect measures. *Psychological Assessment*, 25(4), 1146–1153. https://doi.org/10.1037/a0033326

Seto, M. C. (2012). Is pedophilia a sexual orientation? *Archives of Sexual Behavior*, 41(1), 231–236. https://doi.org/10.1007/s10508-011-9882-6

Seto, M. C. (2017). The puzzle of male chronophilias. *Archives of Sexual Behavior*, 46(1), 3–22. https://doi.org/10.1007/s10508-016-0799-y

Seto, M. C. (2018). *Pedophilia and sexual offending against children: Theory, assessment, and intervention* (2nd ed.). American Psychological Association.

Seto, M. C. (2019). The motivation-facilitation model of sexual offending. *Sexual Abuse*, 31(1), 3–24. https://doi.org/10.1177/1079063217720919

Silverman, J., & Wilson, D. (2002). *Innocence betrayed: Paedophilia, the media and society*. Polity Press.

Stiels-Glenn, M. (2010). The availability of outpatient psychotherapy for paedophiles in Germany. *Recht & Psychiatrie*, 28(1), 74–80.

Tozdan, S., & Briken, P. (2015). The earlier, the worse? Age of onset of sexual interest in children. *The Journal of Sexual Medicine*, 12(7), 1602–1608. https://doi.org/10.1111/jsm.12927

Viki, G. T., Fullerton, I., Raggett, H., Tait, F., & Wiltshire, S. (2012). The role of dehumanization in attitudes toward the social exclusion and rehabilitation of sex offenders. *Journal of Applied Social Psychology*, 42(10), 2349–2367. https://doi.org/10.1111/j.1559-1816.2012.00944.x

Walton, J., & Hocken, K. (2019). Compassion and acceptance as interventions for paraphilic disorders and sexual offending behaviour. In G. Akerman, D. Perkins, & R. Bartels (Eds.), *Assessing and managing deviant sexual interest and arousal*. https://www.researchgate.net/publication/325746252_Compassion_and_Acceptance_as_Interventions_for_Paraphilic_Disorders_and_Sexual_Offending_Behaviour

Ward, T., & Stewart, C. A. (2003). The treatment of sex offenders: Risk management and good lives. *Professional Psychology: Research and Practice*, 34(4), 353–360. https://doi.org/10.1037/0735-7028.34.4.353

Williams, K. M., Cooper, B. S., Howell, T. M., Yuille, J. C., & Paulhus, D. L. (2009). Inferring sexually deviant behavior from corresponding fantasies: The role of personality and pornography consumption. *Criminal Justice and Behavior*, 36(2), 198–222. https://doi.org/10.1177/0093854808327277

9

Passivity Paraphilias

Understanding Necrophilic and Somnophilic Interest

Mark Pettigrew and Elizabeth T. Deehan[1]

[1] *School of Psychology, University of Lincoln, UK*

Introduction

> *The old saying, "death is the brother of sleep" [has significance] insofar as a corpse is likened to a sleeping person. I have known of more than one sleep fetishist for whom only sleeping people had any sexual attraction... One of the most gruesome of the sexual anomalies, necrophilia, may well be based on this.* (Hirschfeld, 1947, p. 228)

Sleep and death share an intertwined history of romanticism. Sleep is commonly regarded as a peaceful state, the dead are at peace; tombstones commonly refer to a person as having fallen asleep, whilst a child can be commonly referred to as sleeping like an angel. Even the classic fairy tale of Sleeping Beauty embodies necrophilic fantasy (Rosman & Resnick, 1989). However, the relationship of sleep and death is more than just cultural; they, in fact, lie on the same behavioral spectrum. When the body sleeps, voluntary speech, movement, and thought are inhibited, response to external stimuli is reduced, and the sensory threshold increases. At the opposite end of the same spectrum, upon death all voluntary actions cease, and the body becomes permanently unresponsive to all external forces and stimuli. Somewhere between sleep and death, lying on that spectrum, are those states in which the level of response fluctuates by degrees, such as unconsciousness and coma for example. The difference is found in the permanence of the passive state. Death and sleep, and those states in between, are passive states in which the person/the body is utterly defenseless to the actions of someone else, including those of a sexual nature. It is death, however, that presents the greatest opportunity for engaging in sexual behaviors with a completely passive partner (i.e., a corpse). This is the primary interest of people with necrophilia. Assumed to be rare, sexual attraction to corpses (necrophilia) and sexual attraction to those who are sleeping (somnophilia) have long been under-researched sexual paraphilias. This chapter collates the most pertinent research on both topics and, in so doing, we suggest that necrophilia and somnophilia share enough characteristics to be grouped together as what we term "passivity paraphilias."

Sexual Deviance: Understanding and Managing Deviant Sexual Interests and Paraphilic Disorders,
First Edition. Edited by Leam A. Craig and Ross M. Bartels.
© 2021 John Wiley & Sons, Ltd. Published 2021 by John Wiley & Sons, Ltd.

Necrophilia

The most recent version of the Diagnostic and Statistical Manual of Mental Disorders (DSM 5: APA, 2013) lists necrophilia as a Paraphilia Not Otherwise Specified (PNOS). Similarly, the World Health Organization in its International Statistical Classification of Diseases and Related Health Problems (ICD 10) classifies necrophilia under "Other Disorders of Sexual Preference." The practice of sexually abusing the dead has been reported for centuries. Indeed, according to legend, King Herod had sex with his wife for several years after he killed her (Rosman & Resnick, 1989). Historic accounts of necrophilia can be traced as far back as Ancient Greece (Drzazga, 1960) and reports of the phenomenon have been found across Europe ever since. However, the relatively small amount of scholarly interest has only occurred, predominantly, from the 20th century onwards (Burg, 1982).

Necrophilia stems from the Greek "*nekros*" (corpse) and "*philia*" (love). Thus, necrophilia has been defined as a "sexual attraction to corpses" (Rosman & Resnick, 1989, p. 153)[1]. The behavioral manifestation of necrophilia (i.e., the sexual violation of a corpse) is differentiated from other related but distinct behaviors such as vampirism (consuming/drinking blood), necrophagia (eating the flesh of corpses), and necrozoophilia (attraction to animal corpses). There may, however, be some overlap with other behaviors that can be paraphilic or sexually motivated, such as sarxenthymiophilia (collection of flesh souvenirs) and osteoenthymiophilia (collection of bone souvenirs; Dimcock & Smith, 1997).

According to Rosman and Resnick (1989), necrophilia can be divided into two groups: (1) true or genuine necrophilia, where the sexual attraction to corpses is persistent; and (2) pseudonecrophilia, where the sexual attraction to corpses is only transient. Thus, people with pseudonecrophilia have a preference for sexual contact with the living (for a detailed discussion of a case of pseudonecrophilia see Meloy, 1996). Although those with true/genuine necrophilia have a primary and persistent attraction to corpses, it is probable that the majority will never actually sexually abuse a corpse. Instead, they are more likely to confine their necrophilic interest to private sexual fantasies and perhaps, for some, the use of pornographic material. Indeed, Knafo (2015) reports that there are over 80,000 websites dedicated to necrophilia and concomitant behaviors. Some people with true/genuine necrophilia may go even further and visit cemeteries or funeral parlors for sexual stimulation, possibly even masturbating in the presence of corpses (Aggrawal, 2009a).

Rosman and Resnick (1989) divided true/genuine necrophiles into two categories: regular necrophiles and homicidal necrophiles. The former will abuse dead bodies they negotiate access to (e.g., by working in morgues or funeral parlors), while the latter will kill in order to secure a corpse. Aggrawal (2009a), however, goes further and offers, in total, 10 different varieties of necrophile. Although the Aggrawal classifications are not without their problems, and somewhat excessively and unnecessarily subdivide necrophilic behavior (Pettigrew, 2019a), there are two distinct varieties of necrophile described by Aggrawal that complement the classification offered by Rosman and Resnick (1989), namely, romantic necrophiles and necromutilomaniacs. The romantic necrophile is unable to cope with the death of a loved one and may keep the body, or part of it, which becomes a source of psychosexual stimulation (for a detailed discussion of such a case see Foraker, 1976). The necromutilomaniac, however, will not relate to corpses in an overtly sexual manner. Instead, sexual gratification is achieved through the mutilation of dead bodies (for a detailed discussion of necromutilomania see Boureghda et al., 2011). One final noteworthy variety of necrophile, missed in both the Aggrawal and Rosman and Resnick classifications is the "necrofetishist." First described by Hickey (2006), necrofetishists enjoy more than sexual activity with corpses, they also enjoy being in their presence, conversing with them, dining with them, sleeping with them, and treating them as sentient. Case study results indicate that the necrofetishist believes they are in a relationship with the corpses they acquire (Pettigrew, 2019b).

At present, the true scale of necrophilia and necrophilic acts is unknown. Criminologists refer to the amount of crime which goes undetected and unreported as the dark figure of crime. The sexual abuse of corpses is likely to have such a (dark) figure as it would be a prime example of an offense(s) not accurately reflected in the statistics. In some jurisdictions, necrophilic acts are not even criminalized and so, when discovered, instances are neither logged nor recorded. In the United States, for example, only four States have specific laws prohibiting acts of necrophilia, approximately one-fifth of States do not have laws prohibiting the practice, and the remaining States offer a patchwork of "crimes against nature" laws (Troyer, 2008, p. 134). Even where the sexual abuse of a corpse is criminalized, as in England and Wales under section 70 of the 2003 Sexual Offences Act (sexual penetration of a corpse), when there is no living victim, detection rates are low. Moreover, when the sexual abuse of a corpse is discovered, incidents will not always be reported to authorities for fear of the consequential damage to the reputation of the funeral home, morgue, or hospital (Heasman & Jones, 2006; Morton, 1990; Price, 1963).

There is currently no fixed or prevailing etiological theory of necrophilia. This is likely due to its assumed rarity and low detection rates, and the fact that the available evidence is largely based on individual case studies and reports. An examination of the existing suggested theories, explanations of necrophilia include: unconscious suppressed hostility towards a parental figure, as well as a sadistic impulse to explore the mother's body (Pomer, 1959); coping with the death of a love object (Rapoport, 1942); low self-esteem arising from severe disturbance or upbringing (Dimcock & Smith, 1997); castration anxiety (Smith & Braun, 1978); compensation for inherent physical weakness and lack of sex drive and virility (Dimcock & Smith, 1997); and/or a fear of death and the dead (with necrophilia being the means of conquering that fear; Rosman & Resnick, 1989). Indeed, these are just a selection of theories as to the development of necrophilic interests. None of them conclusively explains the etiology of necrophilia in all its forms and instances.

The various explanations of the origins of necrophilia notwithstanding, there is a commonality amongst various reports of necrophilic behavior. That is, the person with necrophilia has complete dominion over the corpse, the corpse cannot resist or reject them, the corpse cannot argue, retaliate, or defend themselves, and the corpse cannot demand anything of the person with necrophilia. Indeed, this rationale has been indicated by numerous case study results for over half a century. For example, in an early case, Brill (1941) noted a person with necrophilia as saying: "If they were dead, they could not object to my company and my behaviour ... if you were dead, I could kiss and hug you as much as I liked, and you could not refuse" (p. 23). Similarly, Segal (1953) describes the case of a man who would relish the feelings of power and security he felt when sexually abusing a corpse: "It is there when you wanted, you put it away when finished with it, it makes no demands, it is never frustrating, never unfaithful, never reproachful" (p. 98). In their study of 122 people with necrophilia, Rosman and Resnick (1989) found the most common rationale for necrophilic acts was to possess an unresisting partner. This finding was underscored more recently by Franzini and Grossberg:

> They [necrophiliacs] frequently mention the desirability of a partner who is helpless, unresistant and completely at their mercy. The dead lover never rejects caresses and is always available when required; makes no demands, is never unfaithful, and never rejects you. This lover does not compare your love-making skills with others, will go along with any sort of kinky sex, and, if things go too far, cannot be harmed and will never file a complaint against you. (Franzini & Grossberg cited in Nobus, 2002, p. 178)

Of course, dead bodies are not readily available for those with a sexual interest in the dead. When such access to corpses is not possible, and the compulsion is strong enough, the commission of homicide has been observed in a number of people with necrophilia (Stein et al., 2010). If not apprehended, those who resort to homicide are likely to become serial offenders (Hickey, 2015). Indeed, some of the most infamous serial killers of recent years have engaged in necrophilic behavior, including Ed Gein, Edmund Kemper, Jeffrey Dahmer, Dennis Nilsen, Gerald Brudos, and Andre Chikitalio (Hickey, 2015). However, from the necrophilic fantasizer to the homicidal necrophile, there is a unifying attraction to passivity and the control/dominion over the body of another person. Therein, we contend, lies a key similarity to another under-researched and assumed to be rare paraphilia: somnophilia.

Somnophilia

As with necrophilia, somnophilia is classified in the DSM-5 as a "Paraphilia Not Otherwise Specified" (PNOS). In the ICD-10, somnophilia is classified as "Paraphilia, Unspecified," which incorporates behaviors such as paraphilias involving a non-consenting individual. Originally identified and labeled by Money (1984) as "a gentle and nonviolent stealing of caresses" (p. 170), the various definitions of somnophilia have come to be somewhat contradictory and, paradoxically, overly precise. For example, Aggrawal (2009b) defines somnophilia as fondling or having sex with one's partner whilst they are asleep. Money (1984), however, asserted that a person with somnophilic interests "breaks and enters" into the home of a person for the purpose of finding a sleeping person, while Oeverland (2018) stipulates that somnophilia involves intruding on a stranger and awakening them with sexual contact (including oral sex) but without any threat or violence. From these definitions, the relationship between the individual with somnophilia and the sleeping target (i.e., whether they are a partner or a stranger) has become unclear. However, we assert that this relationship is irrelevant and, thus, propose a clearer definition of somnophilia: namely, the attraction, and consequent sexual arousal, to a sleeping person.

The lack of a satisfactory definition has undoubtedly been aided by the terms "somnophilia" and "Sleeping Beauty syndrome" being used interchangeably when referring to the desire to engage in sexual activity with a sleeping person. The term Sleeping Beauty syndrome (proposed by Calef & Weinshel, 1972), as well as the comparable "sleeping-princess syndrome" offered by Money (1984), refers to the classic fairy tale of Sleeping Beauty, in which a princess is awoken from a 1,000-year sleep by a kiss. We agree with Oeverland (2018) who notes that "classical somnophilia" (i.e., sex with someone who is asleep) is distinct from Sleeping Beauty syndrome, as the latter refers to sexual arousal that is dependent upon the sleeping person awakening during the sexual activity. Recent research has shed some insight on this distinction. Specifically, Deehan and Bartels (2019b) questioned a sample of 232 people with self-reported somnophilic interests as to what their somnophilic sexual fantasies contained. It was found that a partner staying asleep and a partner waking up were reported separately (and in relatively equal amounts) within the sample, suggesting that they are distinct sources of sexual arousal, that the term somnophilia encompasses. As such, this finding lends support to the distinction between "true" somnophilia and Sleeping Beauty syndrome. Also, given that the participants identified as having somnophilia, it can be argued that some may be unaware of the distinction between these two forms of sleep-related sexual interests. While these findings lend support to the distinction, they also provide some context to the different functions of the behavior—one is to have a truly passive, unresponsive partner while the other hope their partner wakes and is surprised by the situation they find themselves in. Arguably, this could be classed as an atypical form of seduction, hoping that the partner will be pleasantly surprised and engage in the behavior upon waking up; however, there was a smaller subset of participants in the Deehan and Bartels (2019b) research who reported the waking participant's fear and confusion as a source of arousal (indicating further need for research into the function of somnophilic offending behavior and its functions).

Whilst the distinction between "true" somnophilia and Sleeping Beauty syndrome is clear, it is unclear how they differ from the phenomenon known as "sleepysex." Sleepysex is a term used by fetish communities to describe sexual activity that occurs when one party is in a semi-conscious state, such as when they are falling asleep or waking up. Sexual arousal in such instances occurs as a result of the cosiness and intimacy of those situations. Research into sleepysex is, so far, limited. However, just as there are many pornographic websites dedicated to necrophilia, somnophilia, and Sleeping Beauty syndrome, there also are indications that the category of "sleepysex" is also increasing in popularity (Oeverland, 2018).

One thing to note about sleepysex is that it seems to occur within the context of consenting sexual partners by virtue of the intimacy and proximity it necessitates. This raises the question of whether "true" somnophilia can be acted upon within the context of consent. This was examined by Deehan and Bartels (2019a) using an online, non-offending sample of 425 individuals. They found that both consensual and non-consensual somnophilia were reported within the sample. Although the idea of consensual somnophilia may be paradoxical, individuals who practice somnophilic behavior within relationships disclose how they consider this to be consensual, as they have agreed limits beforehand. Some have reported going to the extent of creating contracts between each other. This behavior is termed "consensual somnophilia" due to the passive partner giving consent to the active partner to engage in sexual activity whilst they are asleep, even though this contradicts the common understanding of consent (i.e., an individual cannot consent when asleep or unconscious). Fundamentally, however, both parties know what is going to happen in advance and come to an agreement with a partner they trust. Oeverland (2018) made the assumption that the practice of somnophilia is likely (albeit not exclusively) carried out with strangers. This statement is disputed by the findings of Deehan and Bartels (2019a). While non-consensual somnophilia may be enacted with strangers, as per the statement made by Oeverland (2018), consensual somnophilia depends on a pre-existing relationship between the two parties based in trust.

As discussed above, internet searches for sleep-related pornography have reportedly increased (Oeverland, 2018). However, the prevalence of somnophilia has been relatively unexplored until recently. Joyal et al. (2015) found that an interest in sexually abusing a person who is drunk, asleep, or unconscious was present in 22.6% and 10.8% of their male and female sample, respectively. As Joyal et al. (2015) note, the prevalence of this interest within the female sample was statistically unusual (<16%), whereas this was not the case for men. Although this indicates that the interest in sexual activity with a drunk, sleeping, or unconscious person is not unusual in men, it is important to consider how the question was put to participants. This item was framed in offending terms—"abusing a person who is drunk, asleep or unconscious," as opposed to neutral or consensual terms. Had neutral or consensual terms been used, the results might have been different and perhaps provided a different picture of the prevalence of somnophilic interest per se. Further to this, the question was not specific to sleep and included two other states. As such, individuals with fantasies about sex with a drunk person would also respond to this item, further skewing the picture of prevalence. This was addressed in an online study by Deehan and Bartels (2019b) using a non-forensic, online sample of 232 people. They found that 17.8% of the sample identified as someone with somnophilic interests, and 20.8% reported having fantasized about somnophilic behavior. While these figures are similar to those noted by Joyal et al. (2015), they represent a more accurate reflection of the prevalence of somnophilia as the questions were directed towards a specific interest in sleeping partners and was not framed in terms of abuse. On the basis of these findings, somnophilic interests appear to be not unusual within the general population.

As yet, there is no etiological theory underpinning a sexual interest in somnophilic behavior due to the lack of research in the area. However, there have been some insights, drawn from case studies, into the motivations behind this behavior. For example, Fedoroff et al. (1997) proposed four motivations for somnophilic behavior:

1. Fulfilment of sadistic or paraphilic fantasies
2. Bypassing rejection and/or observing of paraphilic fantasies
3. Sexual opportunism
4. Sex while sleeping (sexsomnia)—which is not applicable to somnophilia

The conclusions that Fedoroff et al. (1997) came to indicate that there are a wide variety of functions behind engaging in sexual activity with a sleeping, passive partner. Just as with necrophilia, the control of another person's body, the ability to manipulate them, and the lack of resistance appears to underpin somnophilia.

Empirical research on somnophilia is greatly lacking. However, Deehan and Bartels (2019a) have examined the nature and correlates of somnophilic interests. Drawing upon the motivations proposed by Fedoroff et al. (1997), as well as other relevant sources, they developed the Somnophilia Interest and Proclivity Scale (SIPS). The SIPS requires participants to respond to a series of vignettes depicting somnophilic scenarios that differ in terms of motivation. In their first study, Deehan and Bartels (2019a) found that males scored higher on somnophilic interest than females. For this reason, males and females were analyzed separately to discover if (and how) the relationship between somnophilia and other constructs differs for each gender.

Across both genders, Deehan and Bartels (2019a) found an association between somnophilia and biastophilic (rape) fantasies, with consensual somnophilia being associated to a lesser degree than non-consensual somnophilia. This finding supports the view that somnophilia is linked to an interest in non-consensual sexual activity (e.g., Lauerma, 2016; Pettigrew, 2019a). Although the association between biastophilia and non-consensual somnophilia is unsurprising, the concept of consensual somnophilia being associated with biastophilia is an interesting one. It arguably has links with the practice of "consensual non-consent" within the dynamics of BDSM practices, wherein one partner gives consent to another to act out a non-consensual scenario (e.g., being kidnapped and engaging in rape play). A common "consensual non-consent" scenario is one partner drugging another and engaging in sexual activity (which can also be considered consensual somnophilia if a somnophilic interest is present). Both consensual and non-consensual somnophilia being associated with biastophilic fantasies suggests that an underlying attraction to non-consensual (or seemingly non-consensual) behavior is something that motivates somnophilic interests. It is vital to note that not all individuals with somnophilic interests will be aroused by biastophilic fantasies, just as not all individuals who assault a sleeping victim will be interested in somnophilia. A distinction must be made between those who, for example, use date rape drugs to create an opportunity for rape, and those whose arousal is dependent upon the unconscious and unresponsive state of their victim.

Pertinently, Deehan and Bartels (2019a) also found that necrophilic fantasies were associated with non-consensual somnophilia, but only in the male participants. While further exploration of this relationship is required, empirical evidence of this association supports the concept of a continuum between somnophilia and necrophilia, fueled by a desire to possess a person that cannot resist or reject the individual. These findings support the suggestion that somnophilia and necrophilia are motivated by an underlying interest in "passivity, power, and the elimination, in degrees, of the possibility of rejection" (Pettigrew, 2017, p. 353).

Although Deehan and Bartels (2019a) found that sadistic fantasies and dominance were positively associated with somnophilia, the results of a hierarchical regression indicated that using sadistic fantasies *less* frequently was a significant independent variable of non-consensual somnophilia in both genders. This would suggest that an interest in more aggressive sexual acts is not linked to non-consensual somnophilia. Thus, it could be proposed that non-consensual somnophilia may be driven more by sexual interactions with a passive, unresisting partner. This is partially supported by the findings of Deehan and Bartels' (2019b) second study where individuals with somnophilia were invited to share what they found arousing about their somnophilic fantasies. Participants reported a variety of factors that aroused them, such as having control or power over their sexual partner, a lack of resistance or pressure, and no chance of being rejected by their sexual partner. These findings also reflect the motivations posited by Fedoroff et al. (1997), further supporting the wide variety of motivations for somnophilia. The studies of Deehan and Bartels (2019a, b) have built on the published case studies exploring somnophilia and developed the picture of the consensual and non-consensual forms. By laying this foundation for understanding what drives somnophilia, more questions have been brought to light about the etiological factors of the paraphilia requiring further research.

Dormaphilia

It is not uncommon for there to be a paraphilia that mirrors another. For example, acrotomophilia (arousal to people with amputations) appears to be mirrored by apotemnophilia (arousal around being an amputee). Somnophilia is no exception to this idea, with the mirrored paraphilia being what Deehan and Bartels (2019a) have coined "*dormaphilia*" (from the Latin "*dorma*" meaning "to be asleep/inactive"). Dormaphilia can arguably be considered the ultimate passivity-related paraphilia, as it involves sexual arousal stemming from being the passive (sleeping) party during sexual activity. Indeed, Deehan and Bartels (2019a) found that a dormaphilic interest positively correlated with the use of masochistic fantasies and the need for sexual submission. Although under-researched, this paraphilia/interest has been discussed at length in online forums between people who experience it but are unable to give it a name. Whilst dormaphilia does not fit into the continuum between somnophilia and necrophilia (as it is self-related), it does raise interesting questions surrounding the relationship between sleep and sexual activity. Deehan and Bartels (2019b) began unpacking this relationship by inviting those with dormaphilia to discuss their dormaphilic fantasies. The most common themes that emerged included being considered "irresistible to their partner" and "feeling helpless or used." The former appears to correspond with the romanticism of sleep noted at the beginning of this chapter.

A Spectrum of Passivity Paraphilias?

Somnophilia and necrophilia have long been linked within the research literature. Fedoroff et al. (1997) noted the similarities of both paraphilias, providing clinical examples of somnophilia and necrophilia being both sequential and comorbid. The sexologist William Arndt has asserted that situations involving a person that is asleep or drugged are akin to necrophilia (Arndt, 1991). Similarly, Cantor et al. (2009) asserted that extreme forms or necrophilia involve obtaining corpses "for rendering an unwilling victim unconscious" (p. 530). However, it would seem incongruous for someone with true/genuine necrophilia to be satisfied with a body that is simply unconscious. For example, one individual with necrophilia noted, "the cold, the aura of death, the smell of death, the funeral surroundings, it all contributes" (Morton, 1990, p. 29). All such trappings associated with the corpse would be absent in a somnophilic encounter. Moreover, there are a variety of practical and pragmatic differences between the sexual abuse of a corpse and the sexual abuse of a person who is asleep or unconscious. Firstly, a person with necrophilia can return to the corpse consistently. Gary Ridgway, for example, is reported to have returned to the bodies of women he had killed to perpetrate necrophilic acts, even after decay had begun to the extent of putrefaction (Dutton, 2007, p. 131). Secondly, the time afforded with a corpse is longer than that with someone who is unconscious. Thus, there is more time to act out sexual fantasies and role-play activities. Thirdly, there is less risk of detection, as the corpse cannot wake up and report the abuse to the authorities. Finally, there is absolutely no risk of the corpse rejecting the person with necrophilia as there would be with someone who was alive. For these reasons, it is unlikely that someone with necrophilia would be satisfied with a somnophilic situation (i.e., a sleeping target).

The same reasons may also account for why someone with somnophilia may progress to enacting necrophilic behaviors. Thus, somnophilia can be either a standalone paraphilia or a bridging paraphilia to necrophilia. We do not suggest that all, or even the majority of people with somnophilia, will graduate into developing necrophilia. However, when we remember that sleep and death are opposite poles on the same spectrum, with varying degrees of unconsciousness between the two, we can envisage movement along that spectrum. Moving further down that spectrum, the individual is afforded more time with the person/body, more time to explore sexual fantasies, and more opportunity to engage in more extreme sexual practices. Moving along the spectrum, the benefits increase and the risks decrease. As Heasman and Jones (2006) noted, considering paraphilias have "a tendency to escalate" (p. 277), it is not unreasonable to assume that cases of somnophilia escalating into necrophilia may be found. Such an assumption is reinforced by case evidence. For example, Bartholomew et al. (1978) present a case in which a necrophile would fantasize of having another man wholly in his power, drunk, or drugged, unconscious, powerless in the stocks, or "best of all" dead (p. 30). There is, in that case, a graduation in preference from unconsciousness and helplessness to the complete passivity of a corpse. The possibility of comorbidity of the two paraphilias cannot be ruled out, but similar case study research has demonstrated that the more common scenario is progression from somnophilic fantasies and acts to necrophilic fantasies and acts (Calef & Weinshel, 1972; Fedoroff et al., 1997; Pettigrew, 2017). As such, we believe that progression is one way and that, without some therapeutic intervention, it is highly unlikely that the person with necrophilia would transition into preferring somnophilia. The existing research base does, however, include one such case.

In his treatment of a person with necrophilic fantasies, Lazarus (1977) described guiding the patient away from necrophilic images in stages, from a dead female to an unconscious female, then to an anaesthetized female, to a female having passed out from excessive alcohol consumption, then to a semi-conscious female, and finally to a prostitute "whose attention was diverted while he was engaging in sex" (p. 583). The patient's masturbatory fantasies kept pace with the progression of these mental images, moving further away from the corpse as an object of sexual arousal until he concentrated exclusively on semi-conscious females. Contemporarily, such a treatment process is, of course, dangerous, as it involves conditioning a person to become sexually aroused by what is a rape scenario. However, the case is useful in understanding death, unconsciousness, and sleep on the same spectrum of arousal.

Conclusions

The difference between somnophilia and necrophilia is confined to the permanence of the passive state. The motivations underlying the two have a significant overlap, namely: dominion and passivity; power and defenselessness; and the elimination, in degrees, of the possibility of rejection. Although somnophilia and necrophilia lie on the same continuum, they can be difficult to identify in individuals who do not wish to share their sexual interests. This can be particularly difficult with regards to individuals convicted of sexual offences, as disclosing specific paraphilic interests may increase their risk and prevent progression through their sentence. This is particularly concerning as men with these interests will require paraphilia-specific work in order to reduce the risk that they pose to the public, as well as future partners. It is hoped that by increasing the research base and theoretical understanding of these paraphilias, clinicians will have additional and valuable resources to assess and identify passivity-related paraphilias when case evidence is ambiguous and offenders do not disclose their sexual interests.

Note

1. Others, however, have focused on the behavioral act when defining necrophilia. For example, Aggrawal (2009a) defines necrophilia as "sexual gratification by having sex with the dead" (p. 316).

References

Aggrawal, A. (2009a). A new classification of necrophilia. *Journal of Forensic and Legal Medicine, 16*, 316–320.

Aggrawal, A. (2009b). *Forensic and medico-legal aspects of sexual crimes and unusual sexual practices*. CRC Press.

APA (American Psychiatric Association) (2013). *Diagnostic and statistical manual of mental disorders* (5th ed.). American Psychiatric Publishing.

Arndt, W. (1991). *Gender disorders and the paraphilias*. International Universities Press.

Bartholomew, A., Milte, K. L., & Galbally, F. (1978). Homosexual necrophilia. *Medicine, Science and the Law, 18*, 29–35.

Boureghda, S. S. T., Retz, W., Philipp-Wiegmann, F., & Rosler, M. (2011). A case report of necrophilia: A psychopathological view. *Journal of Forensic and Legal Medicine, 18*, 280–284.

Brill, A. A. (1941). Necrophilia. *Criminal Psychopathology, 2*, 433–443.

Burg, B. R. (1982). The sick and the dead: The development of psychological theory on necrophilia from Krafft-Ebing to the present. *Journal of the History of the Behavioural Sciences, 18*, 242–254.

Calef, V., & Weinshel, E. M. (1972). On certain neurotic equivalents of necrophilia. *International Journal of Psychoanalysis, 53*, 67–75.

Cantor, J. M., Blanchard, R., & Barbaree, H. (2009). Sexual disorders. In P. H. Blaney & T. Millon (Eds.), *Oxford textbook of psychopathology* (2nd ed.) (pp. 527–548). Oxford University Press.

Deehan, E. T., & Bartels, R. M. (2019a). Somnophilia: Examining its various forms and associated constructs. Sexual Abuse, Advance online version.

Deehan, E. T., & Bartels, R. M. (2019b, June). *Further exploring somnophilia and dormaphilia*. Paper presented at the Division of Forensic Psychology Conference, June, 2019, Liverpool, UK.

Dimcock, J., & Smith, S. (1997). Necrophilia and antisocial acts. In L. B. Schlesinger & E. Revitch (Eds.), *Sexual dynamics of antisocial behaviour.* (pp. 241 – 251). Charles C Thomas Publications.
Drzazga, J. (1960). *Sex crimes and their legal aspects.* Charles C Thomas # Publications.
Dutton, D. G. (2007). *The psychology of genocide, massacres, and extreme violence.* Praeger.
Fedoroff, J. P., Brunet, A., Woods, V., Granger, C., Chow, E., Collins, P., & Shapiro, C. M. (1997). A case controlled study of men who sexually assault sleeping victims. In C. Shapiro & A. McCall Smith (Eds.), *Forensic aspects of sleep* (pp. 87–98). Wiley.
Foraker, A. G. (1976). The romantic necrophiliac of Key West. *Journal of the Florida Medical Association, 63,* 642–645.
Heasman, A., & Jones, E. (2006). Necrophilia. In E. Hickey (Eds.), *Sex crimes and paraphilia.* (pp. 273–280). Pearson Prentice Hall.
Hickey, E. (2006). *Sex crimes and paraphilia.* Pearson Prentice Hall.
Hickey, E. (2015). *Serial murderers and their victims* (7th ed.). Cengage Learning.
Hirschfeld, M. (1947). *Sexual pathology: A study of derangements of the sexual instinct.* Emerson Publishing.
Joyal, C. C. (2015). Defining "normophilic" and "paraphilic" sexual fantasies in a population-based sample: On the importance of considering subgroups. *Sexual Medicine, 3*(4),321–330.
Joyal, C. C., Cossette, A., & Lapierre, V. (2015). What exactly is an unusual sexual fantasy? *The Journal of Sexual Medicine, 12,* 328–340.
Knafo, D. (2015). For the love of death: Somnophilic and necrophilic acts and fantasies. *Journal of the American Psychoanalytic Association, 63,* 857–886.
Lazarus, A. A. (1977). A case of pseudonecrophilia treated by behavior therapy. In J. Fischer & H. L. Gochros (Eds.), *Handbook of behavior therapy with sexual problems, Vol. 2.* (pp. 581–584). Pergamon.
Lauerma, H. (2016). Somnophilia and sexual abuse using vaginal administration of Triazolam. *Journal of Forensic Sciences, 61,* 862–863. https://doi.org/10.1111/1556-4029.13050
Meloy, J. R. (1996). Pseudonecrophilia following spousal homicide. *Journal of Forensic Sciences, 41,* 706–708.
Money, J. (1984). Paraphilias: Phenomenology and classification. *American Journal of Psychotherapy, 38,* 164–179.
Morton, J. (1990). The unrepentant necrophile. In A. Parfrey (Eds.), *Apocalypse culture* (pp 28–35). Feral House.
Nobus, D. (2002). Over my dead body: On the histories and cultures of necrophilia. In R. Goodwin & D. Cramer (Eds.), *Inappropriate relationships: The unconventional, the disapproved, and the forbidden* (pp 171–189). Lawrence Erlbaum.
Oeverland, S. (2018). Somnophilia and the sleeping beauty syndrome: The unknown patterns of arousal. *Journal of Psychology and Clinical Psychiatry, 9,* 409–411.
Pettigrew, M. (2017). Comorbid, sequential, or different desires? Exploring the relationship between somnophilia and necrophilia. *Journal of Sexual Aggression, 23,* 351–359.
Pettigrew, M. (2019a). Fantasy, opportunity, homicide: Testing classifications of necrophilic behaviour. *Journal of Police and Criminal Psychology, 34,* 14–22.
Pettigrew, M. (2019b). Corpse dismemberment and a necrofetishist. *Journal of Forensic Sciences, 64,* 934–937.
Pettigrew, M. (2019c). Biastophilia, raptophilia, and somnophilia: The blurred distinctions and comorbidity of sexual paraphilias in a homicidal offender. *The Journal of Forensic Psychiatry & Psychology, 30,* 401–408.
Pomer, S. L. (1959). Necrophilic fantasies and choice of specialty in medicine. *Bulletin of the Philadelphia Association for Psychoanalysis, 9,* 54–55.

Price, D. E. (1963). Necrophilia complicating a case of homicide. *Medicine, Science and the Law, 3,* 121–131.

Rapoport, J. (1942). A case of necrophilia. *Criminal Psychopathology, 4,* 277–289.

Rosman, J. P., & Resnick, P. J. (1989). Sexual attraction to corpses: A psychiatric review of necrophilia. *The Bulletin of the American Academy of Psychiatry and the Law, 17,* 153–163.

Smith, S. M. Braun, C. (1978) Necrophilia and Lust Murder: Report of a Rare Occurrence, *Bulletin of the American Academy of Psychiatry and the Law,* 6(3), 259–68

Segal, H. (1953). A necrophilic fantasy. *International Journal of Psychoanalysis, 34,* 98–101.

Stein, M. L., Schlesinger, L. B., & Pinizzotto, A. J. (2010). Necrophilia and sexual homicide. *Journal of Forensic Sciences, 55,* 443–446.

Troyer, J. (2008). Abuse of a corpse: A brief history and re-theorization of necrophilia laws in the USA. *Mortality, 13,* 132–152.

10

Measures of Male Sexual Interest

Pamela M. Yates[1]

[1] *Cabot Consulting and Research Services, and Saint Mary's University Psychology Department, Canada*

Measures of Male Sexual Interest

Virtually all theories of occurrence and recurrence of sexual offending emphasize the role of deviant sexual interest as an important contributing factor, and the majority of treatment programs include components designed to understand and address the role of deviant interests in offending (McGrath et al., 2010). Deviant sexual interests, or paraphilias, are defined as an intense, recurrent, and unusual sexual interest in atypical sexual activities or objects (American Psychiatric Association, 2013). In addition to its theoretical importance regarding the etiology of sexual offending, deviant sexual interest is well-established as a predictor of recidivism among convicted sexual offenders (Hanson & Bussière, 1998; Hanson & Morton-Bourgon, 2005) and, thus, is a common factor included in risk assessment measures (e.g., Hanson et al., 2015).

There have been, and continue to be, developments in attempts to measure sexual interest for purposes of assessment and treatment. This chapter reviews and provides an overview of the research support for various measures of sexual interest. This review does not provide detailed procedural information related to the use in practice of the various measures, as this is beyond the scope of the present chapter. Instead, the aim is to comment on the empirical support for these measures in the assessment of sexual interests for the purpose of contributing to assessment, diagnosis, and treatment. This is particularly important given the likelihood of negative consequences of a finding of deviant sexual interest, ranging from stigma (Cantor & McPhail, 2016; Jahnke, 2018) to a lack of access to treatment or psychological services (Jahnke et al., 2015) to lifelong or indeterminate detention or incarceration.

It should be noted here that sexual interest is a complex process involving affective, cognitive, and physiological components. Equally important is research that demonstrates that not all sexual offenders are motivated by deviant sexual interests. For example, among sexual offenders against children, it is estimated that between 20% to 60% are pedophilic (Seto, 2008), so not all individuals with pedophilia commit offenses against children, and many offenders against children would not meet diagnostic criteria for pedophilia (Camilleri & Quinsey, 2008; Cantor & McPhail, 2016; Seto, 2008). Furthermore, among men in the community, some self-report sexual interest in children (e.g., Dombert et al., 2013). Lastly, research has not always been able to differentiate between individuals with a history and those without. For example, research has found that nonoffending, normal males do show deviant interest (e.g., Finkelhor, 1984) or a propensity to engage in rape or coercive sex (Malamuth, 1983; Yates, 1996).

It is also clear that other factors, such as intimacy deficits, cognitive schema and social information processing, and general and sexual self-regulation, among others, are also factors that motivate sexual offending and that are predictive of recidivism among detected offenders

Sexual Deviance: Understanding and Managing Deviant Sexual Interests and Paraphilic Disorders,
First Edition. Edited by Leam A. Craig and Ross M. Bartels.
© 2021 John Wiley & Sons, Ltd. Published 2021 by John Wiley & Sons, Ltd.

(Hanson et al., 2015; Hanson & Yates, 2013; Yates, 2013). Lastly, although actual practice varies, it has been argued that assessment is the foundation of intervention, which in evidence-based practice means tailoring treatment and ensuring it targets research-based criminogenic factors that are relevant in an individual case (Andrews & Bonta, 2010; Yates & Kingston, 2016). It goes without saying that measures of dynamic risk factors and other treatment needs, such as sexual interest, must be psychometrically sound in order to be useful.

Assessment of Sexual Interest

Given the aforementioned importance of deviant sexual interest as a predictor of recidivism and its importance in assessment, diagnosis, and treatment, various measures of sexual interest have been developed over the years. Measures of sexual interest include both direct (i.e., self-report) and indirect measures, with the validity of direct measures significantly impacted by impression management and faking (Banse et al., 2010). It is widely acknowledged that individuals who have committed sexual offenses may have a vested interest in concealing sexual interest due to fear, consequences of the label, or other reasons (Thornton et al., 2018; Yates, 2009). To address these concerns, indirect measures of sexual interest have been developed. Empirical support for various self-report and diagnostic rating scales, physiological (i.e., phallometric) assessment and viewing time measures, and indirect (associative) measures are reviewed in the next sections, followed by a summary of overall findings and recommendations for future practice.

Rating Scales and Self-Report

Self-report measures of sexual interest are direct measures in that they assess individuals' explicit cognition, i.e., the admission of deviant sexual interests. However, as noted above, it is well-acknowledged that individuals may be highly motivated to be non-disclosive about the presence of deviant interests. Similarly, rating scales rely on self-report and file information and, therefore, also run the risk of missing or incomplete data.

Perhaps the most commonly used rating scale is the Diagnostic and Statistical Manual of Mental Disorders (currently DSM-V; American Psychiatric Association, 2013), which sets out the criteria that must be met in order for an individual to be diagnosed with a paraphilia. One of the many concerns with these criteria is that they are categorical and, therefore, view sexual interest as taxometric rather than dimensional (Thornton et al., 2018). Furthermore, some diagnoses, such as sexual sadism, lack predictive validity and so are not useful in the assessment of this paraphilia (Kingston et al., 2007, 2010; Marshall et al., 2002). Diagnosis is further complicated by the fact, as mentioned earlier, that not all individuals meeting the criteria for a diagnosis of paraphilia will go on to act in a sexually abusive manner. In general, it has been concluded that the DSM is lacking in support as a reliable and valid measure of sexual interest (Camilleri & Quinsey, 2008; Moser, 2019; O'Donohue, 2016). For a comprehensive review of the multiple issues concerning diagnosis using the DSM-V, the reader is referred to Moser (2019).

Another rating scale, the Screening Scale for Pedophilic Interest (SSPI; Seto & Lalumière, 2001), a four-item measure comprised of offense history items, reliably identified sexual offenders against children with pedophilic interests and predicted sexual recidivism among adult sexual offenders with child victims in some research (Helmus et al., 2015; Seto et al., 2004). However, this latter finding was not replicated in other studies (e.g., Canales et al., 2009), and the measure was not found to add to prediction over and above the Static-99R

(Hanson & Thornton, 1999). Subsequently, the Screening Scale for Pedophilic Interest-2 (SSPI-2; Seto et al., 2017) was developed to improve the measure via the addition of a fifth item pertaining to viewing child pornography. Results indicated that the SSPI-2 demonstrated convergent validity and was significantly associated with sexual arousal to children (superior to the SSPI) and provided greater discrimination than the SSPI (Seto, Sandler et al., 2017; Seto, Stephens et al., 2017).

Another way to measure sexual interest is via self-report. There are numerous self-report measures of sexual interest, some of which are used for research purposes and some applied in practice (Ó Ciardha et al., 2018). Examples include the Multiphasic Sex Inventory (Nichols & Molinder, 1984), Clarke Sexual History Questionnaire (Paitich et al., 1977), and the Sexual Interest Cardsort Questionnaire (Abel & Becker, 1979), each of which has acceptable psychometric properties and some measure of discriminant validity in terms of differentiating between known groups (e.g., sexual offenders vs. no-offenders; Holland et al., 2000). However, as with any self-report measure, these measures of sexual interest and history are dependent upon adequate file information and are subject to social desirability and impression management, thereby limiting confidence in their use.

Indirect Measures of Sexual Interest

While self-report measures assess explicit cognition, measures such as the Implicit Association Test (IAT; Greenwald et al., 1998) assess the strength of relationships between concepts and categories in an attempt to tap into implicit, rather than explicit cognition. For example, an individual may be asked to associate attributes such as *sexy* or *not sexy* with the concept of *adult* or *child* (Babchishin et al., 2013, 2014). Theoretically, the measure is based on the assumption that words/images associated with a topic that a person views favorably will be more accessible than words that are unrelated (Camilleri & Quinsey, 2008). As an example, an individual who is sexually interested in children will more quickly associate words such as *sex* in response to child stimuli than a person who is not sexually interested in children. Sexual interest is inferred from response times, with shorter response times indicating stronger associations between the concepts. Due to the concerns associated with more direct measures of sexual interests, there has recently been attention paid to IAT measures to assess sexual interest in children. This is because indirect measures are thought to be less susceptible to faking and impression management than more direct measures (Banse et al., 2010; Kalmus & Beech, 2005). As with phallometric assessment and viewing time measures (see below), IAT procedures used vary across studies, with different stimuli, implementation procedures, and scoring methods.

Research has found that IAT measures are able to distinguish sexual offenders against children from other comparison groups. Babchishin et al. (2013) found the strongest discrimination between sexual offenders against children and non-offenders, with significant but more modest differences found between sexual offenders against children and non-sexual offenders, and between sexual offenders against children and those who offended against adults. Numerous studies have found that sexual offenders against children, as compared to other groups, show greater associations between children and sex than adults and sex (Babchishin et al. 2014; Babchishin, Malcom et al., 2015; Bartels et al., 2018; Gray et al., 2005). Furthermore, construct validity, as measured by correlations with phallometric assessment, viewing time measures, and sexual offense history, were moderate, although the relationship between IAT and risk measures was unclear (Babchishin et al., 2013). However, IAT measures were also found to have lower discrimination as compared to other indirect measures, such as viewing time (Babchishin et al., 2013), although the addition of self-report measures can improve classification (Banse et al., 2010).

IAT measures are a relatively recent addition to the cadre of measures of sexual interest and show potential in discriminating between sexual offenders against children and others. However, their relationship to risk and predictive accuracy have yet to be demonstrated, and research support for the use of IAT measures is somewhat mixed due to methodological issues (e.g., Babchishin et al., 2015). It has been suggested that, with additional research, IATs show potential as an approach to measuring deviant sexual interest (Babchishin et al., 2015; Camilleri & Quinsey, 2008).

Phallometric Assessment

Phallometric assessment, or penile plethysmography (PPG), is a physiological, rather than cognitive, measure of sexual interest, or, more specifically, sexual arousal, from which sexual interest or preference is inferred. The procedure was developed in 1957 by Kurt Freund (Freund, 1963) to measure penile response to erotic stimuli as a measure of sexual preference and which continues to be used today to measure sexual deviance and to evaluate treatment effectiveness (Marshall, 2014; Marshall & Laws, 2003). Briefly, phallometric assessment involves presenting stimulus materials to subjects while they wear a device that measures changes in the penis in response to the content of the presented stimuli. Responses are evaluated to assess sexual interest in, or preference for, specific age and gender categories or for sadomasochistic violence. In some cases, the degree of deviant arousal (i.e., to violent or age-inappropriate stimuli) is compared to the degree of non-deviant arousal (i.e., consensual, age-appropriate) and/or to arousal to neutral stimuli. Over time, treatment protocols using phallometry were developed, such as aversive conditioning, satiation, and arousal reconditioning, in order to train individuals to control or modify their arousal to deviant stimuli and increase sexual arousal to appropriate stimuli (Marshall & Laws, 2003).

Phallometric assessment is not a standardized measure but is rather a procedure that varies substantially between laboratories (Clegg & Fremouw, 2009; Laws, 2009; Marshall, 2014; O'Donohue & Letourneau, 1992). Stimulus materials used during assessment also vary and may include pictures, video, audio, or some combination of these. Models are typically nude, and the stimulus materials include male and female children of various ages, adults, and depictions of sexual violence. Assessment varies in how arousal is measured, with some methods employing volumetric measurement (changes in air volume using a cylinder) and some employing circumferential (changes associated with penile engorgement) measurement, which differ in how they measure arousal and also differ in terms of sensitivity (see Wilson & Miner, 2016, for a detailed description). Furthermore, neither scoring nor interpretation is standardized, cutoff scores differentiating deviant from non-deviant responding vary, and the measure is subject to high levels of social desirability and response suppression (i.e., faking and dissimulation; Clegg & Fremouw, 2009; Marshall & Fernandez, 2000; Thornton et al., 2018; Wilson & Miner, 2016). This lack of standardization has been highlighted for decades, as a major shortcoming of phallometric assessment that leads to low reliability, conflicting research findings, lack of generalizability of findings, and an absence of normative data against which to compare individuals (Marshall & Fernandez, 2000; Marshall & Laws, 2003; McPhail et al., 2019).

As indicated above, most theories of sexual offending against children include pedohebephilic interests as a potential motivation for behavior. As a result, phallometric assessment utilizes materials designed to measure sexual interest in children, most often relative to sexual arousal to adults. Sexual interest or preference is determined based on interpreting the pattern of responding and (usually) demonstrating arousal that exceeds a predetermined cutoff score.

There is an extensive body of research that provides detailed information on studies conducted to apply and validate phallometric assessment and there are several excellent reviews of these findings. The reader is referred to McPhail et al. (2019), Clegg and Fremouw (2009), and Wilson and Miner (2016) for this more detailed information. The section below summarizes the empirical support for phallometric assessment of individuals who have committed sexual offenses.

To begin, low reliability has been, and remains, an ongoing concern with phallometric assessment (Marshall, 2014; Marshall & Laws, 2003). Studies examining internal consistency suffer from methodological constraints that prohibit definitive conclusions, and test-retest reliability has not been convincingly demonstrated and is problematic due to habituation to stimuli over repeated presentations (Marshall & Fernandez, 2000). In addition, if phallometric assessment has validity, it should be able to accurately identify individuals who have deviant sexual interests (i.e., sensitivity) and to discriminate between individuals with certain sexual interests and those without, or between those who have sexually offended and those who have not (although, as mentioned earlier, not all sexual offenders are motivated by a deviant sexual interest). However, research has been mixed with regard to discriminant validity, likely as a result of the lack of standardization as described earlier. One consistent finding is that the sensitivity of phallometric assessment varies across studies and, in some studies, varies in expected ways with known risk factors, with individuals who have a greater number of victims, male victims, unrelated victims, and younger victims being more likely to demonstrate pedophilic interests (Seto & Lalumière, 2001; see also Marshall, 2014; McPhail et al., 2019). Research has also found that discriminant validity can be improved when a semantic task to reduce faking is added (Harris et al., 1999). Research has also found that using audio and visual stimuli together, rather than using either alone, consistently differentiates between individuals who have sexually offended against adults and those who have offended sexually against children (Blanchard et al., 2001; Cantor & McPhail, 2015; Freund & Blanchard, 1989; Marschall-Lévesque et al., 2018) and that *z*-scores are superior measures than raw scores or percent full erection values (McPhail et al., 2019).

Phallometric assessment requires expensive equipment and can be time-consuming to implement. Furthermore, its stimulus materials are ethically concerning (Gress, 2005; Marschall-Lévesque et al., 2018), as these are "unstandardized images of questionable provenance" (Laws & Gress, 2004, p. 187). As a result, some jurisdictions prohibit the use of phallometry and others have not made use of the procedure at all, and there has been movement toward developing virtual stimuli rather than using real images (e.g., Marschall-Lévesque et al., 2018).

The research described above applies predominantly to individuals who have offended against children and provides some support for the use of PPG with these offenders when certain methodologies are followed. However, the motivations of offenders against adults is less well understood and, as with offenders against children, not all offenders of adults demonstrate either sexual preference for rape or deviant arousal to coercive sexual stimuli (Clegg & Fremouw, 2009; Marshall & Fernandez, 2003). Comparatively less research has been undertaken with this group, and the majority of these studies have not been conducted to validate PPG but for other purposes, such as to test the sexual preference hypothesis (see Clegg & Fremouw, 2009, for a review). In their review, Clegg and Fremouw (2009) found that rapists did not show significantly greater arousal to coercive stimuli than to consenting materials. However, consistent with previous meta-analyses (Hall et al., 1993; Lalumière & Quinsey, 1994), offenders against adults were found to have significantly greater arousal to rape stimuli than non-sexual offenders and community controls.

Unlike PPG with offenders against children, assessment with offenders of adults is less variable with respect to implementation procedures. For example, it is typically conducted using audio-only stimuli in order to effectively convey sexual aggression, although these stimuli are not standardized. However, as is the case with phallometric assessment more generally, faking, impression management, and lack of standardization, and its predictive validity have not yet been demonstrated (Clegg & Fremouw, 2009; Kalmus & Beech, 2005; Looman & Marshall, 2005; Marshall & Fernandez, 2003).

Viewing Time Measures

Viewing time measures represent a less intrusive method of measuring sexual interest and may address some of the ongoing problems associated with phallometric assessment (see Fischer, 2000; Laws & Gress, 2004 for reviews of the history and early research). In viewing time assessment, individuals view various stimuli similar to those used in PPG—ranging from nude to clothed, posed erotically or not, and varying in age and gender. Time spent viewing the stimulus is indicative of interest, with longer viewing times indicative of greater interest (Laws & Gress, 2004). As with PPG, administration procedures for viewing time measures vary in terms of what is measured and how measurement is conducted (e.g., time spent viewing, response latency, and pupil dilation). Viewing time assessment may be less susceptible to dissimulation than self-report measures, and may be comparable to PPG in the assessment of offenders against children in terms of reliability and concurrent and criterion validity and modest effect sizes (Mokros et al., 2013). Two VT measures are presently commercially available: the Abel Assessment for Sexual Interest (AASI; Abel et al., 2004) and the Affinity (Glasgow et al., 2003).

When used in practice, the viewing time portion (Visual Reaction Time™/VRT™) of the AASI is combined with other measures, subjected to analysis, and interpretation is provided back to the user, so the data are not widely available for peer review (Laws & Gress, 2004; Wilson & Miner, 2016). The measure further does not provide normative data against which to compare individuals' responses, as the score that is calculated (termed a *z*-score) uses ipsative scoring (where an individual's responses are compared to their own grand mean scores) and does not provide a measure of actual level or degree of arousal (Fischer, 2000). The AASI is proprietary and, although research has been supportive, it has been subject to few independent evaluations, which have methodological shortcomings. Nonetheless, taken together, research suggests that that both the VRT™ and viewing time generally are a reliable and valid predictor of sexual interest in men, can discriminate between known groups of offenders against children, and are similar to phallometric assessment with regard to their discriminant validity (Gray et al., 2015; Laws & Gress, 2004; Wilson & Miner, 2016).

Affinity (Glasgow et al., 2003) is computer-based, and aims to achieve standardization across stimuli (Laws & Gress, 2004). Like other measures, Affinity uses various types of stimuli to assess sexual interest in various age and gender categories, which the individual rates in terms of sexual attractiveness while response time is measured. As with the AASI, much of the research into Affinity has been conducted by the development group or those associated with them, and empirical support remains mixed. For a detailed description of the development of the Affinity and its technical elements, see Glasgow (2009). As it is a relatively new measure, there is less research available on the Affinity and that which exists shows mixed results in terms of its discriminative validity (Wilson & Miner, 2016).

A recent meta-analysis of viewing time research found that the measure discriminated between sexual offenders against children and other groups, with an effect size similar to IAT measures, although validity increased and surpassed IAT measures when difference scores were used (Schmidt et al., 2017). Nude depictions were found to be superior to clothed depictions. Like other measures, viewing time measures each use different methodologies, which can substantially impact results (Schmidt et al., 2017). Finally, little research has been done pertaining to the susceptibility of viewing time measures to faking and dissimulation (Kalmus & Beech, 2005).

Computer Generated Images and Virtual Reality

Ethical concerns noted earlier regarding the use of depictions of real individuals as stimulus materials have led to the development of computer-generated materials for phallometric and viewing time assessments (Gress, 2001, as cited in Laws & Gress, 2004; Marschall-Lévesque et al. (2018).

Renaud et al. (2013) used interactive virtual immersion technology while measuring arousal using circumferential PPG. Similar to the AASI described earlier, ipsative scoring was applied and converted to within-subject z-scores. Stimuli were computerized nude virtual characters, and visual gazing was recorded. Results from this small study showed distinct arousal profiles associated with different sexual age preferences. Renaud et al. (2014) found that virtual reality in conjunction with the use of computer-generated characters differentiated between sexual offenders against children and non-deviant adult males. Classification accuracy was superior for the virtual reality presentation than an auditory presentation.

Due to a dearth of research, little can yet be concluded regarding the reliability and validity of such computerized measures and stimuli and their potential use in practice as alternatives within phallometric assessment or viewing time measures.

Conclusions and Future Directions

As this review highlights, the majority of measures that have been developed are designed to assess sexual interest in children (i.e., pedophilia) specifically. Diagnostic ratings schemes such as the DSM-V are not predictive and are problematic in how paraphilias are conceptualized (Moser, 2019). Other rating scales, such as the SSPI-2 (Seto et al., 2017), adequately differentiate between individuals who have offended against children and those who have not, but are ideally best used to supplement other measures, such as phallometric assessment. Similarly, indirect measures, designed to mitigate issues such as faking and impression management by measuring more automatic responding based on favorable and unfavorable associations, show potential as an approach to measuring deviant sexual interest (Babchishin et al., 2015; Camilleri & Quinsey, 2008).

Phallometric assessment, which measures physiological arousal rather than cognition, has been the most widely used measure of sexual interest, although most research has been conducted with sexual offenders against children or those with pedohebephilic interests rather than with offenders against adults. Phallometric assessment can be a reliable and objective measure of deviant sexual arousal and, as described above, sexual interest in children as measured by PPG is a significant predictor of recidivism among known sexual offenders (Hanson & Bussière, 1998; Hanson & Morton-Bourgon, 2005). Conversely, the measure is intrusive, requires expensive equipment, and lacks standardization, and stimulus materials using real individuals are ethically questionable.

Viewing time may be superior to phallometric assessment and other indirect measures of sexual interest. However, comparatively less research has been conducted on viewing time assessment, which also suffers from some lack of standardization of materials and procedures, and which may also require nudity in order to produce the most accurate assessment. Finally, computerized stimulus materials and interactive virtual reality measures have been developed to avoid the use of real persons in phallometric and viewing time measures, although these computerized measures are not yet ready for implementation.

As this review has shown, measurement of sexual interests is complicated by a number of factors, not the least of which are different approaches to sexual offending and hypotheses about how information is processed. For example, diagnostic measures rely on self-report with arbitrarily defined criteria that focus on an individual's behavior, and measures of implicit cognition rely on attentional factors and response times, thereby highlighting the role of sexual interest. Still other methods, specifically phallometric assessment and viewing time measures, rely on physiological sexual arousal. As indicated above, sexual interests, preferences, and arousal are complex processes involving emotions, cognition, personal history, context, and a multitude of other factors. As such, it is not surprising that there is variability in research across different measures.

In terms of application in practice, it is first recommended that a multi-method approach to assessment be undertaken that includes static and dynamic risk and treatment-relevant risk factors, including sexual interest. Phallometric assessment or viewing time measures are both suited to this purpose, although more so for the assessment of offenders against children. In agreement with Thornton et al. (2018), assessment should also include ratings scales, such as the SSPI-2 (Seto et al., 2017) to capture sexual interests that may represent processes other than paraphilic interest (e.g., aggression). Finally, attempts to standardize materials should continue, and computerized methods should be subject to further research to determine whether the use of real people can be eliminated in practice.

References

Abel, G., Jordan, G., Rouleau, A., Emerick, J., Barboza-Whitehead, L., & Osborn, R. (2004). Use of visual reaction time to assess male adolescents who molest children. *Sexual Abuse: A Journal of Research and Treatment, 16*(3), 255–265. https://doi.org/10.1023/B:SEBU.0000029136.01177.51

Abel, G. G., & Becker, J. V. (1979). The sexual interest card sort. Unpublished manuscript.

American Psychiatric Association. (2013). *Diagnostic and statistical manual of mental disorders: DSM-5* (5th ed.). American Psychiatric Association Publishing.

Andrews, D. A., & Bonta, J. (2010). *The psychology of criminal conduct* (5th ed.). Lexis Nexis/ Anderson Pub.

Babchishin, K., Nunes, K., & Hermann, K. (2013). The validity of implicit association test (IAT) measures of sexual attraction to children: A meta-analysis. *Archives of Sexual Behavior, 42,* 487–499. https://doi.org/10.1007/s10508-012-0022-8.

Babchishin, K., Nunes, K., & Kessous, N. (2014). A multimodal examination of sexual interest in children: A comparison of sex offenders and nonsex offenders. *Sexual Abuse: A Journal of Research and Treatment, 26*(4), 343–374. https://doi.org/10.1177/1079063213492343.

Babchishin, K., Nunes, K., Hermann, C., & Malcom, J. (2015). Implicit sexual interest in children: Does separating gender influence discrimination when using the implicit association test? *Journal of Sexual Aggression, 21,* 194–208. https://doi.org/10.1080/13552600.2013.836575.

Banse, R., Schmidt, A., & Clarbour, J. (2010). Indirect measures of sexual interest in child sex offenders: A multimethod approach. *Criminal Justice and Behavior, 37*(3), 319–335. https://doi.org/10.1177/0093854809357598.

Bartels, R., Beech, A., Harkins, L., & Thornton, D. (2018). Assessing sexual interest in children using the go/no-go association test. *Sexual Abuse: A Journal of Research and Treatment, 30*(5), 593–614. https://doi.org/10.1177/1079063216686119.

Blanchard, R., Klassen, P., Dickey, R., Kuban, M., & Blak, T. (2001). Sensitivity and specificity of the phallometric test for pedophilia in nonadmitting sex offenders. *Psychological Assessment, 13*(1), 118–126. https://doi.org/10.1037/1040-3590.13.1.118.

Camilleri, J. A., & Quinsey, V. L. (2008). Pedophilia: Assessment and treatment. In D. R. Laws & W. O'Donohue (Eds.), *Sexual deviance: Strengths and weaknesses theory, assessment, and treatment* (pp. 183–212). Guilford.

Canales, D., Olver, M., & Wong, S. (2009). Construct validity of the Violence Risk Scale—Sexual Offender Version for measuring sexual deviance. *Sexual Abuse: A Journal of Research and Treatment, 21*(4), 474–492. https://doi.org/10.1177/1079063209344990.

Cantor, J., & McPhail, I. (2015). Sensitivity and specificity of the phallometric test for hebephilia. *Journal of Sexual Medicine, 12*(9), 1940–1950.

Cantor, J., & McPhail, M. (2016). Non-offending pedophiles. *Current Sexual Health Reports, 8*(3), 121–128. https://doi.org/10.1007/s11930-016-0076-z.

Clegg, C., & Fremouw, W. (2009). Phallometric assessment of rapists: A critical review of the research. *Aggression and Violent Behavior, 14*(2), 115–125. https://doi.org/10.1016/j.avb.2009.01.001.

Dombert, B., Mokros, A., Brückner, E., Schlegl, V., Antfolk, J., Bäckström, A., Zappalà, A., Osterheider, M., & Santtila, P. (2013). The virtual people set: Developing computer-generated stimuli for the assessment of pedophilic sexual interest. *Sexual Abuse: A Journal of Research and Treatment, 25*(6), 557–582. https://doi.org/10.1177/1079063212469062.

Finkelhor, D. (1984). *Child sexual abuse: New theory and research.* Free Press.

Fischer, L. (2000). The Abel screen: A nonintrusive alternative? In D. R. Laws, S. M. Hudson, & T. Ward (Eds.), *Remaking relapse prevention with sex offenders: A sourcebook* (pp. 303–318). Sage.

Freund, K. (1963). A laboratory method for diagnosing predominance of homo- or hetero- erotic interest in the male. *Behaviour Research and Therapy, 1*(1), 85–93. https://doi.org/10.1016/0005-7967(63)90012-3.

Freund, K., & Blanchard, R. (1989). Phallometric diagnosis of pedophilia. *Journal of Consulting and Clinical Psychology, 57*(1), 100–105. https://doi.org/10.1037/0022-006X.57.1.100.

Glasgow, D. V. (2009). Affinity: The development of a self-report assessment of paedophile sexual interest incorporating a viewing time validity measure. In D. Thornton & D. R. Laws (Eds.), *Cognitive Approaches to the Assessment of Sexual Interest in Sexual Offenders.* (pp. 59–84). Wiley.

Glasgow, D., Osborne, A., & Croxen, J. (2003). An assessment tool for investigating paedophile sexual interest using viewing time: An application of single case methodology. *British Journal of Learning Disabilities, 31*(2), 96–102. https://doi.org/10.1046/j.1468-3156.2003.00180.x.

Gray, N. S., Brown, A. S., MacCulloch, M. J., Smith, J., & Snowden, R. J. (2005). An implicit association test of the associations between children and sex in pedophiles. *Journal of Abnormal Psychology, 114,* 304–308. https://doi.org/10.1037/0021-843X.114.2.304.

Gray, S., Abel, G., Jordan, A., Garby, T., Wiegel, M., & Harlow, N. (2015). Visual Reaction Time™ as a predictor of sexual offense recidivism. *Sexual Abuse: A Journal of Research and Treatment, 27*(2), 173–188. https://doi.org/10.1177%2F1079063213502680.

Greenwald, A. G., McGhee, D. E., & Schwartz, J. L. (1998). Measuring individual differences in implicit cognition: the implicit association test. *Journal of Personality and Social Psychology, 74*(6), 1464.

Gress, C. (2005). Viewing time measures and sexual interest: Another piece of the puzzle. *Journal of Sexual Aggression, 11*(2), 117–125. https://doi.org/10.1080/13552600500063666.

Hall, G., Shondrick, D., & Hirschman, R. (1993). The role of sexual arousal in sexually aggressive behavior: A meta-analysis. *Journal of Consulting and Clinical Psychology, 61*(6), 1091–1095. https://psycnet.apa.org/doi/ https://doi.org/10.1037/0022-006X.61.6.1091.

Hanson, R., & Bussière, M. (1998). Predicting relapse: A meta-analysis of sexual offender recidivism studies. *Canadian Journal of Human Sexuality, 7*(2), 161–162. doi: 10.1037/0022-006X.66.2.348.

Hanson, R., Helmus, L., & Harris, A. (2015). Assessing the risk and needs of supervised sexual offenders: A prospective study using STABLE-2007, Static-99R, and Static-2002R. *Criminal Justice and Behavior, 42*(12), 1205–1224. https://doi.org/10.1177%2F0093854815602094.

Hanson, R., & Morton-Bourgon, K. (2005). The characteristics of persistent sexual offenders: A meta-analysis of recidivism studies. *Journal of Consulting and Clinical Psychology, 73*(6), 1154–1163. https://doi.org/10.1037/0022-006X.73.6.1154.

Hanson, R., & Thornton, D. M. (1999). *Static 99: Improving actuarial risk assessments for sex offenders* (User report; 1999–02). Solicitor General Canada.

Hanson, R., & Yates, K. (2013). Psychological treatment of sex offenders. *Current Psychiatry Reports, 15*(3), 1–8. https://doi.org/10.1007/s11920-012-0348-x.

Harris, G., Rice, T., Chaplin, M., & Quinsey, E. (1999). Dissimulation in phallometric testing of rapists' sexual preferences. *Archives of Sexual Behavior, 28*(3), 223–232. https://doi.org/10.1023/A:1018732225435.

Helmus, L., Ó Ciardha, C., & Seto, M. (2015). The Screening Scale for Pedophilic Interests (SSPI): Construct, predictive, and incremental validity. *Law and Human Behavior, 39*(1), 35–43. https://psycnet.apa.org/doi/10.1037/lhb0000099.

Holland, L., Zolondek, S., Abel, G., Jordan, A., & Becker, J. (2000). Psychometric analysis of the Sexual Interest Cardsort Questionnaire. *Sexual Abuse: A Journal of Research and Treatment, 12*(2), 107–122. https://doi.org/10.1023/A:1009538107396.

Jahnke, S. (2018). The stigma of pedophilia. *European Psychologist, 23*(2), 144–153. https://doi.org/10.1027/1016-9040/a000325.

Jahnke, S., Philipp, K., & Hoyer, J. (2015). Stigmatizing attitudes towards people with pedophilia and their malleability among psychotherapists in training. *Child Abuse & Neglect, 40*, 93–102. https://doi.org/10.1016/j.chiabu.2014.07.008.

Kalmus, E., & Beech, A. R. (2005). Forensic assessment of sexual interest: A review. *Aggression and Violent Behavior, 10*(2), 193–217. https://doi.org/10.1016/j.avb.2003.12.002.

Kingston, D., Firestone, A., Moulden, P., & Bradford, H. (2007). The utility of the diagnosis of pedophilia: A comparison of various classification procedures. *Archives of Sexual Behavior, 36*(3), 423–436. https://doi.org/10.1007/s10508-006-9091-x.

Kingston, D., Seto, M., Firestone, P., & Bradford, J. (2010). Comparing indicators of sexual sadism as predictors of recidivism among adult male sexual offenders. *Journal of Consulting and Clinical Psychology, 78*(4), 574–584. https://doi.org/10.1037/a0019734.

Lalumière, M., & Quinsey, V. (1994). The discriminability of rapists from non-sex offenders using phallometric measures: A meta-analysis. *Criminal Justice and Behavior, 21*(1), 150–175. https://doi.org/10.1177%2F0093854894021001010.

Laws, D. R. (2009). Penile plethysmography: Strengths, limitations, innovations. In D. Thornton & D. R. Laws (Eds.), *Cognitive approaches to the assessment of sexual interest in offenders* (pp. 7–29). Wiley-Blackwell.

Laws, D. R., & Gress, C. L. Z. (2004). Seeing things differently: The viewing time alternative to penile plethysmography. *Legal and Criminological Psychology, 9*, 183–196. https://doi.org/10.1348/1355325041719338.

Looman, J., & Marshall, W. (2005). Sexual arousal in rapists. *Criminal Justice and Behavior, 32*(4), 367–389. https://doi.org/10.1177%2F0093854805276402.

Malamuth, N. (1983). Factors associated with rape as predictors of laboratory aggression against women. *Journal of Personality and Social Psychology, 45*(2), 432–442. https://psycnet.apa.org/https://doi.org/10.1037/0022-3514.45.2.432.

Marschall-Lévesque, S., Rouleau, J., & Renaud, P. (2018). Increasing valid profiles in phallometric assessment of sex offenders with child victims: Combining the strengths of audio stimuli and synthetic characters. *Archives of Sexual Behavior, 47*(2), 417–428. https://doi.org/10.1007/s10508-017-1053-y.

Marshall, W. (2014). Phallometric assessments of sexual interests: An update. *Current Psychiatry Reports, 16*(1), 1–7. https://doi.org/10.1007/s11920-013-0428-6.

Marshall, W., Kennedy, P., Yates, P., & Serran, G. (2002). Diagnosing sexual sadism in sexual offenders: Reliability across diagnosticians. *International Journal of Offender Therapy and Comparative Criminology, 46*(6), 668–677. https://doi.org/10.1177/0306624X02238161.

Marshall, W., & Laws, D. (2003). A brief history of behavioral and cognitive behavioral approaches to sexual offender treatment: Part 2. The modern era. *Sexual Abuse: A Journal of Research and Treatment, 15*(2), 93–120. https://doi.org/10.1177/107906320301500202.

Marshall, W. L., & Fernandez, Y. M. (2000). Phallometric testing with sexual offenders: Limits to its value. *Clinical Psychology Review, 20*(7), 807–822. https://doi.org/10.1016/S0272-7358(99)00013-6.

Marshall, W. L., & Fernandez, Y. M. (2003). Sexual preferences: Are they useful in the assessment and treatment of sexual offenders? *Aggression and Violent Behavior, 8*(2), 131–143. https://doi.org/10.1016/S1359-1789(01)00056-8.

McGrath, R. J., Cumming, G. F., Burchard, B. L., Zeoli, S., & Ellerby, L. (2010). *Current practices and emerging trends in sexual abuser management: The safer society 2009 North American survey*. Safer Society Press.

McPhail, I., Hermann, C., Fernane, S., Fernandez, Y., Nunes, K., & Cantor, J. (2019). Validity in phallometric testing for sexual interests in children: A meta-analytic review. *Assessment, 26*(3), 535–551. https://doi.org/10.1177%2F1073191117706139.

Mokros, A., Gebhard, M., Heinz, V., Marschall, R., Nitschke, J., Glasgow, D., ... Laws, D. (2013). Computerized assessment of pedophilic sexual interest through self-report and viewing time: Reliability, validity, and classification accuracy of the Affinity program. *Sexual Abuse: A Journal of Research and Treatment, 25*(3), 230–258. https://doi.org/10.1177%2F1079063212454550.

Moser, C. (2019). DSM-5, paraphilias, and the paraphilic disorders: Confusion reigns. *Archives of Sexual Behavior, 48*(3), 681–689. https://doi.org/10.1007/s10508-018-1356-7.

Nichols, H., & Molinder, I. (1984). Manual for the multiphasic sex inventory. *Tacoma, WA: Crime and Victim Psychology Specialists, 24.*

Ó Ciardha, C., Attard-Johnson, J., & Bindemann, M. (2018). Latency-based and psychophysiological measures of sexual interest show convergent and concurrent validity. *Archives of Sexual Behavior, 47*(3), 637–649. https://doi.org/10.1007/s10508-017-1133-z.

O'Donohue, W. (2016). Problems with the classification and diagnosis of the paraphilias: What is the evidence that the DSM warrants use? In D. R. Laws & W. O'Donohue (Eds.), *Treatment of sex offenders: Strengths and weaknesses in assessment and intervention*. Springer. https://doi.org/10.1007/978-3-319-25868-3_1.

O'Donohue, W., & Letourneau, E. (1992). The psychometric properties of the penile tumescence assessment of child molesters. *Journal of Psychopathology and Behavioral Assessment, 14*(2), 123–174. https://doi.org/10.1007/BF00965172.

Paitich, D., Langevin, R., Freeman, R., Mann, K., & Handy, L. R. R. D. R. (1977). The Clarke SHQ: A clinical sex history questionnaire for males. *Archives of Sexual Behavior, 6*(5), 421–436. https://doi.org/10.1007/BF01541185.

Renaud, P., Chartier, S., Rouleau, J., Proulx, J., Goyette, M., Trottier, D., ... Bouchard, S. (2013). Using immersive virtual reality and ecological psychology to probe into child molesters' phenomenology. *Journal of Sexual Aggression, 19*(1), 102–120. https://doi.org/10.1080/13552600.2011.617014.

Renaud, P., Trottier, D., Rouleau, J., Goyette, M., Saumur, C., Boukhalfi, T., & Bouchard, S. (2014). Using immersive virtual reality and anatomically correct computer-generated characters in the forensic assessment of deviant sexual preferences. *Virtual Reality, 18*(1), 37–47. https://doi.org/10.1007/s10055-013-0235-8.

Schmidt, A., Babchishin, F., & Lehmann, K. (2017). A meta-analysis of viewing time measures of sexual interest in children. *Archives of Sexual Behavior, 46*(1), 287 300. https://doi.org/10.1007/s10508-016-0806-3.

Seto, M. (2008). *Pedophilia and sexual offending against children: Theory, assessment, and intervention* (1st ed.). American Psychological Association.

Seto, M., Harris, C., Rice, G., & Barbaree, T. (2004). The screening scale for pedophilic interests predicts recidivism among adult sex offenders with child victims. *Archives of Sexual Behavior, 33*(5), 455–466. https://doi.org/10.1023/B:ASEB.0000037426.55935.9c.

Seto, M., & Lalumière, M. (2001). A brief screening scale to identify pedophilic interests among child molesters. *Sexual Abuse: A Journal of Research and Treatment, 13*(1), 15–25. https://doi.org/10.1023/A:1009510328588.

Seto, M., Sandler, J., & Freeman, N. (2017). The revised screening scale for pedophilic interests: Predictive and concurrent validity. *Sexual Abuse: A Journal of Research and Treatment, 29*(7), 636–657. https://doi.org/10.1177%2F1079063215618375.

Seto, M., Stephens, S., Lalumière, M., & Cantor, J. (2017). The revised screening scale for pedophilic interests (SSPI–2): Development and criterion-related validation. *Sexual Abuse: A Journal of Research and Treatment, 29*(7), 619–635. https://doi.org/10.1177%2F1079063215612444.

Seto, M. C., & Kuban, M. (1996). Criterion-related validity of a phallometric test for paraphilic rape and sadism. *Behaviour Research and Therapy, 34*(2), 175–183. https://doi.org/10.1016/0005-7967(95)00056-9.

Thornton, D., Ambroziak, G., Kahn, R., & Mundt, E. (2018). Advances in the assessment of sexual deviance. *Current Psychiatry Reports, 20*(8), 1–8. https://doi.org/10.1007/s11920-018-0918-7.

Wilson, R. J., & Miner, M. H. (2016). Measurement of male sexual arousal and interest using penile plethysmography and viewing time. In D. R. Laws & W. O'Donohue (Eds.), *Treatment of sex offenders: Strengths and weaknesses in assessment and intervention* (pp. 107–131). Springer. https://doi.org/10.1007/978-3-319-25868-3_5

Yates, P. M. (1996). *An investigation of factors associated with definitions and perceptions of rape, propensity to commit rape, and rape prevention.* Carleton University, doctoral dissertation.

Yates, P. M. (2009). Is sexual offender denial related to sex offence risk and recidivism? A review and treatment implications. *Psychology, Crime & Law, 15*(2–3), 183–199. https://doi.org/10.1080/10683160802190905.

Yates, P. M. (2013). Treatment of sexual offenders: Research, best practices, and emerging models. *nternational Journal of Behavioral Consultation and Therapy, 8*(3–4), 89–95. http://dx.doi.org/10.1037/h0100989.

Yates, P. M., & Kingston, D. A. (2016). Shortcomings of sex offender treatment. In D. R. Laws & W. O'Donohue (Eds.), *Treatment of sex offenders: Strengths and weaknesses in assessment and intervention* (pp. 261–279), Springer.

Part IV

Sexual Deviance and Offending Behavior

11

Non-contact Paraphilic Disorders and Offending

Leah Kaylor[1] *and Elizabeth L. Jeglic*[2]

[1,2] *Saint Louis University, Missouri, USA and John Jay College of Criminal Justice, USA*

Introduction

Sexual offenses fall into two broad categories: contact (hands-on) and non-contact (hands-off) offenses (Kaylor & Jeglic, 2018; MacPherson, 2003). Exhibitionism and voyeurism are considered to be non-contact or hands-off offenses, since the perpetrator does not come into contact with or touch the victim during the commission of the act. In contrast, contact or hands-on offenses entail physical contact by the perpetrator with the victim during the commission of rape or another form of sexual assault (McNally & Fremouw, 2014). Both exhibitionism and voyeurism are recognized by the American Psychiatric Association as sexual paraphilias that involve sexual arousal derived from non-consenting individuals (American Psychiatric Association, 2013). This chapter will focus on the DSM-5 definition of exhibitionistic and voyeuristic disorder. The changes made from DSM-IV-TR (2000) to DSM-5 (2013) revised the diagnostic criteria for various paraphilias to differentiate between paraphiliac behaviors and paraphilic disorders (Balon, 2016). Specifically, paraphilic disorders are defined as either: (1) acting on one's urges and fantasies; or (2) one's urges or fantasies cause clinically significant distress or impairment in social, occupation, or other important areas of functioning. Paraphilic behaviors encompass the paraphilic act but do not cause significant distress or impairment or do not occur frequently enough to warrant a diagnosis. Thus, when referring to the research conducted prior to the DSM-5 we will call them exhibitionism and voyeurism. Further, when describing voyeuristic or exhibitionistic acts that do not meet criteria for a diagnosis, we will refer to them as voyeuristic or exhibitionistic behavior(s). This chapter will present what is known about Exhibitionistic Disorder and Voyeuristic Disorder in terms of diagnostic criteria, prevalence, gender differences, developmental influences/comorbidity, etiological theories, and recidivism/escalation and will conclude with recommendations for future research.

Diagnostic Criteria

Exhibitionistic Disorder

Exhibitionism was first described as a disorder by French physician Ernest-Charles Lasègue in 1877 (Långström, 2010). However, evidence of exhibitionistic behavior dates back to writings from the 5th century B.C. (Herodotus, 1998). It was only in 1965 that a revision of German psychiatrist Richard von Krafft-Ebing's classic tome *Psychopathia sexualis* included exhibitionism that the disorder became more widely acknowledged (Krafft-Ebing, 1965). Exhibitionism first

Sexual Deviance: Understanding and Managing Deviant Sexual Interests and Paraphilic Disorders,
First Edition. Edited by Leam A. Craig and Ross M. Bartels.
© 2021 John Wiley & Sons, Ltd. Published 2021 by John Wiley & Sons, Ltd.

appeared in the *Diagnostic and Statistical Manual of Mental Disorders* [DSM: American Psychiatric Association] in the DSM-III in 1980, where it was defined as recurrent, intense sexual urges and sexually arousing fantasies involving intense sexual arousal from exposing one's genitals to an unsuspecting stranger for a period of at least six months (APA, 1980). In the DSM-III-R (APA, 1987) a qualifying B criterion was added, indicating that the individual has acted on the urges or is markedly distressed by them. Very little was changed in the DSM-IV except that the statement "the person has acted on these urges" was removed, and the B criterion was changed to read: "The fantasies, sexual urges or behaviors cause clinically significant distress or impairment in social, occupational, or other important areas of functioning" (APA, 1994). However many then interpreted that to mean that in the absence of clinically significant distress or impairment the disorder could not be diagnosed, so in the DSM-IV TR (APA, 2000) the B criterion was once again revised to read: "The person has acted on these sexual urges or the sexual urges or fantasies cause marked distress or interpersonal difficulty."

In the current version of the DSM—the DSM 5 (APA, 2013)—exhibitionism was changed to Exhibitionistic Disorder and criteria include recurrent and intense sexual fantasies, urges, or behaviors derived from exposing one's genitals to an unsuspecting person for a period of at least six months. As in the DSM-IV TR, criterion B stipulates that the person must have "acted on these sexual urges with a nonconsenting person, or the sexual urges or fantasies have caused clinically significant distress or impairment in social, occupational, or other important areas of functioning" (APA, 2013, p. 689). In the DSM-5, the specifiers include whether the person prefers to expose themselves to prepubescent children, adults, or both (APA, 2013). Unlike voyeurism, a minimum age is not required. Both exhibitionistic and voyeuristic disorder can apply to individuals who freely disclose their actions as well as those who deny arousal despite objective evidence (APA, 2013). If a person denies distress in the form of guilt, shame, or anxiety about their paraphilic impulses, is not impaired in important areas of their functioning due to this interest, and their legal and psychiatric history proves that these urges are not acted upon, then they would not meet criteria for exhibitionistic or voyeuristic disorder (APA, 2013).

According to the *International Classification of Diseases* 10th revision [ICD-10] exhibitionism is defined as "recurrent or persistent tendency to expose one's genitals, without desiring or attempting to obtain closer contact" (World Health Organization, 1992). In the ICD-10 (WHO, 1992), these exposures may be limited to times of emotional distress and may disappear for long periods of time (Hanafy et al., 2016; WHO, 1992).

Voyeuristic Disorder

The term "voyeur" is derived from the French verb *voir*, meaning "to see," and dates back to the late 1800s (Janssen, 2018). Voyeurism was not included in the DSM until the second edition in 1968, where it was listed, but not defined until DSM-III (Janssen, 2018; Långström, 2010). The most recent version of the DSM-5 defines voyeuristic disorder as "recurrent and intense sexual arousal derived from observing an unsuspecting individual who is naked, engaging in disrobing, or sexual activity as manifested by urges, behaviors, or fantasies for a period of at least six months" (APA, 2013, p. 686). In order to meet criteria for voyeuristic disorder, the individual has either acted on these urges with a non-consenting person or the fantasies cause clinically significant distress or impairment (APA, 2013). The six-month window is a guideline, not a strict threshold, whereby viewing non-consenting persons is not a transient interest.

Another important change to the fifth edition of the DSM is the addition of an age requirement: criterion C states that the perpetrator must be at least 18 years old (Balon, 2016). Adolescence is a period marked by curiosity and sexual exploration (Kaylor et al., 2016; Sadhu, 2012) and to avoid the risk of pathologizing normative sexual development and interest, the

DSM-5 added a minimum age requirement for the diagnosis of voyeuristic disorder as 18 years of age (APA, 2013). However, one retrospective study of individuals who engaged in voyeurism found that 50% of voyeurs reported that the urge to engage in voyeuristic behavior began before the age of 15 (Hopkins et al., 2016; Kaplan & Krueger, 1997; Mathis, 1972). Some researchers have criticized the updated language of criterion B of voyeuristic disorder in DSM-5, whereby "this paraphilically motivated behavior is causing harm to others," as critics question whether the act of voyeurism causes harm to those who do not know they are being watched (APA, 2013, p. 687; Balon, 2016).

The clinical information for voyeuristic disorder is very similar in the ICD-10 with a slight variation in wording. The ICD-10 describes voyeuristic disorder as a "paraphilia characterized by repetitive looking at unsuspecting people, usually strangers, who are either naked, in the act of disrobing, or engaging in sexual activity, as the method for achieving sexual excitement" (World Health Organization, 1992, p. 328).

Subtypes

Exhibitionistic Disorder

There are three specifiers in the DSM-5 for Exhibitionistic Disorder including preferred exposure to prepubescent children, adults, or both. There is little empirical evidence to support these subtypes (Långström, 2010); however, research suggests that there is overlap between the paraphilic disorders (Abel et al., 1988; Bradford et al., 1992; Fedora et al., 1992; Freund et al., 1997) and thus giving a specifier of preferred exposure to prepubescent children may help the diagnostician consider or rule out co-occurring pedophilia (Långström, 2010).

In addition, various behaviors have been described as types of exhibitionism, but there is little to no research on these typologies. These include anasyrma, which is the lifting of the skirt when one is not wearing underwear; candaulism, which is the exposure of one's partner in a sexually provocative manner; flashing, which is the brief display of a woman's breasts or female or male genetalia; mooning, the brief exposure of the buttocks by pulling down the pants; and streaking, which is running naked through a public place (Baunach, 2010).

Voyeuristic Disorder

Stereotypical portals of a voyeur often depict a man hiding in the bushes peering into the home of an unsuspecting person (Hopkins et al., 2016). However, voyeuristic behavior can be thought of as an umbrella term with various subtypes, such as scoptophilia, which refers to the viewing of people engaged in sexual intercourse; scopophilia, which is the preference for watching individuals undress; troilism, which is the preference of watching one's significant other engage in intercourse with another person; coprophilia, which is viewing individuals eliminating or defecating; and pictophilia, which is the dependence on looking at pornographic images or videos (Hopkins et al., 2016; Kaplan & Krueger, 1997; Smith, 1976). There is debate as to whether watching pornography is considered a form of voyeurism. The DSM-III explicitly stated that "watching pornography, filmed or live causes excitement, however, the people who are being observed are willingly in view, even though in fantasy the observer may imagine (but knows better) that the people are unsuspecting" (APA, 1980, p. 273; Balon, 2016). Despite the much wider availability of pornography, DSM-5 does not make reference to whether viewing pornography falls into the category of voyeuristic behavior.

Prevalence

Historically, non-contact offenses such as exhibitionism and voyeurism were considered to be "nuisance behaviors" rather than sexual offenses (Davis & Davis, 1976; Firestone et al., 2006; Kaylor & Jeglic, 2018; Långström, 2010; Morin & Levenson, 2008; Murphy & Page, 2008). As such, non-contact sexual offenses have received little empirical attention, contributing to the dearth of literature in this area. Compared to contact offenses, a significant challenge in studying non-contact offenses is the scarcity of reliable estimates of the frequency and prevalence of such behaviors, since exhibitionistic and voyeuristic behaviors are rarely brought to the attention of law enforcement (Clark et al., 2016).

Exhibitionistic Disorder

It is estimated that the maximum prevalence of exhibitionistic disorder ranges between 2% and 4% of the general population (APA, 2013). Very little is known about exhibitionistic disorder as the majority of the research is conducted with those in clinical or forensic samples (Långström & Seto, 2006). Långström and Seto (2006) examined the prevalence of exhibitionistic behavior in a large representative sample of Swedish adults. Overall, survey respondents (n = 2,433) reported a lifetime prevalence of 3.1% of exhibitionistic behavior (4.1% for males and 2.1% for females). Given that they did not have information about the intensity, frequency, or persistence of the sexual fantasies or behaviors, the authors estimated that these findings would represent an upper limit to the prevalence of exhibitionistic disorder in a general population sample.

While the exact prevalence of exhibitionistic disorder remains elusive, exhibitionistic behavior it not uncommon (Firestone et al., 2006; Rabinowitz-Greenberg et al., 2002). Exhibitionistic acts are the most commonly reported sex crime accounting for between one-third (Rooth, 1973) and two-thirds of all reported sexual offenses (Abel et al., 1988; Firestone et al., 2006; Gebhard et al., 1965; McNally & Fremouw, 2014).

Voyeuristic Disorder

The prevalence of voyeuristic disorder is unknown as many perpetrators avoid detection. Similar to exhibitionism, existing research on voyeurism has been completed on individuals who come to the attention of law enforcement or therapeutic entities. Based on non-clinical samples, the maximum possible lifetime prevalence for males is 12% and 4% for females (APA, 2013). Långström and Seto (2006) also studied the prevalence of voyeuristic behavior in the same sample of Swedish adults. Their results showed that of the randomly selected individuals who responded (n = 2,433) 11.5% of men and 3.1% of women endorsed at least one incidence of becoming sexually aroused by watching another person engage in intercourse. A possible explanation for the low reporting rates and unreliable estimates of voyeuristic disorder is that voyeurism is an easily relatable concept and therefore does not provoke the same negative reactions as other deviant sexual behaviors (Långström, 2010).

Gender Differences

Exhibitionistic Disorder

There may be gender differences in the prevalence of Exhibitionistic Disorder and behaviors. As noted earlier, Långström and Seto (2006) found that about twice the number of men compared to women (4.3% of men and 2.1% of women) reported that they had exposed their genitals to a stranger and became sexually aroused. While these findings suggest that some women are engaging in exhibitionistic behavior, the large majority of individuals arrested for exhibitionistic behavior are male (Blair & Lanyon, 1981; Gebhard et al., 1965; McGrath, 1991; Swindell et al., 2011) and Långström and Seto (2006) found that male sex was related to exhibitionistic behavior. While some researchers have gone as far as to suggest that exhibitionism is an exclusively male disorder (Rickles, 1955), others highlight that it may just be rare among females (Schneider, 1982; Stekel, 1952).

One explanation for the gender difference in prevalence rates could be the way exhibitionistic acts are viewed by society. For example, in one study of women and men in treatment for sexual addiction, Carnes (2001) found that the proportion of women who reported exhibitionistic behavior was higher than that of males. However, as compared to the men, the women reported receiving fewer legal consequences for the exhibitionistic acts, and instead indicated that their exhibitionistic behavior was often rewarded as they garnered sexual attention from others (Carnes, 2001; Hopkins et al., 2016). Similarly, in another study which compared women and men in treatment for problematic sexual behavior, women reported that they engaged in illegal exhibitionistic behaviors at a greater frequency than the men, but that the men were much more likely to be arrested for sexual offenses (Hopkins et al., 2016). Hopkins and colleagues accounted for these differences by highlighting differential laws (e.g., it is not illegal to show breasts in certain jurisdictions), gender bias (i.e., men are considered to be more dangerous), or low reporting rates against women by men who view the exhibitionistic acts as seductive behavior (Hopkins et al., 2016).

Voyeuristic Disorder

As with Exhibitionistic Disorder, there is more research on male voyeurs as they are more likely to come to the attention of the authorities compared to females (Rye & Meaney, 2007). Hopkins et al. (2016) estimated that 90% of people who engage in voyeuristic behavior are male, thus very little of the existing research looks at females (Fedoroff et al., 1999). Like exhibitionism, it is theorized that female voyeurs are less likely to be prosecuted as a function of sexual stereotypes (Rye & Meaney, 2007). Moreover, studies have shown that men are more likely to engage in risky behavior, thereby increasing the likelihood of criminal justice involvement (David & Brannon, 1976; Eagly et al., 2000; Rye & Meaney, 2007; Thompson & Pleck, 1986). Rye and Meaney (2007) postulated that while both men and women may view voyeurism as equally risky, it may be that men are more willing to take the risk.

Another possible theory accounting for the gender differences in the prevalence of voyeurism could be social conditioning. For example, the vast majority of sexually explicit images in the media are marketed toward heterosexual men (Archer et al., 1983; Hall & Crum, 1994; Rye & Meaney, 2007). Leitenberg and Henning (1995) hypothesize that female fantasies are usually not as sexually explicit or focused on nudity as those of men. There is also research to suggest that women are less likely to view non-consenting people in sexual situations as it may feel "degrading" to those unknowingly being watched; consequently there may be fewer female voyeurs (Cowan & Dunn, 1994; Dio Bleichmar, 1995; Rye & Meaney, 2007).

Comorbidity and Developmental Influences

According to Långström and Seto (2006), both exhibitionistic and voyeuristic behaviors are associated with being male, having psychological problems, drug and alcohol use, and lower life satisfaction. Compared to a control group, individuals diagnosed with exhibitionistic and voyeuristic disorder were found to have lower self-esteem, social skills, and assertiveness as well as poor marital relationships (Blair & Lanyon, 1981; Dwyer, 1988; Hopkins et al., 2016; Kaplan & Krueger, 1997). Further, exhibitionism and voyeurism are frequently comorbid with each other and frotteurism (Abel & Rouleau, 1990; Långström & Zucker, 2005; Price et al., 2002; Rye & Meaney, 2007).

Exhibitionistic Disorder

Childhood emotional and sexual abuse as well as a preoccupation with sex/hypersexuality have been cited as risk factors for developing exhibitionistic disorder (APA, 2013). Acting on exhibitionistic impulses goes against social norms as well as criminal law, thus a risk factor for engaging in exhibitionistic behavior may be a propensity for risk-taking (Långström & Seto, 2006; Quinsey et al., 2004). An inclination for risk-taking behavior may be explained by sex differences, drug and alcohol usage, and antisocial tendencies (Lalumière et al., 2005; Långström & Seto, 2006; Quinsey et al., 2004; Seto & Barbaree, 1997).

Much of the information on known comorbidities for exhibitionism is largely based on research involving individuals who have been convicted for exposing themselves. Therefore, these comorbidities may not apply to everyone meeting criteria for exhibitionistic disorder. According to the DSM 5, exhibitionistic disorder is highly comorbid with anxiety, depression, substance use, bipolar disorder, attention-deficit/hyperactivity disorder, other sexual paraphilias, hypersexuality, and antisocial personality disorder (APA, 2013). Moreover, characteristics most often seen in individuals with exhibitionistic disorder are poor social skills and difficulty controlling anger and hostility (Bader et al., 2008; Lee et al., 2001; Raymond et al., 1999). A study by Bader et al. (2008) found that based on police reports from 106 exhibitionists: 37 were thought to have been abusing illegal drugs, 29 were suspected of abusing alcohol, 26 individuals showed symptoms of a mental disorder, and four perpetrators showed signs of developmental disabilities at the time they were arrested for exposing themselves.

Exhibitionism is highly comorbid with other sexual paraphilias (Bader et al., 2008; Kafka & Hennen, 1999; Price et al., 2001). In a study of 241 individuals with exhibitionistic disorder, 32% also engaged in voyeurism and 30% also engaged in frotteurism (Bader et al., 2008; Freund, 1990). Another study of 142 exhibitionists found that 93% of the sample also engaged in pedophilia, rape, or voyeurism (Abel et al., 1988; Bader et al., 2008).

Voyeuristic Disorder

Voyeurs were found to engage in higher rates of gambling, be attracted to same-sex partners, and have comorbid mental health disorders (Långström & Seto, 2006). As such, hypersexuality, depression, substance use, anxiety, bipolar, attention-deficit/hyperactivity and conduct disorder as well as antisocial personality disorder frequently co-occur with voyeuristic disorder (APA, 2013). With regard to sexual risk factors, individuals with voyeuristic disorder were found to have greater interest in sex, more sexual partners, increased sexual arousal, greater pornography use, increased sexual activity, higher frequency of masturbation, and greater likelihood of having a same-sex partner (Kafka & Hennen, 1999, 2002; Kafka & Prentky, 1992; Långström & Seto, 2006).

Childhood sexual abuse, substance misuse, and sexual preoccupation/hypersexuality are also risk factors related to the development of voyeurism (APA, 2013). Childhood sexual abuse was found to be a stronger predictor of voyeurism in men compared to women (Långström & Seto, 2006). There is also research that voyeurs had a higher rate of unusual fantasies, including bestiality, and began engaging in sexual activity at a later age compared to the norm (Hopkins et al., 2016; Smith, 1976).

Etiological Theories

Courtship Disorder Hypothesis

A popular explanation for the development of various sexual paraphilias is the Courtship Disorder Hypothesis, suggesting that both Exhibitionistic Disorder and Voyeuristic Disorder are a part of a larger chain of sexually deviant behaviors that are thought to function in a way similar to normal dating behaviors (Freund, 1990; Hopkins et al., 2016). A normal courtship begins with visually selecting an attractive partner, leading to non-physical interactions, followed by physical touching, concluding in sexual intercourse (Freund & Watson, 1990). Voyeurism is the first behavior in this series, which can be conceptualized as a deviation from the typical visual selection process. Exhibitionism is the deviation from the typical non-physical stage of courtship. Frotteurism and toucherism are disturbances in the touching stage and, lastly, rape is the final non-consensual stage of this model (Clark et al., 2016; Freund, 1990; Freund & Watson, 1990; Hopkins et al., 2016; Kaylor & Jeglic, 2018). This model postulates that exhibitionism, voyeurism, toucherism, frotteurism, and rape may be better conceptualized as various expressions of the same disorder (Freund & Watson, 1990). Each step of this model deviates from the normal sexual template in that it is pathological rather than adaptive in the development of a relationship (Freund & Watson, 1990; Hopkins et al., 2016). The courtship disorder model is commonly cited as an explanation for the high comorbidity rates amongst sexual paraphilias as well as the escalation toward more serious sexual offending behavior (McNally & Fremouw, 2014). While research on the courtship theory of development for paraphilias remains relatively sparse, some studies suggest exhibitionistic acts are an invitation for sexual contact (Freund et al., 1988; Hopkins et al., 2016; Lang et al., 1987).

Psychoanalytic Theory

Exhibitionistic Disorder

According to psychoanalytic theory, exhibitionistic behavior is a defense against castration anxiety. It is postulated that by engaging in exhibitionistic behavior and receiving a response from the victim, the individual confirms that in fact his penis exists and he has not been castrated (Blair & Lanyon, 1981; Enelow, 1969; Fenichel, 1946; Freud, 1905, 1914; Holtzman & Kulish, 2012. Among women the exposure of breasts is viewed as a defense against the narcissistic wound that is created by castration thereby detracting from her lack of penis (Blair & Lanyon, 1981; Freud, 1905, 1914; Holtzman & Kulish, 2012).

Voyeuristic Disorder

Freud proposed that every child goes through a series of stages in normal libidinal development. Psychoanalytic approaches to the explanation of voyeurism revolve around the desire to resolve internal conflict (Freund & Blanchard, 1986). Freud argued that at some point, the child will see their mother disrobing, or their parents engaged in intercourse, which signifies the threat of castration (Metzl, 2004). According to psychoanalytic theory, voyeuristic behaviors are an attempt to reassure oneself against castration anxiety, and watching others distracts from their fear. This theory also cites a deficit of control over sexual behaviors, leaving the voyeur unable to appreciate the gravity of being caught as well as the willingness to engage in risky behavior in spite of the possibility of being punished (Meyer, 1995; Rye & Meaney, 2007).

Evolutionary Theory

Very little has been written on evolutionary theory and exhibitionism. While there was some likening of exhibitionism to animal behaviors regarding courtship, Mester (1984) argues that the belief that exhibitionism developed as a way for males to advertise their sexuality would be a misunderstanding of the etiology of the disorder. More, however, has been written on evolutionary theory as it pertains to voyeurism, as much of the research on voyeurism contends that viewing others is an inane curiosity and a crucial piece of the normative sexual experience. Evolutionary psychology posits that voyeuristic behavior is an extension to the process of visually selecting a mate for reproductive purposes (Hopkins et al., 2016; Kaplan & Krueger, 1997). Evolution may contribute to, specifically, men's proclivity toward engaging in voyeurism, to the extent that it aids in mating and reproductive success (Buss, 1998; Rye & Meaney, 2007). This theory proposes that males viewing others is an adaptive trait when looking for specific cues, such as youth and hip-to-waist ratio, which will allow for the selection of a suitable partner (Buss, 1998; Rhodes et al., 2005).

Evolutionary theory also serves to explain the gender differences in the rates of voyeurism. The inclination toward voyeurism is considered to be more adaptive for men, as they can pursue various short-term sexual relationships, allowing for a greater number of offspring. As such, women are less likely to engage in voyeurism because short-term sexual encounters are not nearly as beneficial. Thus, evolutionary psychology speculates that there is a genetic predisposition toward voyeurism; however, the degree to which people act on such behaviors may be modulated by social constraints (Buss, 1998; Rye & Meaney, 2007).

Behavioral and Social Learning Theory

Exhibitionistic Disorder

While behavioral interventions have been the treatment of choice for those with exhibitionistic disorder, relatively little has been written on the specific etiology of exhibitionism from a behavioral perspective (Blair & Lanyon, 1981). Initially it was postulated that a single pairing, often accidental, of sexual exposure and arousal caused exhibitionism; however, this theory did not account for the vast majority of individuals who had such experiences and did not go on to develop exhibitionism (McGuire et al., 1964). Using case histories of 45 exhibitionists, McGuire et al. (1964) then theorized that exhibitionism could be explained by conditioning theory in which an initial deviant experience is fantasied about and then masturbated to, thus making it increasingly sexually exciting. Others, such as Bandura (1969), Barlow (1973), and Barlow and Abel (1976), have put forth frameworks for the development of deviant sexual behavior in which they highlight the idiosyncratic nature of the development of deviant sexual behavior for each individual; however, little to no research exists supporting these frameworks (Blair & Lanyon, 1981).

Voyeuristic Disorder

Social learning theory hypothesizes that exhibitionistic and voyeuristic acts, like many other behaviors, are learned via operant and classical conditioning as well as modeling. With regard to operant conditioning, viewing someone disrobing or engaging in sexual behavior is rewarded with arousal (Rye & Meaney, 2007). On the other hand, social controls serve as a form of punishment or negative reinforcement, thereby inhibiting one's engagement in voyeurism. As such, social learning theory (Bandura, 1969) predicts that people will engage in voyeuristic behaviors when: (1) there is an opportunity to do so; (2) when the viewing has previously been rewarded; and (3) the benefits of viewing outweigh the costs of possible punishment (Rye & Meaney, 2007). While evolutionary psychology suggests that men are more likely to take part in exhibitionism and voyeurism, social learning posits that men and women are equally likely to develop both exhibitionistic and voyeuristic tendencies.

Further, according to social learning theory, there is research to suggest that voyeuristic tendencies may be a common occurrence. To illustrate this phenomenon, Kutchinsky (1976) completed a study on police records in Copenhagen before and after the legal restrictions on sexually explicit material were relaxed. Reports of traditional voyeurism to the police were greatly reduced once individuals could legally replace these desires with acceptable forms of consensual voyeurism through pornography and live sex shows. It appears as though there is some psychological motivation to take part in risky behavior when no safer option exists, thus, acts of voyeurism may be controlled by the threat of punishment which leads people to engage in less risky alternatives (Kutchinsky, 1976; Rye & Meaney, 2007). In other words, many people may be interested in viewing such behavior; however, they may only do so when the costs do not outweigh the benefits. Thus, the way voyeuristic behaviors are expressed and interpreted may be a function of the social controls in place at that point in time (Rye & Meaney, 2007).

Technology

Exhibitionistic Disorder

As the world is becoming increasingly electronic, there are now also variants of the paraphilias online. While traditionally exhibitionistic behavior has occurred in public areas where the perpetrator exposes themselves to the victim in person, now the internet, webcams and smartphones have given individuals with exhibitionistic disorder new electronic methods by which they can engage in exposures (Hanafy et al., 2016; Kaylor et al., 2016). There is evidence that individuals, especially adolescents and emerging adults, are sending nude or semi-nude pictures to others as part of a courtship ritual also known as sexting (Kaylor et al., 2016). Kaylor et al. (2016) studied technological exhibitionism in a sample of 959 emerging adults and found that while a small proportion of those sending nude pictures in this age group may be engaging in exhibitionistic behavior, the majority were doing it as part of normal adolescent/young adult sexual exploration and courtship. Relatively little is known about how those with exhibitionistic disorder are utilizing digital forums to expose themselves and how this may impact future diagnostic criteria, although researchers believe that the reach and anonymity of the internet and digital communication lowers the chance of detection and may be appealing to perpetrators (Kaylor et al., 2016).

Voyeuristic Disorder

The traditional definition of voyeurism involves peering into the windows of a stranger's home, otherwise known as being a "Peeping Tom;" however, this definition has been expanded through the development of technology (Bell et al., 2006). A voyeur no longer has to hide behind bushes to peer into someone's home; with advances in technology an individual may achieve the same goal by simply connecting to the internet (Hopkins et al., 2016; Metzl, 2004). Not only has the internet allowed for consensual live sexual behaviors to be broadcast over the internet (e.g., Chatroulette, Snapchat; Hopkins et al., 2016), it has also led to the development of video voyeurism websites (e.g., voyeurlounge.com; Metzl, 2004). These websites allow for the observation of unsuspecting people engaging in everyday activities as well as intimate actions such as disrobing and sexual behaviors.

The number of websites offering voyeuristic content has dramatically increased (Metzl, 2004). According to the latest Google search, the number of websites offering video voyeurism currently stands at approximately 8,670,000, and this number increases daily. Some of these websites are operated by individuals who voluntarily choose to broadcast their personal lives over the internet; however, other voyeurism websites specialize in hidden camera footage, where the subject(s) is unaware that their image is being broadcast via the internet to the world. This type of hidden camera footage is typically obtained when small cameras are placed in areas where there is a reasonable expectation for privacy, such as inside a person's home, public bathrooms, locker rooms, hotel rooms, or other places where people are engaging in intimate acts (Stalking Resource Center, 2003).

A more recent phenomenon involves hacking and gaining control over personal webcams, without permission, in order to watch individuals without detection (Zinni, 2012). By tricking users into downloading spyware disguised as trustworthy software, hackers can gain access and control over webcams (Zinni, 2012). Once hacked, users are unaware that they are being filmed secretly from their webcams. However, unlike other video voyeurism websites where the victims are typically strangers, this type of voyeurism enables the perpetrator to target and observe specific people whom they have sought out (Sophos Press Release, 2008). For example, former Miss Teen USA, Cassidy Wolf, had her privacy violated when individuals hacked into her personal webcam and observed her in intimate moments unbeknownst to her, through her personal webcam (Weber, 2013; Zinni, 2012).

According to the Federal Bureau of Investigation, webcam hacking is a widespread and growing problem with over half a million victims around the world (Perez et al., 2014). Cameras used to secretly film individuals are becoming smaller and easier to hide. As technology further develops, so too does the software used to hack into webcams without detection, making it easier for online voyeurs to take advantage of unsuspecting victims.

Escalation and Recidivism

Exhibitionistic Disorder

Exhibitionism was long thought to be a nuisance behavior (Clark et al., 2016). However, research has shown that not only can exhibitionistic behavior cause long-term distress for victims, but a proportion of those who engaged in exhibitionistic acts go on to perpetrate contact sexual offenses (Clark et al., 2016; McNally & Fremouw, 2014). In a review of the literature on exhibitionistic behavior, McNally and Fremouw (2014) found that between 5 and 10% of offenders who have a history of exhibitionism will go on to have a contact sexual offense, while about 25% will recidivate with another non-contact offense.

When examining factors that were associated with escalation to contact sexual behavior, McNally and Fremouw (2014) found that a more extensive criminal history as measured by criminal charges for other sex offenses—both contact and non-contact—as well physical assaults best differentiated between those exhibitionists who went on to engage in contact sexual offenses and those that did not. Others have found that individuals who masturbated during the exhibitionistic act and touched or spoke to victims were more likely to engage in future contact offenses (Bader et al., 2008; Petri, 1969; Sugarman et al., 1994). Finally, exposure to children, low intelligence, and features of conduct or personality disorders were also related to contact escalation (McNally & Fremouw, 2014; Mohr et al., 1962).

Voyeuristic Disorder

The paucity of research on recidivism and voyeuristic behavior may be due to the view that it too is viewed as a harmless nuisance behavior. However, there is research to suggest that in adolescents, exhibitionistic and voyeuristic behavior should not be confused with normative young adult behavior. Although the majority of individuals convicted of sexual offenses do not show an escalation in sex crimes, a small portion (as high as 35%) progress from non-violent sex crimes during adolescence to more serious sexual offending in adulthood (Longo & Groth, 1983). Based on a sample of 84 adult rapists and child sexual abusers, Longo and McFadin (1981) found that 45% had a history of voyeuristic behavior as juveniles, with a mean age of onset at 13 years old. This study also revealed that rapists more often had a history of voyeuristic behavior compared to individuals who sexually abuse children.

Building upon that study, Longo and Groth (1983) examined a sample of 231 individuals convicted of sex offenses to specifically study the progression from non-contact offending as a juvenile (i.e., exhibitionistic and voyeuristic behavior) to serious sexual crimes in adulthood. Those who engage in voyeuristic behavior may eventually sexually assault the victim of their spying; however, the majority fantasize about the victim and engage in masturbation. The rapists in this study recalled that their voyeuristic behavior was often accompanied by rape fantasies that were aggressive in nature. The researchers stress that it may be possible to hinder escalation in juveniles with early detection and intervention of problematic exhibitionistic and voyeuristic behavior.

Conclusions and Future Directions

Exhibitionistic and voyeuristic behaviors have been identified as sexually deviant behaviors for centuries; however, the research on these disorders is scarce. This chapter reviewed the diagnostic criteria and the changes for the most recent version of the DSM. While it is widely acknowledged that men engage in exhibitionistic and voyeuristic behavior at far higher rates compared to women, the prevalence rates for both of these disorders are limited due to various factors, such as the long-standing perspective that these behaviors are "nuisance behaviors" and consequently are rarely brought to the attention of authorities. Additionally, specifically measuring voyeuristic behavior can be difficult, as this action is more covert and the perpetrator may be able to avoid detection. Both disorders are in need of large population-based studies to gain a better understanding of the incidence, prevalence, and scope.

Exhibitionistic and voyeuristic behaviors frequently occur together as well as with other mental health issues such as depression, substance use, anxiety, hypersexuality, bipolar disorder, attention-deficit/hyperactivity disorder, and antisocial personality disorder. Moreover, exhibitionistic and voyeuristic behaviors are highly comorbid with other sexual paraphilias, which provides support for the courtship disorder hypothesis. This etiological theory is the most popular explanation for the overlap of various sexual paraphilias. The courtship disorder hypothesis posits that deviant sexual behavior follows the template of normal dating behaviors, such as visually selecting a partner (voyeuristic behavior), non-physical interactions (exhibitionistic behavior), physical touching (toucherism/frotteurism), and intercourse (rape). The courtship disorder model is favored in the field as it explains the high comorbidity rates amongst sexual paraphilias as well as the escalation toward more serious sexual offending behavior. By gaining a better understanding of the etiology of these behaviors, clinicians can better tailor interventions.

With the advances in technology, exhibitionists and voyeurs have a much wider reach. A voyeur can observe people engaging in everyday activities as well as intimate actions, such as disrobing and sexual behaviors, by connecting to video voyeurism websites. Moreover, with the use of spyware a voyeur can trick an unsuspecting user into downloading spyware disguised as trustworthy software to gain access and control over webcams. Voyeurs also have the option to hide small cameras to secretly film individuals of their choosing. In order to protect oneself from voyeuristic victimization, people should be encouraged to cover their webcams when not in use to avoid online hackers. Further, downloading software to protect computers against hackers can prevent online victimization. Additionally, people should be wary of areas or locations where small cameras can be placed to record intimate actions for video voyeurism websites.

Similarly, those who wish to engage in exhibitionistic behavior can simply expose themselves using the internet or a smartphone. With these new avenues for exposure, exhibitionists can use the anonymity of the internet to decrease their chances of detection. The general public can be protected by raising awareness that receiving unwanted sexual photographs or sexually explicit images from unknown sources should be reported to the police. Given the limited research on sexual paraphilias and the near total lack of research on sexual paraphilias in a technological realm, future exploratory studies would benefit from gaining an understanding of the frequency and motivations behind engaging in both exhibitionistic and voyeuristic behaviors in a technological and traditional sense.

Studies on recidivism and escalation from exhibitionistic and voyeuristic behaviors to more serious sexual offending is scarce. While there is some evidence that points to increased likelihood for escalation (e.g., exhibitionistic behavior toward children, rape fantasies that accompany voyeuristic behavior), the field would benefit from studies devoted to determining the risk for recidivism and escalation to contact offenses. Researchers have suggested early detection and intervention for juveniles exhibiting problematic sexual behaviors. Despite the common perspective that exhibitionistic and voyeuristic behavior are nuisance behaviors, increased attention to the treatment of these paraphilias is needed in an effort to protect potential victims, prevent recidivism and escalation to more serious sexual offending.

References

Abel, G. G., Becker, J. V., Cunningham-Rathner, J., Mittelman, M., & Rouleau, J. (1988). Multiple paraphilic diagnoses among sex offenders. *Bulletin of the American Academy of Psychiatry and the Law, 16*(2), 153–168. https://www.researchgate.net/publication/19760035_Multiple_paraphilic_diagnoses_among_sex_offenders.

Abel, G. G., & Rouleau, J. L. (1990). The nature and extent of sexual assault. In W. L. Marshall, D. R. Laws, & H. E. Barbaree (Eds.), *Handbook of sexual assault: Issues, theories, and treatment of the offender* (pp. 9–21). Plenum.

American Psychiatric Association. (1980). *Diagnostic and statistical manual of mental disorders* (3rd ed.). Author.

American Psychiatric Association. (1987). *Diagnostic and statistical manual of mental disorders* (3rd ed., revised). Author.

American Psychiatric Association. (1994). *Diagnostic and statistical manual of mental disorders* (4th ed.). Author.

American Psychiatric Association. (2000). *Diagnostic and statistical manual of mental disorders* (4th ed., text rev.). Author.

American Psychiatric Association. (2013). *Diagnostic and statistical manual of mental disorders* (5th ed.). Author.

Archer, D., Iritani, B., Kimes, D. D., & Barrios, M. (1983). Face-ism: Five studies of sex differences in facial prominence. *Journal of Personality and Social Psychology, 45*(4), 725–735. https://doi.org/10.1037/0022 3514.45.4.725

Bader, S. M., Schoeneman-Morris, K. A., Scalora, M. J., & Casady, T. K. (2008). Exhibitionism: Findings from a Midwestern police contact sample. *International Journal of Offender Therapy and Comparative Criminology, 52*(3), 270–279. https://doi.org/10.1177/0306624X07307122

Balon, R. (2016). Lack of clarity in the DSM-5 criteria of voyeuristic disorder. *Journal of Sex & Marital Therapy, 42*(5), 391. https://doi-org.ez.lib.jjay.cuny.edu/10.1080/0092623X.2016.1158760

Bandura, A. (1969). *Principles of behavior modification.* Holt, Rinehart, & Winston.

Barlow, D. H., & Abel, G. G. (1976). Sexual deviation. In *Behavior modification: Principles, issues, and applications.* (pp. 26–48). Houghton Mifflin Boston.

Barlow, W. (1973). *The Alexander principle.* Gollancz.

Baunach, D. M. (2010). Exhibitionism. In P. Bernabeo (Ed.), *Sex and society.* Marshall Cavendish.

Bell, V., Hemmens, C., & Steiner, B. (2006). Up skirts and down blouses: A statutory analysis of legislative responses to video voyeurism. *Criminal Justice Studies: A Critical Journal of Crime, Law & Society, 19*(3), 301–314. https://doi.org/10.1080/14786010600921746

Blair, C., & Lanyon, R. I. (1981). Exhibitionism: Etiology and treatment. *Psychological Bulletin, 89*(3), 439–463. https://doi.org/10.1037/0033-2909.89.3.439

Bradford, J., Boulet, J., & Pawlak, A. (1992). The paraphilias: A multiplicity of deviant behaviours. *Canadian Journal of Psychiatry, 37*(2), 104–108. https://doi-org.ez.lib.jjay.cuny.edu/10.1177/070674379203700206

Buss, D. M. (1998). Sexual strategies theory: Historical origins and current status. *Journal of Sex Research, 35*(1), 19–31. https://www.jstor.org/stable/3813162?seq=1

Carnes, P. J. (2001). *Out of the shadows: Understanding sexual addiction.* Hazelden.

Clark, S. K., Jeglic, E. L., Calkins, C., & Tatar, J. R. (2016). More than a nuisance: The prevalence and consequences of frotteurism and exhibitionism. *Sexual Abuse, 28*(1), 3–19. https://doi.org/10.1177/1079063214525643

Cowan, G., & Dunn, K. (1994). What themes in pornography lead to perceptions of the degradation of women? *Journal of Sex Research, 31*(1), 11–22. https://www.jstor.org/stable/3813078?seq=1

David, D. S., & Brannon, R. (1976). The male sex role: Our culture's blueprint of manhood, and what it's done for us lately. In D. S. David & R. Brannon (Eds.), *The forty-nine percent majority: The male sex role* (pp. 1–45). Addison-Wesley.

Davis, S. K., & Davis, P. W. (1976). Meanings and process in erotic offensiveness: An expose of exposees. *Journal of Contemporary Ethnography, 5*(3), 377–396. https://doi.org/10.1177/089124167600500307

Dio Bleichmar, E. (1995). The secret in the constitution of female sexuality: The effects of the adult's sexual look upon the subjectivity of the girl. *Journal of Clinical Psychoanalysis, 4*(3), 331–342. https://www.pep-web.org/document.php?id=jcp.004.0331a

Dwyer, M. (1988). Exhibitionism/voyeurism. *Journal of Social Work & Human Sexuality, 7*(1), 101–112. https://www-tandfonline-com.ez.lib.jjay.cuny.edu/doi/abs/10.1300/J291v07n01_08

Eagly, A. H., Wood, W., & Diekman, A. B. (2000). Social role theory of sex differences and similarities: A current appraisal. In T. Eckes & H. M. Trautner (Eds.), *The developmental social psychology of gender* (pp. 123–174). Erlbaum.

Enelow, M. L. (1969). Public nuisance offenses: Exhibitionism, voyeurism and transvestism. In S. G. Kling (Ed.), *Sexual behavior and the law*. Pocket Books.

Fedora, O., Reddon, J. R., Morrison, J. W., Fedora, S. K., Pascoe, H., & Yeudall, L. T. (1992). Sadism and other paraphilias in normal controls and aggressive and nonaggressive sex offenders. *Archives of Sexual Behavior, 21*(1), 1–15. https://doi.org/10.1007/BF01542713

Fedoroff, J., Fidhell, A., & Fedoroff, B. (1999). A case series of women evaluated for paraphilic sexual disorders. *Canadian Journal of Human Sexuality, 8*(2), 127–140. https://ez.lib.jjay.cuny.edu/login?url=https://www-proquest-com.ez.lib.jjay.cuny.edu/docview/220773485?accountid=11724

Fenichel, O. (1946). On acting. *Psychoanalytic Quarterly, 15*(2), 144–160. https://www-tandfonline-com.ez.lib.jjay.cuny.edu/doi/abs/10.1080/21674086.1946.11925635

Firestone, P., Kingston, D. A., Wexler, A., & Bradford, J. M. (2006). Long-term follow up of exhibitionists: Psychological, phallometric, and offense characteristics. *Journal of the American Academy of Psychiatry and the Law, 34*(3), 349–359. https://www.researchgate.net/publication/6762209_Long-Term_Follow-up_of_Exhibitionists_Psychological_Phallometric_and_Offense_Characteristics

Freud, S. (1905). Three essays on sexuality. SE 7, 130–243.

Freud, S. (1914). On narcissism: An introduction. SE 14, 73–102.

Freund, K. (1990). Courtship disorders. In W. L. Marshall, D. R. Laws, & H. E. Barbaree (Eds.), *Handbook of sexual assault: Issues, theories, and treatment of the offender* (pp. 195–207). Plenum.

Freund, K., & Blanchard, R. (1986). The concept of courtship disorder. *Journal of Sex & Marital Therapy, 12*(2), 79–92. https://doi.org/10.1080/00926238608415397

Freund, K., Seto, M. C., & Kuban, M. (1997). Frotteurism and the theory of courtship disorder. In D. R. Laws & W. T. O'Donohue (Eds.), *Sexual deviance: Theory, assessment, and treatment* (pp. 111–130). Guilford Press.

Freund, K., & Watson, R. (1990). Mapping the boundaries of courtship disorder. *Journal of Sex Research, 27*(4), 589–606. https://www.jstor.org/stable/3812774?seq=1

Freund, K., Watson, R., & Rienzo, D. (1988). The value of self-reports in the study of voyeurism and exhibitionism. *Sexual Abuse: A Journal of Research and Treatment, 1*(2), 244–262. https://journals-sagepub-com.ez.lib.jjay.cuny.edu/doi/pdf/10.1177/107906328800100205

Gebhard, P. H., Gagnon, J. H., Pomeroy, W. B., & Christenson, C. V. (1965). *Sex offenders: An analysis of types.* Heinemann.

Hall, C. C. I., & Crum, M. J. (1994). Women and "body-isms" in television beer commercials. *Sex Roles, 31*(5–6), 329–337. https://doi.org/doi:10.1007/BF01544592

Hanafy, I., Clervoy, L., & Brenot, P. (2016). Exhibitionists, so much inhibition. *Sexologies: European Journal of Sexology and Sexual Health/Revue Européenne de Sexologie et de Santé Sexuelle, 25*(4), e61–e63. https://doi.org/10.1016/j.sexol.2016.03.008

Herodotus (1998). *The histories* (Trans. R. Waterfield). Oxford University Press.

Holtzman, D., & Kulish, N. (2012). Female exhibitionism: Identification, competition and camaraderie. *The International Journal of Psychoanalysis, 93*(2), 271–292. https://doi-org.ez.lib.jjay.cuny.edu/10.1111/j.1745-8315.2011.00510.x

Hopkins, T. A., Green, B. A., Carnes, P. J., & Campling, S. (2016). Varieties of intrusion: Exhibitionism and voyeurism. *Sexual Addiction & Compulsivity, 23*(1), 4–33. https://doi.org/10.1080/10720162.2015.1095138

Janssen, D. F. (2018). "Voyeuristic disorder": Etymological and historical note. *Archives of Sexual Behavior, 47*(5), 1–5. https://doi-org.ez.lib.jjay.cuny.edu/10.1007/s10508-018-1199-2

Kafka, M. P., & Hennen, J. (1999). The paraphilia-related disorders: An empirical investigation of nonparaphilic hypersexuality disorders in 206 outpatient males. *Journal of Sex and Marital Therapy, 25*(4), 305–319. https://doi.org/10.1080/00926239908404008

Kafka, M. P., & Hennen, J. (2002). A DSM-IV Axis I comorbidity study of males (n = 120) with paraphilias and paraphilia related disorders. *Sexual Abuse: A Journal of Research and Treatment, 14*(4), 349–366. https://doi.org/10.1023/A:1020007004436

Kafka, M. P., & Prentky, R. (1992). A comparative study of nonparaphilic sexual addictions and paraphilias in men. *Journal of Clinical Psychiatry, 53*(10), 345–350.

Kaplan, M. S., & Krueger, R. B. (1997). Voyeurism: Psychopathology and theory. In D. R. Laws & W. O'Donohue (Eds.), *Sexual deviance: Theory, assessment, and treatment* (pp. 297–310). Guilford Press.

Kaylor, L., & Jeglic, E. (2018). Exhibitionists. In O'Donohue (Ed.), *Handbook of sexual assault and sexual assault prevention* (pp. 745–760). Springer.

Kaylor, L., Jeglic, E., & Collins, C. (2016). Examining the impact of technology on exhibitionistic behavior. *Deviant Behavior, 37*(10), 1152–1162. http://doi.org/10.1080/01639625.2016.1169828

Krafft-Ebing, R. V. (1965). *Psychopathia sexualis* (12th ed.). Stein & Day. (Original work published in 1886).

Kutchinsky, B. (1976). Deviance and criminality: The case of voyeur in a peeper's paradise. *Diseases of the Nervous System, 37*(3), 145–151.

Lalumière, M. L., Harris, G. H., Quinsey, V. L., & Rice, M. E. (2005). *The causes of rape: Understanding individual differences in male propensity for sexual aggression.* American Psychological Association.

Lang, R. A., Langevin, R., Checkley, K. L., & Pugh, G. (1987). Genital exhibitionism: Courtship disorder or narcissism? *Canadian Journal of Behavioural Science, 19*(2), 216–232. https://doi.org/10.1037/h0080011

Långström, N. (2010). The DSM diagnostic criteria for exhibitionism, voyeurism, and frotteurism. *Archives of Sexual Behavior, 39*(2), 317–324. https://doi-org.ez.lib.jjay.cuny.edu/10.1007/s10508-009-9577-4

Långström, N., & Seto, M. (2006). Exhibitionism and voyeuristic behavior in a Swedish national population survey. *Archives of Sexual Behavior, 35*(4), 427–435. https://doi.org/10.1007/s10508-006-9042-6

Långström, N., & Zucker, K. J. (2005). Transvestic fetishism in the general population: Prevalence and correlates. *Journal of Sex and Marital Therapy, 31*(2), 87–95. https://doi.org/10.1080/00926230590477934

Lee, J. K. P., Pattison, P., Jackson, H. J., & Ward, T. (2001). The general, common, and specific features of psychopathology for different types of paraphilias. *Criminal Justice and Behavior, 28*(2), 227–256. https://journals-sagepub-com.ez.lib.jjay.cuny.edu/doi/pdf/10.1177/0093854801028002005

Leitenberg, H., & Henning, K. (1995). Sexual fantasy. *Psychological Bulletin, 117*(3), 469–496. https://pdfs.semanticscholar.org/0cec/591a75b65e160824d4b0b65a6e4f27431481.pdf

Longo, R. E., & Groth, A. N. (1983). Juvenile sexual offenses in the histories of adult rapists and child molesters. *International Journal of Offender Therapy and Comparative Criminology, 27*(2), 150–155. https://journals-sagepub-com.ez.lib.jjay.cuny.edu/doi/pdf/10.1177/0306624X8302700207

Longo, R. E., & McFadin, J. B. (1981). Sexually inappropriate behavior: Development in the sexual offender. *Law and Order Magazine, 29*(12), 21–23.

MacPherson, G. J. (2003). Predicting escalation in sexually violent recidivism: Use of the SVR-20 and PCL:SV to predict outcome with noncontact recidivists and contact recidivists. *Journal of Forensic Psychiatry & Psychology, 14*(3), 615–627. https://www.tandfonline.com/doi/abs/10.1080/14789940310001615470

Mathis, J. L. (1972). Voyeurism. In *Clear thinking about sexual deviations* (pp. 41–52). Nelson-Hall Company.

McGrath, R. J. (1991). Sex-offender risk assessment and disposition planning: A review of empirical and clinical findings. *International Journal of Offender Therapy and Comparative Criminology, 35*(4), 328–350. https://journals-sagepub-com.ez.lib.jjay.cuny.edu/doi/pdf/10.1177/0306624X9103500407

McGuire, R. J., Carlisle, J. U., & Young, B. G. (1964). Sexual deviations as conditioned behaviour: A hypothesis. *Behaviour Research and Therapy, 2*(2–4), 185–190. https://doi.org/10.1016/0005-7967(64)90014-2

McNally, M. R., & Fremouw, W. J. (2014). Examining risk of escalation: A critical review of the exhibitionistic behavior literature. *Aggression and Violent Behavior, 19*(5), 474–485. https://doi.org/10.1016/j.avb.2014.07.001

Mester, H. (1984). Phenomenology and history of the origin of exhibitionism. *Forensic and Neurological Psychiatry, 52*(7), 237–249. https://doi.org/10.1055/s-2007-1002022

Metzl, J. M. (2004). Voyeur nation? Changing definitions of voyeurism, 1950–2004. *Harvard Review of Psychiatry, 12*(2), 127–131. http://citeseerx.ist.psu.edu/viewdoc/download?doi=10.1.1.630.5864&rep=rep1&type=pdf

Meyer, J. K. (1995). Paraphilias. In H. I. Kaplan & B. J. Sadock (Eds.), *Comprehensive textbook of psychiatry IV* (pp. 1334–1347).

Mohr, J. W., Turner, E. R., & Ball, R. B. (1962). Exhibitionism and pedophilia. *Corrective Psychiatry & Journal of Social Therapy, 8*(4), 172–186.

Morin, J., & Levenson, J. (2008). Exhibitionism: Assessment and treatment. In D. R. Laws & W. T. O'Donohue (Eds.), *Sexual deviance: Theory, assessment, and treatment* (2nd ed., pp. 76–107). Guilford Press.

Murphy, W., & Page, I. (2008). Exhibitionism: Psychopathology and theory. In D. R. Laws & W. T. O'Donohue (Eds.), *Sexual deviance: Theory, assessment, and treatment* (2nd ed., pp. 61–75). Guilford Press.

Perez, E., Prokupecz, S., & Cohen, T. (2014). More than 90 people nabbed in global hacker crackdown. CNN Justice. http://www.cnn.com/2014/05/19/justice/us-global-hacker-crackdown/index.html?hpt=hp_t1

Petri, H. (1969). Exhibitionism: Theoretical and social aspects and treatment with antiandrogens. *Nervenarzt, 40*(5), 220–228.

Price, M., Gutheil, T. G., Commons, M. L., Kafka, M. P., & Dodd-Kimmey, S. (2001). Telephone scatologia: Comorbidity and theories of etiology. *Psychiatric Annals, 31*(4), 226–232. https://doi-org.ez.lib.jjay.cuny.edu/10.3928/0048-5713-20010401-03

Price, M., Kafka, M., Commons, M. L., Gutheil, T. G., & Simpson, W. (2002). Telephone scatological comorbidity with other paraphilias and paraphilia-related disorders. *International*

Journal of Law and Psychiatry, 25(1), 37–49. https://www.dareassociation.org/documents/Telephone%20scatologia2002.pdf
Quinsey, V. L., Skilling, T. A., Lalumière, M. L., & Craig, W. M. (2004). *Juvenile delinquency: Understanding the origins of individual differences*. American Psychological Association.
Rabinowitz-Greenberg, S. R., Firestone, P., Bradford, J. M., & Greenberg, D. M. (2002). Prediction of recidivism in exhibitionists: Psychological, phallometric, and offense factors. *Sexual Abuse: Journal of Research and Treatment, 14*(4), 329–347. https://doi.org/10.1023/A:1019921720366
Raymond, N. C., Coleman, E., Ohlerking, F., Christenson, G. A., & Miner, M. M. (1999). Psychiatric comorbidity in pedophilic sex offenders. *American Journal of Psychiatry, 156*(5), 786–788. https://ajp-psychiatryonline-org.ez.lib.jjay.cuny.edu/doi/pdfplus/10.1176/ajp.156.5.786
Rhodes, G., Simmons, L. W., & Peters, M. (2005). Attractiveness and sexual behavior: Does attractiveness enhance mating success? *Evolution and Human Behavior, 26*(2), 186–201. https://doi.org/10.1016/j.evolhumbehav.2004.08.014
Rickles, N. K. (1955). Exhibitionism. *Journal of Social Therapy, 1*, 168–181.
Rooth, F. G. (1973). Exhibitionism, sexual violence, and paedophilia. *British Journal of Psychiatry, 122*(6), 705–710. https://doi-org.ez.lib.jjay.cuny.edu/10.1192/bjp.122.6.705
Rye, B. J., & Meaney, G. J. (2007). Voyeurism: It is good as long as we do not get caught. *International Journal of Sexual Health, 19*(1), 47–56. https://doi.org/10.1300/J514v19n01_06
Sadhu, J. M. (2012). Sexting: The impact of a cultural phenomenon on psychiatric practice. *Academic Psychiatry, 36*(1), 76–81. https://doi-org.ez.lib.jjay.cuny.edu/10.1176/appi.ap.10100146
Schneider, R. D. (1982). Exhibitionism: An exclusively male deviation? *International Journal of Offender Therapy and Comparative Criminology, 26*(2), 173–176. https://doi.org/10.1177/0306624X8202600210
Seto, M. C., & Barbaree, H. E. (1997). Sexual aggression as antisocial behavior: A developmental model. In D. Stoff, J. Breiling, & J. D. Maser (Eds.), *Handbook of antisocial behavior* (pp. 524–533). Wiley.
Smith, R. S. (1976). Voyeurism: A review of literature. *Archives of Sexual Behavior, 5*(6), 585–608. https://doi.org/10.1007/BF01541221
Sophos Press Release. (2008). *Four years jail for voyeur hacker who spied via webcam*. http://www.sophos.com/en-us/press-office/press-releases/2008/08/webcam.aspx
Stalking Resource Center. (2003). *In partnership with the national center for victims of crime*. New frontiers of stalking-Video voyeurism. National Center for Victims of Crime. http://www.victimsofcrime.org/docs/src/new-frontiers-of-stalking—video-voyeurism.pdf?sfvrsn=2
Stekel, W. (1952). *Patterns of psychosexual infantilism*. Liveright.
Sugarman, P., Dumughn, C., Saad, K., Hinder, S., & Bluglass, R. (1994). Dangerousness in exhibitionists. *Rurnal of Forensic Psychiatry, 5*(2), 287–296. https://www-tandfonline-com.ez.lib.jjay.cuny.edu/doi/abs/10.1080/09585189408412299
Swindell, S., Stroebel, S. S., O'Keefe, S. L., Beard, K. W., Robinett, S. R., & Kommor, M. J. (2011). Correlates of exhibition-like experiences in childhood and adolescence: A model for development of exhibitionism in heterosexual males. *Sexual Addiction & Compulsivity, 18*(3), 135–156. https://doi.org/10.1080/10720162.2011.593432
Thompson, E. H., & Pleck, J. H. (1986). The structure of male role norms. *American Behavioral Scientist, 29*(5), 531–543. https://journals-sagepub-com.ez.lib.jjay.cuny.edu/doi/pdf/10.1177/000276486029005003

Weber, C. (2013). *Miss Teen USA extortion plot foiled, Suspect arrested.* Huffpost. http://www.huffingtonpost.com/2013/09/26/miss-teen-usa-exortortion_n_3997828.html
World Health Organization. (1992). International classification of diseases and related health problems (10th rev., ICD-10). Author.
Zinni, M. (2012). *Hackers gain access to homes through webcams.* Fox 8. http://fox8.com/2012/05/09/hackers-gain-access-to-homes-through-webcams

12

Sexual Sadism and Offending

Tamsin Higgs[1], Jean Proulx[2], Alexandre Gauthier[2], Etienne Garant[2], and Jonathan James[3]

[1] *Department of psychology, University of Montreal, Quebec, Canada*
[2] *School of criminology, University of Montreal, Quebec, Canada*
[3] *Department of psychology, University of Quebec at Three Rivers, Canada*

Introduction

With nearly 35 million print and electronic copies sold in the United States alone by the end of 2019, E. L. James's *Fifty shades* ... erotic novel series topped the list of best-selling books for the last decade (NPD Group, 2019). Notwithstanding the question of the population representativeness of *Fifty shades* ... consumers, is there a reasonable inference to be made that most people indulge at least occasionally in sexual fantasies that might be described as somewhat risqué, atypical—or, even, deviant? Maybe so, according to general population survey data revealing paraphilic (i.e., atypical sexual interests; American Psychiatric Association, 2013) content in the sexual fantasies disclosed by survey respondents in Germany (367 men aged 40 to 79 years; Ahlers et al., 2011) and Canada (717 men and 799 women aged 18 to 77 years; Joyal & Carpentier, 2017). Paradoxically, of the "atypical" sexual fantasies revealed in the two surveys, those including voyeurism and fetishism were relatively common (in the male general population, 35–60% and 30–40%, respectively). Fantasies with masochistic or sadistic content were more atypical, in that they were reported to be experienced by fewer people, although not so infrequently that they may be called rare (16–19% and 9–22% respectively). These findings suggest that deviancy, including sexual sadism, is more present in the sexual fantasy life of the general population than initially estimated by the scientific community. Consequently, this chapter examines sexual sadism as a non-harmful sexual practice (i.e., when acting upon fantasies does not violate the human rights of another individual), in contrast to sadistic sexual offending. Understanding when, how, and why sexual sadism is enacted against a victim rather than a consenting partner is central to the question of the role of sadism in sexual offending.

BDSM Subculture and Practitioners

> *Don't torture yourself. That's my job.*
> Morticia to Gomez, in *The Addams Family* (Wilson et al., 1991)

Prevalence and Definition of BDSM

BDSM (bondage-discipline, dominance-submission, sadism, masochism) can be defined as "physical, psychological and sexual role-play involving power exchange between consensual participants" (De Neef et al., 2019, p. 129), during a scene, which may be defined as a period of

Sexual Deviance: Understanding and Managing Deviant Sexual Interests and Paraphilic Disorders,
First Edition. Edited by Leam A. Craig and Ross M. Bartels.
© 2021 John Wiley & Sons, Ltd. Published 2021 by John Wiley & Sons, Ltd.

time during which agreed-upon activities are enacted (Pitagora, 2013). Explicit consent is a fundamental rule of BDSM interactions, even if there is a dominant and a submissive partner. Alison et al. (2001) identified four clusters of BDSM activities: (1) pain play, such as spanking and caning; (2) humiliation (e.g., verbal abasement); (3) physical restriction (e.g., bondage); and (4) hypermasculinity (e.g., anilingus). Finally, a BDSM scene may or may not include penetrative sexual behaviors (Pitagora, 2013).

While a significant percentage of adult men in the general population have sadistic sexual fantasies, only some of them act on these fantasies and get involved in BDSM activities. In fact, the prevalence rates of men who self-identify as BDSM practitioners varies between 2.2% and 7.6% (De Neef et al., 2019). In addition, while BDSM practitioners often engage in sexually sadistic activities (e.g., body torture: 46.8%; humiliation: 34.6%), their sexual repertoire is not limited to sexual sadism (Connoly, 2006; Stiles & Clark, 2011; Taylor & Ussher, 2001).

Motivations in BDSM Practitioners

Although physical and psychological pain seems to be paramount in BDSM activities, it is the exertion of power that is the genuine essence of the scene (Cross & Matheson, 2006; Wismeijer & Van Assen, 2013). However, the assumption that it is the dominant participant who has all the power is quite open to question. Indeed, the use by submissives of a safe word, which allows them to interrupt the role play when they want, may be considered the ultimate power in BDSM activities (Pitagora, 2013). In addition, in contrast to the presupposition that in BDSM activities the dominant controls the scene to service their own pleasure, there is a "tendency for dominants to focus on the pleasure of their partner, and submissives to focus on their own pleasure" (Pitagora, 2013, p. 33).

In an extensive investigation of BDSM subculture, Stiles and Clark (2011) highlighted "sacrifice and delights" associated with this lifestyle. Their study is based on 73 BDSM practitioners (31 dominants, 42 submissives). They used a qualitative methodology to understand the perspectives of participants in BDSM activities. Although social concealment is the rule for a majority of BDSM participants, since such activities tend to be socially perceived as deviant/pathological, secrecy also has its advantages. First, there is a sense of community (support, companionship) between those involved in a BDSM club or network. Furthermore, there is the "pleasure of concealing secrets from outsiders" (p. 177). Apart from secrecy, BDSM participants experience "limitless opportunities for self-expression and reinvention" (p. 183) and are able to "freely and openly discuss sex" (p. 184). In fact, being part of a BDSM subculture favors, in some participants, the development of a positive social and personal identity. Briefly, the social experience of BDSM practitioners is positive in several ways that go far beyond mere sexual pleasure.

Psychosocial Profile of BDSM Practitioners

Contrary to what may be expected, in BDSM practitioners sexism and acceptance of rape myths is particularly low (Klement et al., 2017). That being so, what kind of person engages in behaviors that share several similarities with those of sadistic sexual aggressors? To answer this question, studies about the psychosocial characteristics of BDSM practitioners are presented here. Specifically, we focus on male BDSM practitioners who assume a dominant role, because this subgroup is of greatest interest if we are ultimately concerned with sadistic sexual offending, which most frequently involves the subjugation of a victim by a male perpetrator.

The sociodemographic profile of male BDSM practitioners indicates that these men are well adapted socially (De Neef et al., 2019). A high proportion (70.1%) of BDSM practitioners have a university degree (Wismeijer & Van Assen, 2013). In addition, the intensity of involvement in BDSM practices is positively correlated with the level of education (Coppens et al., 2020). Finally, a majority (67.7%) of BDSM practitioners work in professional fields (Connoly, 2006).

In terms of relationships, a significant proportion of BDSM practitioners are involved in a stable intimate relationship (Connoly, 2006; Landgraf et al., 2018). Furthermore, they are secure in their relationship and not sensitive to rejection (Wismeijer & Van Assen, 2013). Also, male BDSM practitioners who assume a dominant role have a positive view of their attractiveness (Jozifkova & Kolackova, 2017).

Regarding psychopathology in male BDSM practitioners, most studies have failed to find clinically significant differences between them and non-BDSM practitioners (Connoly, 2006; Cross & Matheson, 2006; Wismeijer & Van Assen, 2013). Connoly (2006) investigated major mental disorders as well as personality disorders in a sample of 132 self-identified BDSM practitioners (73 males, 56 females, 3 non-binary individuals). BDSM practitioners presented non-pathological scores on psychometric measures of personality characteristics (MCMI-III, Millon et al., 1997; MMPI-2; Butcher et al., 2001) and of depression (BDI-II, Beck et al., 1996), and anxiety (BAI, Beck & Steer, 1993)—lower, in fact, than normative samples. Regarding post-traumatic stress disorder, only 1.7% of participants received a clinically significant score on the Posttraumatic Stress Diagnostic Scale (Foa, 1995). Furthermore, none of the participants had a clinically significant score on the sadistic scale of the MCMI-III. However, 10.5% of them had a clinically significant score on the dominance scale of the MMPI-2. Finally, the only personality disorder characteristics (scores of 75 or greater on the MCMI-III scales) that were relatively prevalent were narcissistic (30.2%) and histrionic (19.8%). These results, however, do not necessarily indicate psychopathology, since moderate scores on the narcissistic and histrionic scales may indicate personality strengths and adaptative traits (Millon et al., 1997).

Moving beyond psychopathologies, Wismeijer and Van Assen (2013) carried out an important study on the psychological characteristics of BDSM practitioners. A total of 902 BDSM practitioners (464 males, 438 females) and 434 non-BDSM control participants (129 males, 305 females) were included. Among the BDSM practitioners, 48.3% of men were dominant, as opposed to 8.0% of women. With regard to attachment characteristics, psychometric assessment indicated that the BDSM-dominants felt more secure in intimate relationships than BDSM-submissives and the non-BDSM control participants. Their personality traits were assessed using Costa and McCrae's (Costa & McCrae, 1992) NEO Five Factor Inventory. BDSM-dominants scored higher than the non-BDSM control participants on openness to experience (e.g., creativity, curiosity) and conscientiousness (e.g., organization, competence, ambition). In addition, the BDSM-dominants scored lower than the control participants on neuroticism (e.g., depression, anxiety, low self-esteem) and agreeableness (e.g., altruism, credulity, modesty). The BDSM-dominants scores for extraversion did not differ from those of the non-BDSM control participants. Finally, on a measure of subjective wellbeing, the BDSM-dominants scored higher than the non-BDSM control participants. In brief, the results from this study "suggest that BDSM practitioners are characterized by greater psychological and interpersonal strength and autonomy, rather than by psychological maladaptive characteristics" (Wismeijer & Van Assen, 2013, p. 1949). Consequently, BDSM role play may be considered a recreational activity that favors self-actualization, rather than a pathological self-destructive activity. Thus, the logical question is: Do sadistic sexual aggressors share the positive psychological profile and socially adequate lifestyle seen in BDSM-dominants?

Sadistic Sexual Aggressors

Forensic Evaluation of Sexual Sadism and Clinical Case Formulation

Identifying objective criteria that reliably capture sadistic drives as distinct from other kinds of motivation for sexual aggression has proved highly problematic (Knight et al., 1994). Sexual arousal and the prominence of sexual gratification within offense scripts are not only implicit—meaning that they must often be inferred in the absence of access to the perpetrator's internal world—but also idiosyncratic, meaning that the same objectively observable events can have different subjective significance: one man's mistake is another's game[1]. Thus, while it is accepted that sexual sadism entails the physically painful and/or psychological subjugation of the victim (Brittain, 1970; Gratzer & Bradford, 1995; Groth & Birnbaum, 1979; Proulx et al., 2006; Seto & Kuban, 1996), more specific defining features are still being debated (Marshall & Kennedy, 2003). In addition, cruelty without sexual connotation should not be confounded with sadism. Inflicting deliberate harm is an insufficient condition, regardless of the pain and/or humiliation experienced by the victim, for viewing someone as a sexual sadist; rather, it is the victim's suffering that provides the perpetrator of a sadistic offense with feedback eliciting an eroticized response.

Despite the inherent difficulties in the reliable identification of sexually sadistic behavior in the context of a criminal offense, the Diagnostic and Statistical Manual of Mental Disorders (DSM-5; American Psychiatric Association, 2013) recommends diagnosis of sexual sadism disorder when two conditions are met: (1) the individual discloses or recurrent behavior indicates sadistic sexual interest, meaning persistent "sexual arousal from the physical or psychological suffering of another person" (p. 695), which is "greater or equal to normophilic sexual interests" (p. 685); and (2) these sexual interests have been experienced as distressing, caused impairment in important areas of functioning, or have been acted on with a nonconsenting person. The World Health Organization's International Classification of Diseases uses comparable diagnostic criteria to define its coercive sexual sadism disorder (ICD-11; World Health Organization, 2018).

Whether or not sadism represents a taxonomic phenomenon, as categorical diagnosis assumes, remains an empirical question. Current hypotheses favor a dimensional construction (Longpré, Guay, Knight et al., 2018; Wollert & Frances, 2017), or possibly a trichotomous latent structure whereby diagnostic categories (paraphilic disorder being present or absent) would be valid, but with a third taxon representing non-preferential paraphilic sexual interest (McPhail, 2020). Furthermore, assessors are often limited to criminal-event information and self-reports and are therefore not necessarily able to be confident that a lack of evidence to satisfy DSM or ICD criteria precludes the presence of sadism. Partly in response to general uncertainty of clinical diagnoses in the forensic domain (Mokros et al., 2018) and the variability of assessor agreement on sexual sadism in particular (Nitschke et al., 2013), the Sexual Sadism Scale (SeSaS; Nitschke et al., 2009) was developed. The SeSaS is a structured professional judgment measure focusing on offense-related behavioral elements, comprising one part consisting of 11 items coded for sexually sadistic crime-scene behaviors (including index offense and previous offenses), and a second part consisting of three items relating to offense planning and previous sadistic behavior (Mokros et al., 2014). The use of the SeSaS in the evaluation of forensically relevant sexual sadism offers advantages, by virtue of its scoring procedure, which focuses on behavioral evidence available from the crime scene, and its psychometric properties that suggest that it captures moderate to severe levels of the latent trait of sexual sadism (Stefanska et al., 2019).

Crucially, evaluation in forensic-clinical practice is concerned with the relevance of sexual sadism—whether considered in terms of a categorical diagnosis or a dimensional extremity—to case formulation and subsequent psychological intervention and/or other types of risk management. This requires competency in assessment approaches, but also an evidence-based understanding of the functional role of sadism in specific forms of sexual offending. First, a limitation in the available evidence base must be addressed. Several studies aiming to examine the perpetrators of sadistic sexual offenses and their crimes conflate sadism with a particular type of offending, notably sexual murder and, even more so, serial sexual killing. Sadism is a factor that may favor seriality in sexual murder (James & Proulx, 2014), but it should be noted that very few sexual murderers—approximately 2%—are serial killers (Proulx, Cusson et al., 2007). Indeed, sexual murder is a broad term that captures all homicide where a sexual element may be identified due to: the victim's body being found partially or entirely naked, or evidence of sexual activity including touching the victim's genitals, penetration of the victim vaginally, anally or orally, insertion of foreign objects, mutilation of genitals, or other sexually exploitative activities or sexual contact (Meloy, 2000; Ressler et al., 1988), which may occur at any or all stages before, during, or after the killing, and in some cases evidence of sexual activity might be found near to the victim's body (Meloy et al., 1994; Schlesinger, 2007), or may not be overtly available but sexual motivations may be disclosed by the perpetrator or identified by professionals involved in the case (Clarke & Carter, 2000). Clearly, this definition encompasses both sadistic and non-sadistic crimes. Therefore, an act that may on the surface appear sadistic, as is a common misperception when presented with the crude facts of a crime such as sexual murder, is not necessarily driven by sexual sadism.

Prevalence of Sexual Sadism Among Perpetrators of Sexual Offenses

Sexual Murderers with Adult Victims

Whilst the majority of sexual murderers are driven to kill either by grievance and/or an excessively aggressive response style, rather than sexual sadism, or by situational factors or instrumental motives such as detection avoidance (preventing the victim from being able to identify the perpetrator), a systematic review of the literature concluded that for a certain type of offender there is a functional role of the act of killing which is related to sexual deviancy—which may or may not equate to sexual sadism (Higgs, Carter et al., 2017). Researchers discussing subtypes of sexual murderers tend to refer to sadistic sexual murder (also, lust murder, erotophonophilia, or compulsive murder, all essentially referring to the same phenomenon), due to greater scores or greater frequencies on the researchers' chosen measure of sadism for one group compared to other groups identified. It may be accurate to consider that sadism characterizes this particular type of sexual murder, but given the difficulties associated with the reliable identification of sexual sadism, the issue can be deconstructed: For these perpetrators, taking a life provides a source of sexual stimulation, be it from the act itself, or the infliction of non-fatal injuries during the offending process, or from other planned or opportunistic acts that are enabled through killing, such as post mortem sexual acts. In other words, the act of murder is inherently sexualized; hence, within the overarching term "sexual murder," "Sexualized murder" refers to cases in which killing is functionally related to the sexual element of the offense, while "grievance murder" is driven by angry schemata, and "rape murder" means exactly that—situationally or instrumentally driven fatal violence subsequent to sexual assault (Higgs, Carter et al., 2017). Not all perpetrators of sexualized murders meet DSM or ICD diagnostic criteria for sexual sadism, nor do they necessarily score highly on measures such as the SeSaS, but the conceptualization corresponds closely to the integral features of sexual sadism, and a perpetrator assessed as having sexual sadism disorder is likely to have committed a sexualized murder rather than a grievance or rape murder. Concordantly, sexual sadism is typically found in one-third of all sexual murderers (Briken et al., 2005; Geberth & Turco, 1997; Stefanska et al., 2019), whereas when evidence from the criminal investigation indicates that a murder was indirectly sexual—such as when a conflict arises after consensual sex, or when killing is an instrumental act, or in any other scenario in which violence is not fused with sexual arousal—there is a low probability of finding evidence for sexual sadism when evaluating the perpetrator (Stefanska et al., 2017).

Our understanding of the prevalence and role of sexual sadism in sexual murder relies on research focused on adult male perpetrators and adult female victims, this being the context of most cases of sexual murder (James & Proulx, 2014). We may not glean from the limited empirical literature providing insight into male sexual murder victimization the proportion of these crimes carried out by sexually sadistic perpetrators. However, similarities have been found between male sexual murderers of men and male sexual murderers of women, in that both commit sexualized murders (Beauregard & Proulx, 2007; Geberth, 1996). That is, there is evidence of sexual sadism underlying sexual murder perpetrated against adult men but, as with sexual murder perpetrated against women, there are circumstances of male sexual-murder victimization that are better explained by excessive use of force to commit a sexual assault, violence in reaction to a triggering event occurring during or after sex with a consenting partner or sex worker, or instrumental use of fatal violence.

Sexual Murderers with Child Victims

Sexual sadism was found in one sample of sexual murderers of children at an equal rate to that of a comparison sample of sexual murderers of women (37.1% and 32%, respectively; Spehr et al., 2010), but in only 16.7% of another sample of sexual murderers of children compared to 51.3% of the adult-victim comparison sample (Proulx et al., 2018); these being the only two studies comparing sexual murderers of children to sexual murderers of women, using a measure of sexual sadism. Possibly, the results reported by Spehr and colleagues diverge from those of Proulx and colleagues due to different sample construction. Spehr and colleagues defined children as younger than 18 years, and included murderers with more than one victim, whereas Proulx and colleagues defined children as younger than 14 and excluded murderers with more than one victim. Despite the differences between these studies, their results, together with those of the few other relevant studies published (Firestone et al., 1998, 2000; Langevin, 2006), suggest that sexual sadism is relatively rare among sexual murderers of children. Instead, these offenders are better characterized, as a group, by other paraphilic disorders, particularly pedophilia, and psychopathy.

Non-homicide Sexual Aggressors of Women

Sexual aggressors who have not killed do not differ significantly from sexual murderers in terms of developmental, personality, and mental health factors, and overall criminality (Stefanska et al., 2016). As such, non-homicide sexual aggressors and sexual murderers can be understood by addressing comparable questions in the process of case conceptualization. Indeed, the established typology of sexual murderers mirrors the principal empirically derived types of sexual aggression, notwithstanding fatality. Knight and Prentky's (1990) rapist typology describes the primary motivation of perpetrators as either pervasively angry (generalized anger), vindictive (anger directed specifically toward women), opportunistic (impulsive prioritization of own needs over others'), or sexual—whereby sexual aggression serves to gratify sexual fantasies, these being sadistic for a subgroup of offenders. Proulx and Beauregard (2009, 2014) found three offense pathways in their typology: angry, opportunistic, and sadistic. The sadistic subgroup represented 27% of the sample, in line with the rate of sexual sadism found in most samples of sexual murderers. Within this sample, 60% of the sadistic offenders had killed their victim compared to 40% of the angry offenders and none of the opportunistic ones. However, the prevalence of sexual sadism among sexual offenders is arguably impossible to ascertain, due to the different evaluation methods employed across studies, poor reliability in diagnostic systems, and important variation in sampling strategies. As an illustration, estimates vary from 2% to 5% (Quinsey et al., 1981) to 80% (MacCulloch et al., 1983).

Female Sexual Aggressors

Although very little data is available given the overall lower occurrence of female-perpetrated sexual offending (estimates suggest that around 12% of all perpetrators of sexual offenses are female; Cortoni, 2018), Pflugradt and Allen (2013) found the presence of sexual sadism in seven of their sample of 90 convicted female sexual offenders. Behavioral markers seemed to be similar to those validated for male offenders, in that the SeSaS identified sexual sadism in these female offenders. However, the relative frequency of almost all SeSaS items was significantly lower in the female sample than previously found in male samples and non-significantly different items between male and female samples simply related to characteristics that had low relative frequency among men as well as among women (keeping trophies, mutilation of sexual parts of the victim's body, and insertion of objects into bodily orifices). While a larger female sample would be needed to meaningfully analyze the relative frequencies of behavioral indicators, there is likely gender-specificity in the expression of sexual sadism just as there is in other psycho-criminological phenomena: psychopathy manifests in gender-specific ways (Forouzan & Cooke, 2005) and, more generally, a gendered approach to risk assessment and interventions is recommended (Marshall & Miller, 2018). Indeed, qualitative research indicates that in addition to physical torture and humiliation, female sexual sadists favor certain psychological strategies, such as nurturing victims—who are usually children or adolescents in relation to whom the female offender has a caregiver role—to foster emotional dependence which facilitates control (Pflugradt & Allen, 2012). In addition, according to the same research, female perpetrators often manipulate others to inflict harm (i.e., they act with a co-offender rather than typically offending alone), such that they are able to gain gratification vicariously.

Descriptive Studies of Sadistic Sexual Aggressors

This part of this chapter will focus on male sadistic sexual aggressors against women, since studies on those having adult male (Beauregard & Proulx, 2007) or child victims (Proulx et al., 2018; Spehr et al., 2010) are too rare. Furthermore, the expression and the meaning of sadistic behaviors may be different in sexual aggressors against women than in those having adult men or child victims.

Based on clinical observations, Brittain (1970) presented a portrait of the sadistic sexual murderer. During their childhood, these aggressors were victimized by their parents, in the form of overprotective and controlling behaviors by the mother and excessive discipline by the father. Following these abuses, sexual sadists withdraw from social interaction and develop low self-esteem. As adults, they are shy and socially isolated, and have low self-esteem, a variety of paraphilias (e.g., exhibitionism, voyeurism), and a perception of themselves as sexually incompetent. In addition, they have an intense fantasy world, in which they torture and humiliate women in a sexual context. These fantasies constitute the template for their future sexual aggression.

Following Brittain's seminal paper, MacCulloch and colleagues (1983) carried out a descriptive study based on a sample of 13 sadistic sexual aggressors. As in Brittain's study, their participants reported low self-esteem and social isolation in both childhood and adulthood. Furthermore, they reported sadistic sexual fantasies that became increasingly violent, presumably as a result of habituation. According to MacCulloch et al., these fantasies, as well as actual sexual aggression, compensate for the paucity of the emotional gratification in their social and socio-sexual interactions with peers.

In another descriptive study based on a sample of 34 sadistic sexual aggressors (including 20 sexual murderers), Dietz and colleagues (Dietz et al., 1990; Warren et al., 1996) reported a slightly different portrait for this type of offender. In fact, as in Brittain's paper, the sadistic sexual aggressors reported sadistic sexual fantasies, but—unlike Brittain's sample—reported no other paraphilias. In addition, a majority of them were well integrated into society—they had a job and were socially active and in an intimate relationship. However, half of them had problems with alcohol and drugs.

These three studies provide a relatively consistent portrait of the sadistic sexual aggressor. He is a man who is socially isolated, although he may appear to be a good citizen. In addition, he has low self-esteem and he indulges in deviant-sadistic sexual fantasies. The presence of other paraphilias (e.g., exhibitionism, voyeurism) is not as well established. Finally, he is also likely to be an alcohol and drug user.

Comparative Studies of Sadistic Sexual Aggressors

Langevin et al. (1985) carried out the first empirical study in which sadistic sexual aggressors ($N = 9$) were compared to non-sadistic sexual aggressors ($N = 11$), and to non-sexual and non-violent offenders ($N = 20$). Surprisingly, the three groups did not differ in their phallometric responses (i.e. rape index). These results contrast with those of Proulx (2001) who reported higher rape indexes in sadistic sexual aggressors against women compared to angry or opportunistic offenders. With regard to non-deviant activities, sadistic aggressors had less sexual experience and knowledge that did non-sadistic ones. Furthermore, they perceived themselves to be sexually incompetent and were not at ease in socio-sexual contexts. Finally, although none of the sadistic sexual aggressors showed a psychopathic personality profile, they reported anger toward women.

In another study, Gratzer and Bradford (1995) compared 28 sadistic sexual aggressors (including 20 sexual murderers) to 29 non-sadistic sexual aggressors (including 14 sexual murderers). During childhood, sadistic aggressors were more likely to have been physically abused than non-sadistic ones. As adults, sadistic aggressors reported paraphilias (i.e., transvestism, exhibitionism, voyeurism) more frequently than did non-sadistic ones. Furthermore, a large proportion of sadistic offenders (86%) were diagnosed with antisocial personality disorder

(DSM-III-R criteria). Finally, the modus operandi of sadistic offenders included premeditation and torture of the victims.

Marshall et al. (2002) carried out a comparative study whose results contrast with those from previous studies. Participants in this study were sadistic sexual aggressors (*N* = 41), and non-sadistic sexual aggressors (*N* = 18). In both groups, a quarter of the offenders were sexual murderers. In phallometric assessments a lower proportion of sadistic offenders (17.1%) than nonsadistic ones (44.4%) presented a rape index suggesting a sexual preference for a rape with a high level of physical coercion. Nevertheless, murderous fantasies were only reported in sadistic aggressors (41.5%). With regard to personality disorders, both groups presented antisocial disorder (sadistic: 51.2%; non-sadistic: 66.7%), but only non-sadistic offenders were diagnosed with other personality disorders. Finally, the modus operandi of non-sadistic offenders was more likely to include torture and striking the victims. A possible explanation for some of these unexpected results may be related to the nature of their sample, namely sexual aggressors for whom a psychiatric assessment was conducted. This is uncommon in the Canadian judicial system where this study took place and may indicate that the sample characteristics differed in important ways compared to the samples used in other studies.

Following cluster analysis of modus operandi characteristics of non-serial sexual murderers of women (*N* = 36), Beauregard and Proulx (2002) identified two profiles, which they labeled sadistic (*N* = 16) and angry (*N* = 20). The modus operandi of the murderers in the sadistic profile was more likely than that of non-sadistic murderers to include premeditation (81% vs 5%), humiliation (81% vs 11%), mutilation (44% vs 10%), and moving or hiding the victim's corpse (56% vs 16%). With regard to precipitating factors in the 48 hours prior to the crime, sadistic murderers more frequently reported a positive affect, such as sexual arousal (41.7%), than did angry ones (11.1%), whereas anger was less characteristic of sadistic murderers (33%) than angry ones (83.3%). Loneliness was relatively rare in the hours preceding the murder (sadists = 0%; angry = 22.2%), as well as in the year preceding the assault (sadists = 0%; angry = 27.8%). Alcohol consumption was reported by sexual murderers in the two profiles (82.4%). Finally, deviant sexual fantasies were reported by a higher proportion of sadistic murderers (50%) than angry ones (21.1%).

On the basis of the two sadism scales of the MTC-R-3 (Knight & Prentky, 1990), Proulx et al. (2006, 2007) classified sexual aggressors of women as sadists or not. In total, 43 aggressors were classified as sadists (18 sexual murderers and 25 sexual aggressors against women), and 98 as non-sadists (22 sexual murderers and 76 sexual aggressors). During childhood and adolescence, offenders in both groups had been exposed to displays of physical and psychological violence, and physical victimization was frequent in both types of offenders. However, psychological victimization, such as humiliation, was more prevalent among sadists (62.8%) than among non-sadists (43.3%). In addition, prior to the age of 18, sadists were more likely than non-sadists to have had low self-esteem (46.3% vs. 28.4%), to have experienced social isolation (52.5% vs. 34.7%), to have consumed pornography (35.7% vs. 14.7%), and to have had deviant sexual fantasies (48.8% vs. 18.6%). During adulthood, the criminal activities of offenders in both groups was diversified, not specialized in sexual crimes, and intense, resulting in several convictions. With regard to phallometrically assessed sexual preferences, sadists exhibited higher mean rape indexes for humiliation (1.7 vs. 0.6) and physical violence (1.7 vs. 0.6). These results indicated that these sadistic offenders were almost two times more sexually aroused by rape scenarios than by mutually consenting ones. Turning to personality profile, assessed with the MCMI-I (Millon, 1983), base rate scores higher than 84 were more frequent in sadists than in non-sadists on the schizoid (44.0% vs. 14.3%) and avoidant (33.3% vs. 18.6%) scales. These results indicate that sexually sadistic aggressors had low self-esteem and avoided social interactions because they were afraid of being rejected and criticized. Finally, results from this study indicate that during the pre-crime phase (48 hours), generalized conflicts with women (58.5% vs. 21.1%), anger (65.8% vs. 39.0%) and deviant sexual fantasies (46.5% vs. 17.3%) were more prevalent in sadists than in non-sadists.

In a large mixed sample of sexual offenders against women (59 sexual murderers, 121 non-homicide sexual aggressors), Proulx and Beauregard (2014) identified three offense pathways, using multiple correspondence analysis and cluster analysis: sadistic (27%), angry (41%), and opportunistic (32%). An anxious personality profile (avoidant, schizoid, dependent) was observed in 80% of the offenders following the sadistic pathway, whereas a dramatic profile (antisocial, narcissistic) was observed in 70% of the offenders following the angry pathway and 83% of offenders following the opportunistic one. In addition, sadistic sexual offenders reported having a sexual lifestyle characterized by deviant sexual fantasies, and intense non-deviant sexual activities such as compulsive masturbation, the consumption of pornography, sexual contact with prostitutes, and frequenting strip clubs. Nevertheless, they reported sexual dissatisfaction. The general adult lifestyle of sadistic offenders was characterized by both internal (e.g., low self-esteem, social isolation) and external (e.g., rebelliousness, reckless behavior, outbursts of temper, alcohol and drug abuse) problems. Finally, the life context in the year before the index offense of sadistic offenders was largely defined by conflicts with women and by difficulties in complying with societal rules and authority figures. These core features of sadistic sexual aggressors constitute a pathway: (1) through an avoidant personality profile characterized by low self-esteem and the belief that the people they meet, especially women, will reject and humiliate them; (2) such cognitive distortions trigger negative emotions (i.e., anger, humiliation, anxiety, suffering) that dominate their inner world; (3) in reaction, they isolate themselves and withdraw into a world of sadistic fantasies; (4) the likely function of these fantasies is to allow them to cope with negative emotions that they feel but leave unexpressed in their everyday lives; (5) in addition, deviant sexual fantasies are strong internal constraints that not only constitute a motivation to offend, but also shape their modus operandi; (6) anger and alcohol/drug intoxication may be disinhibiting factors which increase the intensity of the aggressor's deviant sexual arousal; (7) finally, to ensure their sexual crimes match their sadistic fantasies, these aggressors carefully plan their offenses.

On the basis of developmental, criminological, and psychopathological factors, Higgs, Stefanska et al. (2017) compared three groups of non-serial sexual offenders against women: (1) sexual murderers who engaged in post mortem sexual interference, namely, sexual activities and sexual mutilation (PMSI; N = 89); (2) non-post mortem sexual interference sexual murderers (non-PMSI; N = 92); and (3) non-homicide sexual aggressors against women, in other words, rapists (N = 72). PMSI sexual murderers scored higher on a developmental childhood inadequacies scale (e.g., social isolation, cruelty to animals, anxiety disorder, substance abuse, fire setting) than did rapists, but not higher than non-PMSI sexual murderers. In adulthood, PMSI sexual murderers had a higher prevalence of social isolation, sexual inexperience, and sexual sadism than did the other two groups. However, PMSI sexual murderers had lower prevalences of sexual contacts with sex workers, as well as promiscuous behaviors, than did rapists. With regard to criminal history, PMSI sexual murderers had a lower frequency of sexual and of violent crimes than either rapists or non-PMSI sexual murderers. Finally, there was no statistically significant difference between groups on the PCL-SV total score.

As with the descriptive studies, the portrait of the sadistic sexual aggressors is stable across comparative studies. Social isolation and loneliness are among the main characteristics that distinguish sadistic sexual aggressors from non-sadistic ones (Higgs, Carter et al., 2017; Proulx & Beauregard, 2014; Proulx, Blais et al., 2007). Another important feature of sadists is deviant sexual fantasies (i.e., sadistic or murderous; Beauregard & Proulx, 2002; Marshall et al., 2002; Proulx & Beauregard, 2014; Proulx et al., 2006). However, phallometric studies have reported contradictory results for the sexual preferences of sadistic sexual aggressors. Whereas some studies have reported sadists to have higher rape indexes than non-sadists (Proulx, 2001; Proulx & Beauregard, 2014; Proulx, Blais et al., 2007), others have reported that the groups did not differ (Langevin et al., 1985; Seto & Kuban, 1996), or even that sadists had lower rape indexes (Marshall et al., 2002). A possible explanation for these divergent results is that phallometry seems to capture lower levels of sexual sadism, as opposed to the SeSaS, which assesses severe sexual sadism (Longpré et al., 2016). Apart from sexual sadism, sexual sadists also reported other paraphilias, such as exhibitionism and voyeurism (Gratzer & Bradford, 1995; Higgs, Carter et al., 2017). Regarding non-deviant sexual activities, sexual sadists reported less sexual experience than non-sadists (Higgs, Carter et al., 2017; Langevin et al., 1985). In addition, sexual sadists perceived themselves as both sexually and socially incompetent (Langevin et al., 1985; Proulx et al., 2006; Proulx, Blais et al., 2007).

It was commonly believed that sexual sadists were psychopaths (Dietz, 1986). However, the majority of empirical studies indicate a weak association between sexual sadism and psychopathy (Holt et al., 1999; Mokros et al., 2011). The most prevalent personality disorders in sexually sadistic sexual aggressors are avoidant and schizoid (Myers et al., 2010; Proulx & Beauregard, 2014; Proulx, Blais et al., 2007).

Regarding the disinhibitors in the hours preceding a sexual assault, anger (Langevin et al., 1985; Proulx, Blais et al., 2007) and alcohol intoxication (Proulx & Beauregard, 2014; Proulx, Blais et al., 2007) have been reported to be quite prevalent in sexual sadists. Finally, in the modus operandi, torture (Gratzer & Bradford, 1995) and premeditation (Proulx & Beauregard, 2014) are two distinctive characteristics of sexually sadistic sexual aggressors.

Developmental Models of Sexual Sadism

Robertson et al. (2018) investigated the etiology of forensic sexual sadism in a mixed sample of sexual aggressors (N = 219) that included aggressors having adult or child victims, or both. Sexual sadism was defined in terms of behaviors and fantasies that were not limited to the infliction of physical (e.g., cutting, burning) or psychological (e.g., humiliation) pain, and included control over others (e.g., overpowering, tying up, handcuffing). Data were collected with the Multidimensional Inventory of Development, Sex and Aggression (Knight et al., 1994), a computerized self-report inventory. Following structural equation modeling, the multifactorial model they developed explained 42% of the variance in the latent sexual-sadism trait. More precisely, psychological and sexual abuse—but not physical abuse—during childhood contributed to both juvenile externalizing (e.g., fighting, juvenile delinquency) and hypersexuality (e.g., sexual compulsion, sexual preoccupation, and sexual drive). In addition, the presence of these two latent traits in adolescence was strongly associated with the intensity of the sexual-sadism trait in adulthood. Although several aspects of sexual aggressors' adolescent and adult lifestyles have not been considered in this model (e.g., social isolation, low self-esteem), it demonstrates the relevance of developmental factors in building a theory of sexual sadism.

Longpré, Guay, and Knight (2018) developed another developmental model of sexual sadism, based on variables related to different stages of life, namely childhood, adolescence, and adulthood. The main originality of this model is an exhaustive analysis of behaviors and attitudes in adulthood. A total of 518 adult male sexual offenders were included in this study (233 rapists, 190 child molesters, and 95 mixed offenders). The data were collected from files (e.g., clinical, criminal) of offenders incarcerated at the Massachusetts Treatment Center for

Sexually Dangerous Persons. The level of sexual sadism was assessed on the basis of a scale that comprises five dimensions (i.e., control, aggression, cruelty without sexuality, torture and insertion of objects in bodily orifices). Following structural equation modeling, they developed a model of sexual sadism that includes three separate paths in adulthood. These paths, nevertheless, share a common root in childhood (i.e., antisocial father, unstable mother, neglect and abuse, family instability and early conduct problems, such as fights, vandalism, and throwing objects). The schizoid path is followed by sexual aggressors who indulge in deviant sexual fantasies, have low self-esteem, and are socially isolated. These aggressors present schizoid and avoidant personality disorders. In addition, they have paraphilias (i.e., exhibitionism, voyeurism and frotteurism). This portrait of the sexual sadist concords with the one presented in descriptive studies (Brittain, 1970; MacCulloch et al., 1983) as well as comparative studies (Beauregard & Proulx, 2002; Higgs, Carter et al., 2017; Proulx & Beauregard, 2014; Proulx, Blais et al., 2007). The disinhibition path is characterized by substance abuse and externalized behaviors (e.g., criminal activities) in adulthood. Substance abuse, particularly alcohol consumption, serves as a disinhibitor and favors aggressive behavior. The aggressors following this path presented an antisocial personality disorder, which implies a lack of empathy for their victims, as well as highly impulsive aggression and an unstable lifestyle. Although these offenders enacted sadistic behaviors during their sexual crimes, they were not motivated by intense and long-lasting deviant sexual fantasizing. Finally, the offenders in the narcissistic-meanness path were characterized by narcissistic personality disorder. They were obsessed by a quest for power, prestige, and admiration from others. These aggressors exerted domination and power over their victims by inflicting pain and humiliation that the latter could not avoid or escape. These three paths to sexually sadistic crimes are based on three different motivations (sadistic fantasies, disinhibition, and power). Consequently, despite the similarities of the sadistic behaviors enacted in the three paths, a comprehensive model of sexual sadism must go beyond the behaviors to include the motivations behind these sadistic acts.

Convergences and Divergences Between Sadistic Sexual Aggressors and Male BDSM Dominants

According to Pitagora (2013), "While the more physically aggressive BDSM interactions can incorporate activities that appear identical to sexual assault (e.g., punching or choking), they can be experienced as pleasurable (by both parties), or inappropriately violent (by the aggressor) and traumatic (from the perspective of the aggressee) [...] depending on whether there exists a mutually understood psychological mindset, namely whether consent was obtained prior to the interaction" (p. 28). In fact, during BDSM activities, both parties, dominant and submissive, agree on a sexual script, which includes the behaviors of the dominant and the limits of the submissive (e.g., through the use of safe words). In this mutually consenting scene, there is no psychological distress in either the submissive or the dominant partner. In contrast, during a sadistic sexual assault, there is no mutually consented-upon script, and the offender imposes his own script on the victim. Such a situation causes psychological (e.g., fear, anxiety, humiliation) and physical suffering to the victim, and may go as far as fatality.

The psychosocial profile of sadistic sexual aggressors and male BDSM dominants differ in several ways. Whereas BDSM dominants are well adapted socially (e.g., are educated, work in professional fields, are engaged in the community and in intimate relationships), and sexually fulfilled, sadistic sexual aggressors are sexually and socially unfulfilled (e.g., limited sexual experience, sexual dysfunction, social isolation, conflicts with women and difficulties in complying with societal rules). Furthermore, BDSM dominants do not generally have psychopathologies. Rather, they present personality strengths and positive adaptative traits. Among sadistic sexual aggressors, the norm is a diversity of personality disorders, notably schizoid, avoidant, antisocial, and narcissistic. Consequently, beyond the similarities in the sexual behaviors of BDSM dominants and those of sadistic sexual aggressors, the context and the psychological meaning of these behaviors are very different. For BDSM dominants, they are a source of mutual sexual satisfaction in a context in which the submissive's pleasure and limits are central, whereas for the sadistic sexual aggressors, they are desperate attempts to cope with an extended sense of personal failure, with no concern for their powerless victim.

Note

1. The proverb "one man's mistake is another's game" appears first in print in brewer William Ellis's (1736) *The London and Country Brewer.*

References

Ahlers, C. J., Schaefer, G. A., Mundt, I. A., Roll, S., Englert, H., Willich, S. N., & Beier, K. M. (2011). How unusual are the contents of paraphilias? Paraphilia-associated sexual arousal patterns in a community-based sample of men. *Journal of Sexual Medicine, 8*(5), 1362–1370. https://doi.org/10.1111/j.1743-6109.2009.01597.x

Alison, L., Santtila, P., Sandnabba, N. K., & Nordling, N. (2001). Sadomasochistically oriented behavior: Diversity in practice and meaning. *Archives of Sexual Behavior, 30*(1), 1–12. https://doi.org/10.1023/A:1026438422383

American Psychiatric Association. (2013). *Diagnostic and statistical manual of mental disorders* (5th ed.). Author.

Beauregard, E., & Proulx, J. (2002). Profiles in the offending process of nonserial sexual murderers. *International Journal of Offender Therapy and Comparative Criminology, 46*(4), 386–399. https://doi.org/10.1177/0306624X02464002

Beauregard, E., & Proulx, J. (2007). A classification of sexual homicide against men. *International Journal of Offender Therapy and Comparative Criminology, 51*(4), 420–432. https://doi.org/10.1177/0306624X06294432

Beck, A. T., & Steer, R. A. (1993). *Manual for the Beck Anxiety Inventory.* The Psychological Corporation.

Beck, A. T., Steer, R. A., & Brown, G. K. (1996). *Manual for the revised Beck Depression Inventory.* The Psychological Corporation.

Briken, P., Habermann, N., Berner, W., & Hill, A. (2005). The influence of brain abnormalities on psychosocial development, criminal history and paraphilias in sexual murders. *Journal of Forensic Sciences, 50*(5), 1204–1208. https://doi.org/10.1520/JFS2004472

Brittain, R. (1970). The sadistic murderer. *Medicine, Science and the Law, 10*(4), 198–207. https://doi.org/10.1177/002580247001000402

Butcher, J. N., Graham, J. R., Ben-Porath, Y. S., Tellegen, A., Dahlstrom, W. G., & Kaememer, B. (2001). *Minnesota multiphasic personality inventory-2: Manual for administration, scoring, and interpretation* (Rev ed.). University of Minnesota Press.

Clarke, J., & Carter, A. J. (2000). Relapse prevention with sexual murderers. In D. R. Laws, S. M. Hudson, & T. Ward (Eds.), *Remaking relapse prevention with sex offenders* (pp. 389–401). Sage Publications.

Connoly, P. H. (2006). Psychological functioning of Bondage/Domination/Sado-Masochism (BDSM) practitioners. *Journal of Psychology and Human Sexuality, 18*(1), 79–120. https://doi.org/10.1300/J056v18n01_05

Coppens, V., Ten Brink, S., Huys, W., Fransen, E., & Morrens, M. (2020). A survey on BDSM activities: BDSM experience correlates with age of first exposure, interest profile and role identity. *The Journal of Sex Research, 57*(1), 129–136. https://doi.org/10.1080/00224499.2018.1558437

Cortoni, F. (2018). *Women who sexually abuse. Assessment, treatment & management.* Safer Society Press.

Costa, P. T., & McCrae, R. R. (1992). *NEO PI-R: Professional manual.* Psychological Assessment Resources.

Cross, P. A., & Matheson, K. (2006). Understanding sadomasochism: An empirical examination of four perspectives. *Journal of Homosexuality, 50*(2–3), 133–166. https://doi.org/10.1300/J082v50n02_07

De Neef, N., Coppens, V., Huys, W., & Morrens, M. (2019). Bondage-discipline, dominance-submission and sadomasochism (BDSM) from an integrative biopsychosocial perspective: A systematic review. *Sexual Medicine, 7*(2), 129–144. https://doi.org/10.1016/j.esxm.2019.02.002

Dietz, P. E. (1986). Mass, serial and sensational homicides. *Bulletin of the New York Academy of Medicine, 62*(5), 477–491.

Dietz, P. E., Hazelwood, R. R., & Warren, J. (1990). The sexually sadistic criminal and his offenses. *Bulletin of the American Academy of Psychiatry and the Law, 18*(2), 163–178.

Firestone, P., Bradford, J. M., Greenberg, D. M., Larose, M. R., & Curry, S. (1998). Homicidal and non-homicidal child molesters: Psychological, phallometric, and criminal features. *Sexual Abuse: A Journal of Research and Treatment, 10*, 305–323. https://doi.org/10.1023/A:1022146105664

Firestone, P., Bradford, J. M., Greenberg, D. M., & Nunes, K. L. (2000). Differentiation of homicidal child molesters, nonhomicidal child molesters, and nonoffenders by phallometry. *American Journal of Psychiatry, 157*(11), 1847–1850. https://doi.org/10.1176/appi.ajp.157.11.1847

Foa, E. B. C. (1995). *Posttraumatic Stress Diagnostic Scale (PDS) manual.* National Computer Systems.

Forouzan, E., & Cooke, D. J. (2005). Figuring out la femme fatale: Conceptual and assessment issues concerning psychopathy in females. *Behavioral Sciences & the Law, 23*(6), 765–778. https://doi.org/10.1002/bsl.669

Geberth, V. J. (1996). *Practical homicide investigation: Tactics, procedures, and forensic techniques* (3rd ed.). CRC Press.

Geberth, V. J., & Turco, R. N. (1997). Antisocial personality disorder, sexual sadism, malignant narcissism, and serial murder. *Journal of Forensic Sciences, 42*(1), 49–60. https://doi.org/10.1520/JFS14067J

Gratzer, T., & Bradford, J. M. (1995). Offender and offence characteristics of sexual sadists: A comparative study. *Journal of Forensic Sciences, 40*(3), 450–455. https://doi.org/10.1520/JFS13802J

Groth, A. N., & Birnbaum, H. J. (1979). *Men who rape: The psychology of the offender.* Plenum Press.

Higgs, T., Carter, A. J., Tully, R. J., & Browne, K. D. (2017). Sexual murder typologies: A systematic review. *Aggression and Violent Behavior, 35*, 1–12. https://doi.org/10.1016/j.avb.2017.05.004

Higgs, T., Stefanska, E. B., Carter, A. J., & Browne, K. D. (2017). The developmental and criminal histories of subgroups of sexual murderers engaging, or not engaging, in post mortem sexual interference, compared to rapists. *Journal of Criminal Justice, 53*, 92–101. https://doi.org/10.1016/j.jcrimjus.2017.10.001

Holt, S., Meloy, J. R., & Strack, S. (1999). Sadism and psychopathy in violent and sexually violent offenders. *Journal of American Academy of Psychiatry and the Law, 27*(1), 23–32.

James, J., & Proulx, J. (2014). A psychological and developmental profile of sexual murderers: A systematic review. *Aggression and Violent Behavior, 19*(5), 592–607. https://doi.org/10.1016/j.avb.2014.08.003

Joyal, C. C., & Carpentier, J. (2017). The prevalence of paraphilic interests and behaviors in the general population: A provincial survey. *The Journal of Sex Research, 54*(2), 161–171. https://doi.org/10.1080/00224499.2016.1139034

Jozifkova, E., & Kolackova, M. (2017). Sexual arousal by dominance and submission in relation to increased reproductive success in the general population. *Neuroendocrinology Letters, 38*(5), 381–387.

Klement, K. R., Sagarin, B. J., & Lee, E. M. (2017). Participating in a culture of consent may be associated with lower rape-supportive beliefs. *The Journal of Sex Research, 54*(1), 130–134. https://doi.org/10.1080/00224499.2016.1168353

Knight, R. A., & Prentky, R. A. (1990). Classifying sexual offenders: The development and corroboration of taxonomic models. In W. L. Marshall, D. R. Laws, & H. E. Barbaree (Eds.), *Handbook of sexual assault: Issues, theories and treatment of the offender* (pp. 23–52). Plenum.

Knight, R. A., Prentky, R. A., & Cerce, D. D. (1994). The development, reliability, and validity of an inventory for the multidimensional assessment of sex and aggression. *Criminal Justice and Behavior, 21*(1), 72–94. https://doi.org/10.1177/0093854894021001006

Landgraf, S., von Treskow, I., & Osterheider, M. (2018). "Sex in a relationship" versus "sex during a one-night stand": The link between mental representations of consensual sexuality, mating strategies, and sexual experience in heterosexual women and men. *Archives of Sexual Behavior, 47*(3), 725–736. https://doi.org/10.1007/s10508-017-1088-0

Langevin, R. (2006). An actuarial study of recidivism risk among sex killers of adults and children: Could we have identified them before it was too late? *Journal of Forensic Psychology Practice, 6*(1), 29–49.

Langevin, R., Bain, J., Ben-Aron, M. H., Coulthard, R., Day, D., Handy, L., Heasman, G., Hucker, S. J., Purins, J. E., Roper, V., Russon, A. E., Da Wortzman, G. (1985). Sexual aggression: Constructing a predictive equation. In R. Langevin (Ed.), *Erotic preference, gender identity and aggression in men: New research studies* (pp. 39–76). Lawrence Erlbaum.

Longpré, N., Guay, J.-.P., & Knight, R. A. (2018). The developmental antecedents of sexual sadism. In J. Proulx, A. Carter, E. Beauregard, A. Mokros, R. Darjee, & J. James (Eds.), *Routledge international handbook of sexual homicide* (pp. 283–302). Routledge.

Longpré, N., Guay, J.-P., Knight, R. A., & Benbouriche, M. (2018). Sadistic offender or sexual sadism? Taxometric evidence for a dimensional structure of sexual sadism. *Archives of Sexual Behavior,* (47), 403–416. https://doi.org/10.1007/s10508-017-1068-4

Longpré, N., Proulx, J., & Brouillette-Alarie, S. (2016). Convergent validity of three measures of sexual sadism: Value of a dimensional measure. *Sexual Abuse, 30*(2), 192–208. https://doi.org/10.1177/1079063216649592

MacCulloch, M. J., Snowden, P. R., Wood, P. J. W., & Mills, H. E. (1983). Sadistic fantasy, sadistic behaviour and offending. *British Journal of Psychiatry, 143*(1), 20–29. https://doi.org/10.1192/bjp.143.1.20

Marshall, E. A., & Miller, H. A. (2018). Examining gender-specific and gender-neutral risk factors in women who sexually offend. *Criminal Justice and Behavior, 46*(4), 511–527. https://doi.org/10.1177/0093854818796872

Marshall, W. L., & Kennedy, P. (2003). Sexual sadism in sexual offenders: An elusive diagnosis. *Aggression and Violent Behavior, 8*(1), 1–22. https://doi.org/10.1016/S1359-1789(01)00052-0

Marshall, W. L., Kennedy, P., & Yates, P. (2002). Issues concerning the reliability and validity of the diagnosis of sexual sadism applied in prison settings. *Sexual Abuse: A Journal of Research and Treatment, 14*(4), 301–311. 1079-0632/02/1000-0301/0

McPhail, I. V. (2020). Of dimensions, dichotomies, and trichotomies: Comments on the taxometric ghost that haunts Longpré, Guay, Knight, and Benbouriche (2018). *Archives of Sexual Behavior, 49*, 19–23. https://doi.org/10.1007/s10508-019-01530-y

Meloy, J. R. (2000). The nature and dynamics of sexual homicide: An integrative review. *Aggression and Violent Behavior, 5*(1), 1–22. https://doi.org/10.1016/S1359-1789(99)00006-3

Meloy, J. R., Gacono, C. B., & Kenney, L. (1994). A Rorschach investigation of sexual homicide. *Journal of Personality Assessment, 62*(1), 58–67. https://doi.org/10.1207/s15327752jpa6201_6

Millon, T. (1983). *Millon clinical multiaxial inventory manual.* Interpretive Scoring Systems.

Millon, T., Davis, R., & Million, C. (1997). *MCMI-III manual* (2nd ed.). National Computer Systems.

Mokros, A., Habermeyer, E., & Küchenhoff, H. (2018). The uncertainty of psychological and psychiatric diagnoses. *Psychological Assessment, 30*(4), 556–560. https://doi.org/10.1037/pas0000524

Mokros, A., Osterheider, M., Hucker, S. J., & Nitschke, J. (2011). Psychopathy and sexual sadism. *Law and Human Behavior, 35*(3), 188–199. 10.1007/s10979-010-9221-9

Mokros, A., Schilling, F., Weiss, K., Nitschke, J., & Eher, R. (2014). Sadism in sexual offenders: Evidence for dimensionality. *Psychological Assessment, 26*(1), 138–147. https://doi.org/10.1037/a0034861

Myers, W. C., Chan, H. C., Vo, E. J., & Lazarou, E. (2010). Sexual sadism, psychopathy, and recidivism in juvenile sexual murderers. *Journal of Investigative Psychology and Offender Profiling, 7*(1), 49–58. https://doi.org/10.1002/jip.113

Nitschke, J., Mokros, A., Osterheider, M., & Marshall, W. L. (2013). Sexual sadism: Current diagnostic vagueness and the benefit of behavioral definitions. *International Journal of Offender Therapy and Comparative Criminology, 57*(12), 1441–1453. https://doi.org/10.1177/0306624X12465923

Nitschke, J., Osterheider, M., & Mokros, A. (2009). A cumulative scale of severe sexual sadism. *Sexual Abuse: A Journal of Research and Treatment, 21*(3), 262–278. https://doi.org/10.1177/1079063209342074

NPD Group. (2019, December 18). Nonfiction and screen adaptations led U.S. book sales from 2010 to 2019, according to NPD Bookscan. https://www.npd.com/wps/portal/npd/us/news/press-releases/2019/fifty-shades-of-grey-was-the-best-selling-book-of-the-decade-in-the-us-the-npd-group-says

Pflugradt, D., & Allen, B. (2012). A grounded theory analysis of sexual sadism in females. *Journal of Sexual Aggression, 18*(3), 325–337. https://doi.org/10.1080/13552600.2011.597058

Pflugradt, D. M., & Allen, B. P. (2013). Identifying sadists among female sexual offenders using the cumulative scale of severe sexual sadism. *Sexual Offender Treatment, 8*(1), 1–12.

Pitagora, D. (2013). Consent vs. coercion: BDSM interactions highlight a fine but immutable line. *The New School Psychology Bulletin, 10*(1), 27–36.

Proulx, J. (2001). *Sexual preferences and personality disorders of MTC:R3 rapist types. Paper presented at the 19th conference of the Association for the Treatment of Sexual Abusers (ATSA)*, San Antonio, TX.

Proulx, J., & Beauregard, E. (2009). Decision making during the offending process: An assessment among subtypes of sexual aggressors of women. In A. R. Beech, L. A. Craig, & K. D. Browne (Eds.), *Assessment and treatment of sex offenders: A handbook* (pp. 181–197). Wiley.

Proulx, J., & Beauregard, E. (2014). Pathways in the offending process of extrafamilial sexual aggressors against women. In J. Proulx, E. Beauregard, P. Lussier, & B. Leclerc (Eds.), *Pathways to sexual aggression* (pp. 71–109). Routledge.

Proulx, J., Blais, E., & Beauregard, E. (2006). Sadistic sexual aggressors. In W. L. Marshall, Y. M. Fernandez, L. E. Marshall, & G. A. Serran (Eds.), *Sexual offender treatment: Controversial issues* (pp. 61–77). Wiley.

Proulx, J., Blais, E., & Beauregard, E. (2007). Sadistic sexual offenders. In J. Proulx, E. Beauregard, M. Cusson, & A. Nicole (Eds.), *Sexual murderers: A comparative analysis and new perspectives* (pp. 107–122). Wiley.

Proulx, J., Cusson, M., & Beauregard, E. (2007). Sexual murder: Definitions, epidemiology and theories. In J. Proulx, E. Beauregard, M. Cusson, & A. Nicole (Eds.), *Sexual murderers: A comparative analysis and new perspectives* (pp. 9–28). Wiley.

Proulx, J., James, J., Siwic, M., & Beauregard, E. (2018). Sexual murderers of children: Psychopathological and modus operandi factors. In J. Proulx, A. Carter, A. Mokros, E. Beauregard, R. Darjee, & J. James (Eds.), *Routledge international handbook of sexual homicide studies* (pp. 117–132). Routledge.

Quinsey, V. L., Chaplin, T. C., & Varney, G. W. (1981). A comparison of rapists' and non-sex offenders' sexual preferences for mutually consenting sex, rape, and physical abuse of women. *Behavioral Assessment, 3*, 127–135.

Ressler, R. K., Burgess, A. W., & Douglas, J. E. (1988). *Sexual homicide: Patterns and motives.* Lexington.

Robertson, C. A., Graham, F. J., Krstic, S., & Knight, R. A. (2018). The aetiology of forensic sexual sadism: From experiential perturbations to symptomatology. In J. Proulx, A. Carter, E. Beauregard, A. Mokros, R. Darjee, & J. James (Eds.), *Routledge international handbook of sexual homicide* (pp. 269–281). Routledge.

Schlesinger, L. B. (2007). Sexual homicide: Differentiating catathymic and compulsive murders. *Aggression and Violent Behavior, 12*(2), 242–256. https://doi.org/10.1016/j.avb.2006.09.007

Seto, M. C., & Kuban, M. (1996). Criterion-related validity of a phallometric test for paraphilic rape and sadism. *Behavior Research and Therapy, 34*(2), 175–183. https://doi.org/10.1016/0005-7967(95)00056-9

Spehr, A., Hill, A., Habermann, N., Briken, P., & Berner, W. (2010). Sexual murderers with adult or child victims: Are they different? *Sexual Abuse: A Journal of Research and Treatment, 22*(3), 290–314. https://doi.org/10.1177/1079063210374346

Stefanska, E. B., Beech, A. R., & Carter, A. J. (2016). A systematic review of the literature comparing male non-serial sexual killers and sexual aggressors: Examining homogeneous and heterogeneous characteristics of these groups. *Journal of Sexual Aggression, 22*(3), 323–341. https://doi.org/10.1080/13552600.2015.1126657

Stefanska, E. B., Higgs, T., Carter, A. J., & Beech, A. R. (2017). When is a murder a sexual murder? Understanding the sexual element in the classification of sexual killings. *Journal of Criminal Justice, 50*, 53–61. https://doi.org/10.1016/j.jcrimjus.2017.03.004

Stefanska, E. B., Nitschke, J., Carter, A. J., & Mokros, A. (2019). Sadism among sexual homicide offenders: Validation of the sexual sadism scale. *Psychological Assessment, 31*(1), 132–137. https://doi.org/10.1037/pas0000653

Stiles, B. L., & Clark, R. E. (2011). BDSM: A subculture analysis of sacrifices and delights. *Deviant Behavior, 32*(2), 158–189. https://doi.org/10.1080/01639621003748605

Taylor, G. W., & Ussher, J. M. (2001). Making sense of S&M: A discourse analytic account. *Sexualities, 4*(3), 293–314. https://doi.org/10.1177/136346001004003002

Warren, J. I., Hazelwood, R. R., & Dietz, P. E. (1996). The sexually sadistic serial killer. *Journal of Forensic Science, 41*(6), 970–974. https://doi.org/10.1520/JFS14033J

Wilson, L., Thompson, C., & Rudnick, P. (1991). *The Addams family*. The Daily Script. https://www.dailyscript.com/scripts/the_addams_family.pdf

Wismeijer, A. A., & Van Assen, M. A. (2013). Psychological characteristics of BDSM practitioners. *The Journal of Sexual Medicine, 10*(8), 1943–1952. https://doi.org/10.1111/jsm.12192

Wollert, R., & Frances, A. (2017). Use of the DSM-5 paraphilias taxonomy and its residual categories in sexually violent predator evaluations. In D. P. Boer (Ed.), *The Wiley handbook on the theories, assessment, and treatment of sexual offending* (Vol. 2, L. E. Craig & M. Rettenberger, Eds., pp. 903–924). John Wiley & Sons.

World Health Organization. (2018). *International classification of diseases* (11th revision ed.). Author.

13

The Structure and Measurement of Sadism: Implications for Validation

Raymond A. Knight[1] *and Nicholas Longpré*[2]

[1] *Department of Psychology, Brandeis University, Waltham, Massachusetts, USA*
[2] *Department of Psychology, University of Roehampton, London, UK*

Definition and Structure of Sadism

Brief History of Hypotheses about the Nature of Sadism

Although behaviors that represent sexual sadism can be found throughout history, the construct was first named after the Marquis de Sade (1740–1814), whose life and literary works epitomized the merger of eroticism and violence. Krafft-Ebing (1886/1965) generated the first qualitative/medical definition of the construct, focusing on the eroticized infliction of pain and injury in fantasy or behavior. Freud (1905/1949) hypothesized that sadism was the result of algolagnia, a manifestation of the death instinct that seeks sexual pleasure from physical pain. The notion that sadism includes control and arousal to non-consent evolved later, when Karpman (1954) argued that the essence of sadism was the perpetrator's power or control over his victim, a theme that several others have reiterated (e.g., Fromm, 1977; MacCulloch et al., 1983). Although some rating scales of sadism include items that assess both arousal to coercion/control and brutality (e.g., Marshall & Hucker, 2006; Nitschke et al., 2009), control items have been less frequent. Consistent with the emphasis on brutality, McLawsen et al. (2008) found that when clinicians diagnosed the condition, they focused predominantly on the imposition of pain and physical suffering during sex, giving only a nod to controlling, physically restraining, or humiliating the victim.

Despite the emphasis on brutality, these clinical reflections on the nature of sadism imply that sadism comprises aspects of both control/coercion arousal and brutality, but speculation about how these different aspects of sadism interrelate has been lacking. In contrast, the two major organizational models for the paraphilias have proposed that arousal to coercion and arousal to pain should be parsed into two distinct paraphilias. In accord with these theories, some have advocated that separate mental illness diagnoses for paraphilic coercion (PC) and sadism should be included in the Diagnostic and Statistical Manual of Mental Disorders (DSM) paraphilia section.

Organizational Models of the Paraphilias

The two major typological organizations of the paraphilias (Freund et al., 1972; Money, 1986) both distinguished PC and sadism as separate types and argued that they are different in kind. Freund's model proposed that the paraphilias cohere in three overarching clusters: courtship disorders, algolagnic disorders, and anomalous target disorders. The courtship disorders, which are the core of his theory, are hypothesized to be distorted counterparts of the normal

Sexual Deviance: Understanding and Managing Deviant Sexual Interests and Paraphilic Disorders,
First Edition. Edited by Leam A. Craig and Ross M. Bartels.
© 2021 John Wiley & Sons, Ltd. Published 2021 by John Wiley & Sons, Ltd.

process of courtship, which starts with (a) the location and appraisal of potential partners, (b) moves first to pre-tactile and then (c) to tactile interaction, and (d) culminates in sexual intercourse (Freund & Blanchard, 1986; Freund & Seto, 1998; Freund et al., 1972, 1983). Voyeurism (location), scatologia and exhibitionism (pretactile), toucheurism and frotteurism (tactile), and preferential rape (intercourse) were hypothesized to be erotic anomalies for each of these four courtship stages. Algolagnic disorders (sadism and masochism) and anomalous target preferences (pedophilia, fetishism, and transvestism) were hypothesized to be different in kind from the courtship disorders, which were seen as constituting the "same basic disturbance" (Freund et al., 1983, p. 378) and "expressions of a common underlying disturbance" (Freund & Seto, 1998, p. 433).

The data that Freund marshalled in support of his theory were the purported increased comorbidity of the proposed courtship disorders among paraphiliacs. The data were, however, neither strong nor convincing, especially for preferential rape, which was found to co-occur with the other supposed courtship disorders only for a subset of rapists who were selected because they were exhibitionists (Freund & Seto, 1998) or in a methodologically problematic study in which the same interviewer (Freund) determined the undefined discrimination between rape and sadism and simultaneously diagnosed the comorbid paraphilias (Freund & Watson, 1990). Despite its problems, this model was recently given new prominence, when it was used as an overarching organizational scheme for the paraphilias in the DSM-5 (American Psychiatric Association, 2013).

Money (1986) proposed a different theoretical structuring of the paraphilias, developed from his extensive clinical experience. In his lovemap conceptualization of paraphilias, Money (1986) hypothesized that each paraphilic cluster represents a specific vandalization or redesign of lovemaps, which are linguistic schemata that guide the negotiation of achieving sexual satisfaction and adaptation and are manifested in fantasy and actualized in performance. During sexual development distinct paraphilias flow from different compromises between love and lust motivations. He hypothesized that for paraphiliacs sexual activity functions in the service of lust but in accord with specific anomalous transformations of lovemaps. He categorized the redesigns into six thematic clusters: sacrifice and expiation, marauding and predation, mercantile and venal strategies, fetishes and talismans, stigmata and eligibility, and solicitation and allure. Money (1986) proposed that whereas sadism and sadomasochism evolved from the sacrifice and expiation solution, PC, which he called biastophilia, was hypothesized to be a result of the marauding and predation theme, and exhibitionism and voyeurism emerged as part of the solicitation and allure resolution. Money (1986) conceptualized these thematic categories as separate, distinguishable syndromes with different experiential etiologies, but he provided no quantitative studies testing this model.

Both Freund and Money's clinically-derived typologies proposed that PC and sadism constitute syndromes that are different in kind. The major disagreement between the systems is that whereas Freund lumped preferential rape (i.e., PC) with the courtship disorders, Money saw PC as an instantiation of a different lovemap theme (predation) from exhibitionism/voyeurism (solicitation). Both agreed that PC and sadism constitute distinct disorders.

Paraphilic Coercive Disorder and Sadism in the DSMs

The two typological perspectives, but not the earlier clinical speculations, lent support to DSM proposals for a separate mental disorder diagnosis for paraphilic coercive disorder (PCD) that is distinct from sadism. In defense of this proposal, recent advocates of PCD also marshaled plethysmographic data comparing sexual arousal to coercive rape scenarios to arousal to depictions of consensual sex (the rape index) indicating that rapists showed relatively higher rape indices then non-rapist controls. They also argued that the data on the sexual arousal of sadists to coercion was inconsistent, suggesting that their arousal was exclusively to brutality (Thornton, 2010). Opponents questioned the interpretation of the rape index as exclusively an indicator of arousal to coercion (e.g., Janssen & Prause, 2017; Knight, 2010; Lohr et al., 1997), and they pointed out that when studies used reliable, behavior-oriented indices of sadism, sadistic offenders consistently showed high rape indices (Knight, 2010).

Proponents of PCD first proposed a separate paraphilic disorder diagnosis under the label "Sexual Assault Disorder" for the DSM-III (American Psychiatric Association, 1980). It was rejected then, but it has been proposed and rejected in subsequent DSM revisions (DSM-III-R [American Psychiatric Association, 1987]; DSM-5 [American Psychiatric Association, 2013]; Frances & First, 2011). The paraphilia sub-workgroup for the DSM-5 (American Psychiatric Association, 2013) proposed a diagnosis for PCD that defined it as "recurrent and intense sexual arousal focused on sexual coercion." They hypothesized that PCD was a separate mental disorder, distinct from sadism, which continued to be defined as "recurrent and intense sexual arousal from the physical or psychological suffering of another person." After the completion of field trials, consideration of public comment, and significant lack of consensus among workgroup advisors on the empirical support for the diagnosis, the sub-workgroup ultimately decided not to recommend PCD for inclusion either in the DSM-5 or in its Section III, "Conditions for Further Study." Several researchers and clinicians, however, have continued to argue for the validity of PCD as a separate disorder (e.g., Harris et al., 2012; Seto et al., 2012; Zinik & Padilla, 2016), and it continues to be used in civil commitment hearings for sexual offenders under the guise of Other Specified Paraphilic Disorder, non-consent, with no set, standard diagnostic criteria and insufficient reliability (Graham, 2018; consistent with Levenson, 2004).

Empirical Support for an Alternate Model

In contrast to the separate disorders model, Knight (2010) hypothesized an alternative model for sadism and its relation to PC, arguing that the two constructs are distributed along a single continuum, called the Agonistic Continuum, which varies from no coercive fantasies, through fantasies of forcing sexual compliance, to fantasies and behaviors of hurting, humiliating, and torturing during sex. He reported strong correlations between a PC scale that he had created and previously validated sadism scales in data gathered with the Multidimensional Inventory of Development, Sex, and Aggression (MIDSA), a contingency-based, computerized inventory. Table 13.1 presents an exploratory principal axis factor analysis with OBLIMIN rotation of 11 paraphilia-related scales and a measure of hypersexuality (Sexual Preoccupation), calculated on a sample of 529 incarcerated sex offenders. A three-factor solution emerged that was determined by Kaiser's criterion (i.e., eigenvalues >1.00; Kaiser, 1960), by examination of the scree plot, and by consideration of the theoretical cohesion of the factor loadings. As can be seen in the table, three clean factors emerged with no cross-loadings of items on multiple factors—General Paraphilia, Pedophilia, and Agonistic Continuum. It is noteworthy that PC loaded substantially and solely on the Agonistic Continuum factor. Also, Sexual Preoccupation, which is a measure of sexual drive (Knight & Graham, 2017), loads only on the General Paraphilia scale, suggesting that high sexual drive may be important in both their cohesion and etiology. Other research (Longpré et al., 2018b) indicates that the Agonistic Continuum covaries more with Problematic Sexuality, which is measured by sexual coping, sexual compulsivity, and a failure to avoid negative consequences of sexual behavior (Knight & Graham, 2017).

This alternative model for sadism has been tested and corroborated in two studies in our laboratory. The first (Knight et al., 2013) tested a sample of 529 incarcerated sexual offenders, using the MIDSA. Factor analyses of items representing purported levels of the Agonistic

Table 13.1 Exploratory factor analyses of paraphilia and sexual drive.

	Factor		
	Paraphilia	**Pedophilia**	**Agonistic Continuum**
Exhibitionism	**.785**	.090	−.079
Voyeurism	**.716**	.100	.116
Transvestism	**.648**	.000	−.049
Scatologia	**.611**	−.121	.047
Fetishism	**.593**	−.060	.071
Sexual Preoccupation	**.502**	.248	.107
Child Sex Arousal	.051	**.916**	−.051
Cognitive Distortions	−.012	**.805**	.008
Child Pornography	−.013	**.457**	.024
Sadistic Behavior	−.093	−.006	**.929**
Sadistic Fantasy	.104	−.010	**.837**
Paraphilic coercion	.078	.024	**.760**

Note. Extraction method: Principal axis factoring; Rotation method: Oblimin with Kaiser Normalization.

Continuum suggested that PC and sadism did indeed distribute along a single dimension. Item Response Theory analyses indicated further that the items in this dimension were ordered as a probabilistic Guttman scale with PC at the lower end and sadism at the high end. A probabilistic Guttman Scale constitutes a set of items that are ordered in a hierarchy, such that individuals located at each level of the scale would have a high probability of endorsing all items below their level but would be unlikely to endorse items above their level. The ordering of PC and sadism suggested that those high on sadism would always qualify as likely having PC fantasies and behaviors, but there would also be individuals lower on the scale who enjoyed coercing their victims but did not manifest more severe sadistic characteristics.

Finally, Knight et al. (2013) used taxometrics in this study to examine whether the apparent, phenotypic Agonistic Continuum might be masking a latent taxonic structure. Taxometrics, developed by Meehl and his collaborators to address the flaws of prior methods (see Ruscio & Ruscio, 2004, for a review), evaluate whether a psychological construct is categorical (i.e., identifies a nonarbitrary group or taxon) or dimensional (is differentiated by one or more continuous measures). These taxometric algorithms have been widely applied in psychiatry and psychology (Haslam et al., 2012) and constitute the optimal solution to the categorical/dimensional problem (Ruscio et al., 2006). Knight et al. (2013) found evidence only of dimensionality for the Agonistic Continuum and for its PC and sadism subcomponents, consistent with other data derived from archival sources (Longpré et al., 2018a; Mokros et al., 2014). Consistent with the previously presented factor analysis, the results of this first study disconfirmed both the courtship disorder and the lovemaps organizational models for the paraphilias and also provided an empirical answer to the question about how PC and brutality are interrelated along the Agonistic Continuum.

Although these results were promising, data that support such a theoretical shift in the conceptualization of a construct and that have such important practical legal and measurement consequences required replication. Replication studies are central to the integrity and reproducibility of research (Makel et al., 2012; Schooler, 2014). Consequently, Longpré et al. (2020) replicated and extended these results in a new sample of 680 offenders convicted of sexual aggression, comprising both a new research sample tested under conditions of confidentiality and ultimate anonymity and a sample tested in a clinical assessment context. Latent Profile Analysis was also calculated in this replication. The results of the new study yielded a substantial replication of the original study, finding the exact same four factor structure for the Agonistic Continuum, which was best explained as four components of a single dimension that showed no evidence of nonarbitrary cutoffs along its entire continuum. The ordering of the items along this continuum was also comparable to the original study. Moreover, the study found those respondents with the highest endorsement of more severe sadism were significantly higher on self-reported sexual arousal to coercion than those low on the continuum, directly disconfirming hypotheses about sadism proposed in other studies (e.g., Harris et al., 2012; Seto et al., 2012).

Although the results were comparable for participants who were administered the MIDSA either under research or clinical conditions, the research sample results were more tightly congruent with the original study than were the results of the clinical sample, suggesting that moving forward it is essential to corroborate structural issues on research samples, but also to evaluate clinical samples to determine how the research findings generalize to clinical practice. Longpré and Knight (2020) have also replicated the basic findings for the Agonistic Continuum using non-sexual offenders, community controls, and college students.

Implications of the New Agonistic Model

The theoretical and practical implications of the new model are manifold. The results disconfirm the hypothesis that PC and sadism are distinct syndromes, and they strongly support the contention that they are not worthy of separate mental disorder designations in the DSM. They suggest PC is not an erotic distortion of the culmination of a courtship process, but is rather linked to same dynamics that motivate sadism. They challenge Money's differentiation of marauding/predation and sacrifice/expiation themes and suggest either that some integration of these schemas is necessary or alternatively that they need to be melded into or replaced by a more comprehensive overarching motivational schematic.

The results have implications as well about how the construct should be measured. They suggest that one reason that sadism has performed suboptimally in predicting recidivism (e.g., Eher et al., 2016; Knight, 1999) may be the truncation produced by only looking exclusively at the upper end of the Agonistic Continuum. The hypothesis that there is a dimension and not a taxon demands psychometric scrutiny across the entire length of the continuum and requires that cutoffs on the continuum for practical decisions be determined by careful consideration of the categorization errors at each cutoff level. Finally, a mismatch between the type of analytic strategy and the latent structure of a construct (e.g., using extreme group analysis to measure a dimensional construct or the reverse) has been shown to have a deleterious impact on measurement error (Preacher et al., 2005). Consequently, these results argue for the use of dimensional and not categorical research strategies for establishing the nomological network of sexually coercive/brutal behaviors. The data presented indicate further that this network is likely to generalize across offending and non-offending populations.

The Covariates of the Agonistic Continuum/Sadism—Delineating Its Nomological Network

Although the Agonistic Continuum constitutes a new conceptualization of sadism and only a few studies have used this new metric to explore the nomological space it occupies, previous measures of sadism, despite their potential truncation and misconceptualization of sadism as a taxon, nonetheless provide suggestions of where we should look in our search for covariates. The covariates identified in the categorical literature coincide with dimensional studies.

Historically, sadism, which has often been treated categorically, has consistently been associated with other sexual and personality disorders. Its significant similarities to other disorders have led some authors to speculate that sexual sadism may be a by-product of other disorders and not a distinct or comorbid phenomenon (Murphy & Vess, 2003). Recently, however, despite its overlap with other sexual and personality disorders, sexual sadism has emerged in both categorical and dimensional research as a cohesive construct that shares features with psychopathy, hypersexuality, and emotional dysregulation (Kirsch & Becker, 2007; Mokros et al., 2011; Robertson & Knight, 2014). We discuss each in turn.

Psychopathy

Psychopathy is marked by a lack of remorse, callous disregard of others, impulsivity, and chronic antisocial behaviors (Hare, 2003). Across diverse studies and samples, psychopathic traits have been found to be strongly related to sexually coercive behaviors (most consistently against women), both among offenders and in the general population (Knight & Guay, 2006, 2018). Such traits have also been both empirically and theoretically linked to major elements of sexually aggressive behaviors, such as inability to respond to victims' distress cues (Blair et al., 2005), failure to inhibit sexual arousal when faced with victim resistance (Firestone et al., 2000), and hypersexuality (Graham & Knight, 2016).

Sexual sadism and psychopathy have both been theoretically, clinically, and empirically linked to sexual violence (Cardona et al., 2020; Knight & Guay, 2006, 2018). These two constructs covary (Knight & Guay, 2006, 2018; Robertson & Knight, 2014) and share several common features, such as emotional detachment from the suffering of others and a proclivity to inflict severe injuries (e.g., Mokros et al., 2011). Psychopathy is highly prevalent among both sexual offenders and sexual murderers (Porter et al., 2003). Among those who have sexually offended, and especially among rapists and mixed-age-offenders, high base rates of psychopathy have been found (Olver & Wong, 2006; Porter et al., 2000; Rice & Knight, 2019). Among sexual murderers it has been estimated that nearly 85% have moderate to high psychopathy scores, and nearly 48% exceed the PCL-R cut-off score of 30, which has traditionally been proposed as the categorical marker for psychopathy (Hare, 2003; Porter et al., 2003).

Kirsch et al. (2006) also found a higher incidence of psychopathy among sadistic offenders than among non-sadistic sexual offenders. Likewise, Mokros et al. (2011) found that sadistic offenders scored significantly higher than non-sadistic offenders on the PCL-R, especially the Affective and Antisocial facets. Moreover, Robertson and Knight (2014) found that self-reported sadism correlated with the Interpersonal, Lifestyle, and Antisocial facets of the PCL-R, with the Affective facet covarying with sexual violence and abnormal sexual behavior and the Antisocial facet correlating with sexual violence and physical control in the offense. The subtype of offender characterized by the highest Affective and Antisocial facet scores was also most likely to engage in expressive aggression and sadistic assault before, during, and after the commission of sexual crimes (Krstic et al., 2018). Based on these results, it is reasonable to hypothesize that some core components of psychopathy may be inextricably linked to sexual violence and sadistic behaviors.

Hypersexuality

Although sexual preoccupation, one of the measures of the level of sexual drive, did not load on the Agonistic Continuum factor in Table 13.1, partially because of its higher covariation with the other paraphilias in Factor 1, nonetheless, hypersexuality and sadism have been found to be related among both adults and juveniles who have sexually offended and in the general population (Knight & Cerce, 1999; Knight & Sims-Knight, 2003, 2004; Långström & Hanson, 2006). In Knight and Sims-Knight's etiological model of sexual offending against women, which was developed and tested on both offender and community samples, the latent trait Hypersexuality has consistently covaried both with aspects of psychopathy, particularly with the Callous/Manipulative latent trait, and with an analogue of the Agonistic Continuum, which they originally labeled, "Aggressive Sexual Fantasy" (Knight, 2013; Knight & Graham, 2017; Knight & Sims-Knight, 2003, 2004, 2011). Subsequent studies from other laboratories have replicated these covariations between measures of hypersexuality and aspects both of psychopathy (e.g., Baughman et al., 2014; Kastner & Sellbom, 2012) and of sadism (Långström & Hanson, 2006). Given the dimensional nature of all three constructs (Guay et al., 2007; Knight et al., 2013; Walters et al., 2011), and their significant covariation with each other and with sexual coercion, they are prime candidates as cross-temporally stable mediators in etiological models of sexual coercion.

Other Personality Disorders: The Evidence for Emotional Dysregulation

Proulx and colleagues (Proulx & Beauregard, 2014; Proulx et al., 2007) proposed an alternative description of the personality profile of sadistic offenders, describing them as avoidant and schizoid personalities, leading isolated lives, obsessed by violent and sadistic fantasies. Brittain (1970) first hypothesized this purported link between sadism and schizoid personality. He described the sadistic offender as introspective, withdrawn from others, and plagued with feelings of inferiority. Since then, several studies have also reported data supporting the potential presence of schizoid characteristics in sadistic offenders (e.g., Malamuth et al., 1993; Proulx et al., 2007; Warren et al., 1996).

The characterization of the sadist as an introverted schizoid seems, however, contrary to his depiction as an extraverted psychopath. Longpré et al. (2018b) attempted to reconcile the possible covariation of social isolation with psychopathic traits among sadistic offenders, proposing that the seclusion of the sadist may result from the consequences of the emotional dysregulation and callousness that characterize both psychopaths and sadists. Although not regularly assessed, the prevalence of emotional dysregulation is high among sadistic offenders (e.g., Longpré et al., 2018b; Robertson, 2017). Proulx et al. (2007) reported higher levels of borderline traits among sadistic than non-sadistic offenders, and James and Proulx (2014) found that borderline personality disorder (BPD) was more prevalent than either avoidant (APD) or schizoid (SPD) personality disorders among sexual murderers. As Proulx and Beauregard (2014) noted, a higher number of sadistic offenders have had conflicts with both women and the legal system than non-sadistic offenders.

Because BPD has been linked to violence (Grosz et al., 1994; Newhill et al., 2004), especially the externalizing/impulsive components of BPD (Cardona et al., 2020), these results suggest the possibility that emotional dysregulation could contribute to the development of social isolation. Possible manifestations of emotional dysregulation include angry outbursts or explosive behaviors such as throwing objects, aggression, and threats to kill (Harenski et al., 2012). These behaviors have been associated with an overactive amygdala and an underactive frontal region for both sadism and psychopathy (Harenski et al., 2012). Such emotional dysregulation could interfere with a person's social interactions, relationships, and employment and could contribute to the severe aggressive behaviors associated with both sadism and psychopathy. Consequently, what others have described as APD and SPD in sadists may in fact be the result of emotional dysregulation and not causally central to sadism. Preliminary results from a community sample support this theory (Longpré & Knight, 2019).

The Etiology of Sadism

Although the nomological network in which sadism is embedded is becoming clearer, few studies have specifically examined the causal relations among the variables in this network or the developmental factors that contribute to their etiology, and even fewer have validated etiological models (Longpré et al., 2018c; Proulx et al., 2007). This lack of knowledge is surprising considering the severe consequences of sadistic assaults (e.g., physical and psychological trauma, life-threatening injuries). Most knowledge about the etiology of sexual sadism has been generated from case studies of sexual murderers. Although sexual murderers as a group are comparatively high on extreme forms of sadism, not all have been diagnosed as sadists (Stefanska et al., 2019). Moreover, our knowledge of sadism comes from studies that are typically plagued with multiple methodological limitations (for more details, see Longpré et al., 2018a). Consequently, etiological models for sexual sadism have remained elusive (Robertson et al., 2018), and only the broad strokes of sadism's developmental antecedents have empirical support. Knight and Sims-Knight (2003, 2004, 2011) incorporated an assessment of sadistic fantasies into their structural equation model (SEM) of the developmental antecedents of sexual coercion against women, and two empirical SEMs have directly addressed the issue of the etiology of sexual sadism (i.e., Longpré et al., 2018c; Robertson et al., 2018). These models have revealed that sexual sadism appears to be a progressive disorder that begins with abusive experiences in childhood, has negative consequences for adaptation in adolescence, is mediated by cross-temporally stable traits, and eventually manifests as sadistic behaviors in adulthood.

Childhood

Analyses of retrospective data suggest that sadism arises from a series of aversive events during childhood. In the SEM models psychological, physical, and sexual abusive experiences have been found to be developmental antecedents of adolescent conduct problems/juvenile antisocial behavior (Knight & Sims-Knight, 2011; Longpré et al., 2018c; Robertson et al., 2018), hypersexuality (Knight & Sims-Knight, 2011; Robertson et al., 2018), and Callous/Manipulativeness (Knight & Sims-Knight, 2011), all of which are mediators between child abuse experiences and aspects of sadism. Consistent with these findings, parental/caregiver abuse and maltreatment during childhood have consistently been recognized as central in the development of an association between pain and sexual pleasure (Burgess et al., 1986; MacCulloch et al., 2000; Proulx et al., 2007; Robertson, 2014). Associative links between states of sexual arousal and feelings of aggression that arise from abuse are hypothesized to sow the seeds of subsequent sadistic fantasy (MacCulloch et al., 2000; Robertson et al., 2018).

Mothers in such violent and unstable family environments have been described as overprotective and controlling, or absent and neglectful, whereas fathers have been described as absent, authoritarian, and violent (Brittain, 1970; Meloy, 2000). Although neither Robertson et al. (2018) nor Knight and Sims-Knight (2011) scrutinized the differential effects of mothers and fathers, Longpré et al.'s (2018c) SEM model supported these findings about mothers. Abusive parenting has been hypothesized to generate dysfunctional schemas such as hostility and misogynist beliefs (Malamuth et al., 1993; Marshall & Barbaree, 1990) that affect the establishment of interpersonal relationships and lead to intimacy problems (Burgess et al., 1986).

Adolescence

Adolescence can be a demanding period for individuals with vulnerabilities, in whom adverse psychosocial factors play a significant role (e.g., Marshall & Barbaree, 1990). It is not surprising, therefore, that abuse during childhood has been found in various SEM models to covary with behavioral disruptions in adolescence. The link between childhood abuse and externalizing behaviors, such as impulsivity and antisocial behavior, has been well established empirically (e.g., Larsson et al., 2008; Manly et al., 2001). The emergence during adolescence of behavioral problems that include the association with delinquent peers, violent behaviors, juvenile delinquency, and substance abuse has frequently been reported in studies of sexually coercive offenders (Burgess et al., 1986; Malamuth et al., 1993; Meloy, 2000; Robertson, 2014).

Individual personality structure is central in the development of attitudes toward sexuality and sexual preference (Bancroft, 2012). Robertson et al. (2018) and Knight and Sims-Knight (2011) found that abuse during childhood led to Hypersexuality (Sexual Compulsivity, Sexual Preoccupation, and Sexual Drive). Davis and Knight (2019a, 2019b) found that paternal or male caregiver psychological abuse rather than maternal or female caregiver psychological abuse was a particularly potent covariate of subsequent hypersexuality along with sexual abuse. Such data are consistent with the hypothesis that early sexualization may precede both involvement in violent sexual fantasies and a proclivity to view violent pornography, covarying in turn with sexual sadism (Proulx et al., 2007). Knight and Sims-Knight's (2003, 2004, 2011) SEMs have consistently generated strong covariations between Hypersexuality and Aggressive Sexual Fantasies.

Adulthood

Sadistic offenders' adulthoods are also marked with multiple adaptation difficulties. A general antisocial lifestyle with criminal peers and a distorted sense of entitlement characterize many sadistic offenders (e.g., Burgess et al., 1986; Knight & Sims-Knight, 2011; Longpré et al., 2018b; Meloy, 2000; Proulx et al., 2007; Robertson et al., 2018). Such externalizing and emotional dysregulation problems have also been associated with both psychopathy and with sexually coercive behavior in general (Knight & Guay, 2006, 2018). Sadistic offenders have also been found to report feelings of sexual inferiority (Brittain, 1970; Langevin et al., 1988; Proulx & Beauregard, 2014), anger toward women (Meloy, 2000; Proulx & Beauregard, 2014), and social isolation (MacCulloch et al., 2000; Proulx & Beauregard, 2014).

Although the various SEM models converge on several paths that could potentially lead to sadistic behaviors and fantasies, including behavioral disinhibition, externalizing behavior, and substance abuse, as well as narcissism, callous/manipulativeness, and hypersexuality (Knight & Sims-Knight, 2011; Longpré et al., 2018c; Robertson et al., 2018), and although these models suggest that abuse experiences precede these mediating covariates, their data are retrospective and causal inferences require both the validation of prospective longitudinal studies and the more precise measurement specification of the construct that is provided by the Agonistic Continuum.

Conclusion

The data reviewed indicate that sadism should be reconceptualized as a continuum marked by no coercive fantasies at the low end, moving through coercive/control fantasies and behaviors to desires to humiliate and scare sexual victims, and finally arriving at sadistic fantasies and torture. Nowhere along this continuum is there any evidence of a non-arbitrary categorical cutoff that distinguishes those at the upper end of the continuum from the lower end. This restructuring of PC and sadism disconfirms the hypothesized organizational schemas proposed for the paraphilias both in the courtship disorder (Freund et al., 1972) and lovemap (Money, 1986) models. The new model has important implications for measurement, research strategies, and dispositional and legal decisions. Replication of this model is essential in multiple, diverse samples with multimethod measurement strategies (e.g., self-report, archival ratings, both cognitive and affective behavioral/performance measures, and psychophysical/neurological assessments).

Our knowledge both of the nomological network of the Agonistic Continuum and its developmental antecedents is primitive. The improvement in measurement provided by the new psychometric model of the construct should help in this process. For causal specificity prospective longitudinal studies are required.

References

American Psychiatric Association. (1980). *Diagnostic and statistical manual of mental disorders* (3rd ed.). author.

American Psychiatric Association. (1987). *Diagnostic and statistical manual of mental disorders* (3rd ed.-Revised). author.

American Psychiatric Association. (2013). *Diagnostic and statistical manual of mental disorders* (5th ed.). author.

Bancroft, J. (2012). *Human sexuality and its problems* (3rd ed.). Churchill Livingstone Elsevier.

Baughman, H. M., Jonason, P. K., Veselka, L., & Vernon, P. A. (2014). Four shades of sexual fantasies linked to the dark triad. *Personality and Individual Differences, 67*, 47–51. http://dx.doi.org/10.1016/j.paid.2014.01.034

Blair, J. R., Mitchell, G., & Blair, K. (2005). *The psychopath: Emotion and the brain*. Blackwell.

Brittain, R. (1970). The sadistic murderer. *Medicine, Science and the Law, 10*(4), 198–207. https://doi.org/10.1177/002580247001000402

Burgess, A. W., Hartman, C. R., Ressler, R. K., Douglas, J. E., & McCormack, A. (1986). Sexual homicide: A motivational model. *Journal of Interpersonal Violence, 1*(1), 251–272. https://doi.org/10.1177/088626086001003001

Cardona, N., Berman, A., Sims-Knight, J. E., & Knight, R. A. (2020). Covariates of violence perpetrated in sex offenses: Psychopathy and borderline characteristics. *Sexual Abuse, 32*(5), 154–178. https://doi.org/10.1177/1079063218807485

Davis, K. A., & Knight, R. A. (2019a). The relation of childhood abuse experiences to problematic sexual behaviors in male youths who have sexually offended. *Archives of Sexual Behavior, 48*, (7), 2149–2169. https://doi.org/10.1007/s10508-018-1279-3

Davis, K. A., & Knight, R. A. (2019b). Childhood maltreatment experiences and problematic sexual outcomes in adult males who have sexually offended: Further evidence of the potency of male caregiver psychological abuse. *Child Abuse & Neglect, 96*, Advanced online publication. https://doi.org/10.1016/j.chiabu.2019.104097

Eher, R., Schilling, F., Hansmann, B., Pumberger, T., Nitschke, J., Habermeyer, E., & Mokros, A. (2016). Sadism and violent reoffending in sexual offenders. *Sexual Abuse, 28*(1), 46–72. https://doi.org/10.1177/1079063214566715

Firestone, P., Bradford, J. M., Greenberg, D. M., & Serran, G. A. (2000). The relationship of deviant sexual arousal and psychopathy in incest offenders, extrafamilial child molesters, and rapists. *Journal of the American Academy of Psychiatry and Law, 28*(3), 303–308.

Frances, A., & First, M. B. (2011). Paraphilia NOS, Not ready for the courtroom. *Journal of the American Academy of Psychiatry and the Law, 39*(4), 555–561.

Freud, S. (1949). *Three essays on the theory of sexuality*. Imago. (Original work published in 1905).

Freund, K., & Blanchard, R. (1986). The concept of courtship disorder. *Journal of Sex & Marital Therapy, 12*(2), 79–92. https://doi.org/10.1080/00926238608415397

Freund, K., Scher, H., & Hucker, S. (1983). The courtship disorders. *Archives of Sexual Behavior, 12*(5), 369–379. https://doi.org/10.1007/BF01542881

Freund, K., Seeley, H. R., Marshall, W. E., & Glinford, E. K. (1972). Sexual offenders needing special assessment and/or therapy. *Canadian Journal of Criminology & Corrections, 14*(4), 345–365. https://doi.org/10.3138/cjcc.14.4.345

Freund, K., & Seto, M. C. (1998). Preferential rape in the theory of courtship disorder. *Archives of Sexual Behavior, 27*(5), 433–443. https://doi.org/10.1023/A:1018796312289

Freund, K., & Watson, R. (1990). Mapping the boundaries of courtship disorder. *The Journal of Sex Research, 27*(4), 589–606. https://doi.org/10.1080/00224499009551581

Fromm, E. (1977). *The anatomy of human destructiveness*. Penguin.

Graham, F. J. & Knight, R. A. (2016). *The role of psychopathy and externalizing psychopathology in the development of hypersexual traits*. [Poster presentation]. Society for Research in Psychopathology 30th Annual Meeting, Baltimore, Maryland, United States.

Graham, N. (2018). *Examining the use of hebephilia and paraphilia non-consent in sexually violent predator evaluations*. [Paper presentation]. Florida Sexually Violent Predator Program (SVPP) Annual Training, Tallahassee, FL, United States.

Grosz, D. E., Lipschitz, D. S., Eldar, S., Finkelstein, G., Blackwood, N., Gerbino-Rosen, G., Faedda, G. L., & Plutchik, R. (1994). Correlates of violence risk in hospitalized adolescents. *Comprehensive Psychiatry, 35*(4), 296–300. https://doi.org/10.1016/0010-440X(94)90022-1

Guay, J. P., Ruscio, J., Knight, R. A., & Hare, R. (2007). A taxometric analysis of the latent structure of psychopathy: Evidence for dimensionality. *Journal of Abnormal Psychology, 116*(4), 701–716. https://doi.org/10.1037/0021-843X.116.4.701

Hare, R. D. (2003). *The Hare Psychopathy Checklist-revised*. Multi-Health Systems.

Harenski, C. L., Thornton, D. M., Harenski, K. A., Decety, J., & Kiehl, K. A. (2012). Increased frontotemporal activation during pain observation in sexual sadism. *Archives of General Psychiatry, 69*(3), 283–292. https://doi.org/10.1001/archgenpsychiatry.2011.1566

Harris, G. T., Lalumière, M. L., Seto, M. C., Rice, M. E., & Chaplin, T. C. (2012). The sexual arousal of rapists to rape stories: The contributions of sex, nonconsent, and injury. *Archives of Sexual Behavior, 41*(1), 221–229. https://doi.org/10.1007/s10508-012-9940-8

Haslam, N., Holland, E., & Kuppens, P. (2012). Categories *versus* dimensions in personality and psychopathology: A quantitative review of taxometric research. *Psychological Medicine, 42*(5), 903–920. https://doi.org/10.1017/S0033291711001966

James, J., & Proulx, J. (2014). A psychological and developmental profile of sexual murderers: A systematic review. *Aggression and Violent Behavior, 19*(5), 592–607. https://doi.org/10.1016/j.avb.2014.08.003

Janssen, E., & Prause, N. (2017). Sexual response. In J. T. Cacioppo, L. G. Tassinary, & G. G. Berntson (Eds.), *Handbook of psychophysiology* (pp. 284–299). Cambridge University Press.

Kaiser, H. F. (1960). The application of electronic computers to factor analysis. *Educational and Psychological Measurement, 20*(1), 141–151. https://doi.org/10.1177/001316446002000116

Karpman, B. (1954). *The sexual offender and his offenses: Etiology, pathology, psychodynamics and treatment.* Julian.

Kastner, R. M., & Sellbom, M. (2012). Hypersexuality in college students: The role of psychopathy. *Personality and Individual Differences, 53*(5), 644–649. https://doi.org/10.1016/j.paid.2012.05.005

Kirsch, L. G., & Becker, J. V. (2007). Emotional deficits in psychopathy and sexual sadism: Implications for violent and sadistic behavior. *Clinical Psychology Review, 27*(8), 904–922. https://doi.org/10.1016/j.cpr.2007.01.011

Kirsch, L. G., Becker, J. V., Fanniff, A. M., & Martens, A. (2006). *Childhood sexual abuse by a female and the development of sexual sadism.* [Poster presentation]. Association for the Treatment of Sexual Abusers 25th Annual Meeting, Chicago, IL, United States.

Knight, R. A. (1999). Validation of a typology for rapists. *Journal of Interpersonal Violence, 14*(3), 297–323. https://doi.org/10.1177/088626099014003006

Knight, R. A. (2010). Is a diagnostic category for paraphilic coercive disorder defensible? *Archive of Sexual Behavior, 39*(2), 419–426. https://doi.org/10.1007/s10508-009-9571-x

Knight, R. A. (2013, September). *New developments in the structural models of paraphilic coercion and rape.* [Paper presentation]. Society for Research in Psychopathology 27th Annual Meeting, Oakland, CA, United States.

Knight, R. A., & Cerce, D. D. (1999). Validation and revision of the multidimensional assessment of sex and aggression. *Psychologica Belgica, 39*(2/3), 187–213. http://dx.doi.org/doi/10.5334/pb.948

Knight, R. A., & Graham, F. J. (2017). Hypersexuality: Equifinal, cohesive, clinical presentation or symptom cluster with multiple underlying mechanisms? *Archives of Sexual Behavior, 46*(8), 2261–2264. https://doi.org/10.1007/s10508-017-1089-z

Knight, R. A., & Guay, J. (2006). The role of psychopathy in sexual coercion against women. In C. J. Patrick (Ed.), *Handbook of psychopathy* (pp. 512–532). Guilford Press.

Knight, R. A., & Guay, J.-P. (2018). The role of psychopathy in sexual coercion against women: An update and expansion. In C. J. Patrick (Ed.), *Handbook of psychopathy* (Vol. *II*, pp. 662–681). Guilford Press.

Knight, R. A., & Sims-Knight, J. E. (2003). Developmental antecedents of sexual coercion against women: Testing of alternative hypotheses with structural equation modeling. In R. A. Prentky, E. Janus, & M. Seto (Eds.), *Sexual coercion: Understanding and management* (pp. 72–85). New York Academy of Sciences. https://doi.org/10.1111/j.1749-6632.2003.tb07294.x

Knight, R. A., & Sims-Knight, J. E. (2004). Testing an etiological model for male juvenile sexual offending against females. *Journal of Child Sexual Abuse, 13*(3–4), 33–55. http://dx.doi.org/10.1300/j070v13n03_03

Knight, R. A., & Sims-Knight, J. E. (2011). Risk factors for sexual violence. In J. White, M. P. Koss, & A. Kazdin (Eds.), *Violence against women and girls* (Vol. *I*, pp. 125–172). American Psychological Association.

Knight, R. A., Sims-Knight, J. E., & Guay, J.-P. (2013). Is a separate disorder category defensible for paraphilic coercion? *Journal of Criminal Justice, 41*(2), 90–99. https://doi.org/10.1016/j.jcrimjus.2012.11.002

Krafft-Ebing, R. V. (1965). *Psychopathia sexualis.* [Psychopathy of sex]. Stein & Day. (Original work published 1886).

Krstic, S., Neumann, C. S., Roy, S., Robertson, C., Knight, R. A., & Hare, R. D. (2018). Using latent variable- and person-centered approaches to examine the role of psychopathic traits in sex offenders. *Personality Disorders: Theory, Research, and Treatment, 93*(3), 207–216. http://dx.doi.org/10.1037/per0000249

Langevin, R., Ben-Aron, M. H., Wright, P., Marchese, V., & Handy, L. (1988). The sex killer. *Annals of Sex Research, 1*(2), 263–301. https://doi.org/10.1177/107906328800100206

Långström, N., & Hanson, R. K. (2006). High rates of sexual behavior in the general population: Correlates and predictors. *Archives of Sexual Behavior, 35*(1), 37–52. https://doi.org/10.1007/s10508-006-8993-y

Larsson, H., Viding, E., & Plomin, R. (2008). Callous-unemotional traits and antisocial behavior: Genetic, environmental, and early parenting characteristics. *Criminal Justice and Behavior, 35*(2), 197–211. https://doi.org/10.1177/0093854807310225

Levenson, J. S. (2004). Reliability of sexually violent predator civil commitment criteria in Florida. *Law and Human Behavior, 28*(4), 357–368. https://doi.org/10.1023/b:lahu.0000039330.22347.ad

Lohr, B. A., Adams, H. E., & Davis, J. M. (1997). Sexual arousal to erotic and aggressive stimuli in sexually coercive and noncoercive men. *Journal of Abnormal Psychology, 106*(2), 230–242. https://doi.org/10.1037/0021-843X.106.2.230

Longpré, N., Guay, J.-P., & Knight, R. A. (2018c). The developmental antecedents of sexual sadism. In J. Proulx, A. Carter, E. Beauregard, A. Mokros, R. Darjee, & J. James (Eds.), *International handbook of sexual homicide* (pp. 283–30). Routledge.

Longpré, N., Guay, J. P., Knight, R. A., & Benbouriche, M. (2018a). Sadistic offender or sexual sadism? Taxometric evidence for a dimensional structure of sexual sadism. *Archives of Sexual Behavior, 47*(2), 403–416. https://doi.org/10.1007/s10508-017-1068-4

Longpré, N., & Knight, R. A. (2020). *Taxometric analyses of sadism in criminal and non-criminal samples.* Manuscript in preparation.

Longpré, N., Knight, R. A. & Guay, J. P. (2018b, October). *Unpacking the etiology and potential mechanisms underlying the agonistic continuum.* [Paper presentation]. Association for the Treatment of Sexual Abusers 37th Annual Meeting, Vancouver, Canada.

Longpré, N., Sims-Knight, J. E., Neumann, C. S., Guay, J. P., & Knight, R. A. (2020). Is paraphilic coercion a different construct from sadism or simply the lower end of a continuum anchored at the high end by sadism? *Journal of Criminal Justice,* Advanced online publication. https://doi.org/10.1016/j.jcrimjus.2020.101743

MacCulloch, M. J., Gray, N., & Watt, A. (2000). Brittain's sadistic murderer syndrome reconsidered: An associative account of the aetiology of sadistic sexual fantasy. *Journal of Forensic Psychiatry, 11*(2), 401–418. https://doi.org/10.1080/09585180050142606

MacCulloch, M. J., Snowden, P. R., Wood, P. J. W., & Mills, E. W. (1983). Sadistic fantasy, sadistic behaviour and offending. *British Journal of Psychiatry, 143*(1), 20–29. https://doi.org/10.1192/bjp.143.1.20

Makel, M. C., Plucker, J. A., & Hegarty, B. (2012). Replications in psychology research: How often do they really occur? *Perspectives on Psychological Science, 7*(6), 537–542. https://doi.org/10.1177/1745691612460688

Malamuth, N., Heavey, C., & Linz, D. (1993). Predicting men's antisocial behavior against women: The Interaction Model of sexual aggression. In G. Hall, R. Hirschman, J. Graham, & M. Zaragoza (Eds.), *Sexual aggression: Issues in etiology and assessment, treatment and policy* (pp. 63–97). Hemisphere Books.

Manly, J. T., Kim, J. E., Rogosch, F. A., & Cicchetti, D. (2001). Dimensions of child maltreatment and children's adjustment: Contributions of developmental timing and subtype. *Development and Psychopathology, 13*(4), 759–782. https://doi.org/10.1017/S0954579401004023

Marshall, W. L., & Barbaree, H. E. (1990). An integrated theory of the etiology of sexual offending. In W. L. Marshall, D. R. Laws, & H. E. Barbaree (Eds.), *Handbook of sexual assault: Issues, theories, and treatment of the offender* (pp. 257–275). Plenum Press.

Marshall, W. L., & Hucker, S. J. (2006). Issues in the diagnosis of sexual sadism. *Sexual Offender Treatment, 1*(2), 1–4.

McLawsen, J. E., Jackson, R. L., Vannoy, S. D., Gagliardi, G. J., & Scalora, M. J. (2008). Professional perspectives on sexual sadism. *Sexual Abuse: A Journal of Research and Treatment, 20*(3), 272–304. https://doi.org/10.1177/1079063208320250

Meloy, J. R. (2000). The nature and dynamics of sexual homicide: An integrative review. *Aggression and Violent Behavior, 5*(1), 1–22. https://doi.org/10.1016/S1359-1789(99)00006-3

Mokros, A., Osterheider, M., Hucker, S. J., & Nitschke, J. (2011). Psychopathy and sexual sadism. *Law and Human Behavior, 35*(3), 188–199. https://doi.org/10.1007/s10979-010-9221-9

Mokros, A., Schilling, F., Weiss, K., Nitschke, J., & Eher, R. (2014). Sadism in sexual offenders: Evidence for dimensionality. *Psychological Assessment, 26*(1), 138–147. https://doi.org/10.1037/a0034861

Money, J. (1986). *Lovemaps: Clinical concepts of sexual/erotic health and pathology, paraphilia, and gender transposition in childhood, adolescence, and maturity.* Irving Publishers, Inc.

Murphy, C., & Vess, J. (2003). Subtypes of psychopathy: Proposed differences between narcissistic, borderline, sadistic, and antisocial psychopaths. *Psychiatric Quarterly, 74*(1), 11–29. https://doi.org/10.1023/a:1021137521142

Newhill, C. E., Mulvey, E. P., & Pilkonis, P. A. (2004). Initial development of a measure of emotional dysregulation for individuals with cluster B personality disorders. *Research on Social Work Practice, 14*(6), 443–449. https://doi.org/doi:10.1177/1049731504267332

Nitschke, J., Osterheider, M., & Mokros, A. (2009). A cumulative scale of severe sexual sadism. *Sexual Abuse: A Journal of Research and Treatment, 21*(3), 262–278. https://doi.org/10.1177/1079063209342074

Olver, M. E., & Wong, S. C. P. (2006). Psychopathy, sexual deviance, and recidivism among sex offenders. *Sexual Abuse: A Journal of Research and Treatment, 18*(1), 65–82. https://doi.org/10.1007/s11194-006-9006-3

Porter, S., Fairweather, D., Drugge, J., Birt, A., Herve, H., & Boer, D. (2000). Profiles of psychopathy in incarcerated sexual offenders. *Criminal Justice and Behavior, 27*(2), 216–233. https://doi.org/10.1177/0093854800027002005

Porter, S., Woodworth, M., Earle, J., Drugge, J., & Boer, D. (2003). Characteristics of sexual homicides committed by psychopathic and nonpsychopathic offenders. *Law and Human Behavior, 27*(5), 459–470. https://doi.org/10.1023/a:1025461421791

Preacher, K. J., Rucker, D. D., MacCallum, R. C., & Nicewander, W. A. (2005). Use of the extreme groups approach: A critical reexamination and new recommendations. *Psychological Methods, 10*(2), 178–192. https://doi.org/10.1037/1082-989X.10.2.178

Proulx, J., & Beauregard, E. (2014). Pathways in the offending process of extrafamilial sexual aggressors against women. In J. Proulx, E. Beauregard, P. Lussier, & B. Leclerc (Eds.), *Pathways to sexual aggression* (pp. 71–109). Routledge.

Proulx, J., Blais, E., & Beauregard, E. (2007). Sadistic sexual offenders. In J. Proulx, M. Cusson, E. Beauregard, & A. Nicole (Eds.), *Sexual murderers: A comparative analysis and new perspective* (pp. 107–122). John Wiley & Sons.

Rice, J., & Knight, R. A. (2019). Differentiating adults with mixed age victims from those who exclusively sexually assault children or adults. *Sexual Abuse: A Journal of Research and Treatment, 31*(4), 410–430. https://doi.org/10.1177/1079063218759324

Robertson C. A. (2014, October). *Sadism: Historical and developmental roots—Relation with psychopathy and violence.* [Paper presentation]. Association for the Treatment of Sexual Abusers 33rd Annual Meeting, San Diego, CA, United States.

Robertson, C. A. (2017). *Psychopathic and sexually sadistic cognitions, traits, and behaviors: Relations with biomarkers and stress responses.* Unpublished doctoral dissertation, Brandeis University, Waltham, MA.

Robertson, C. A., Graham, F. J., Krstic, S. K., & Knight, R. A. (2018). The etiology of forensic sexual sadism: From experiential perturbations to symptomatology. In J. Proulx, A. Carter, E. Beauregard, A. Mokros, R. Darjee, & J. James (Eds.), *International handbook of sexual homicide* (pp. 269–281). Routledge.

Robertson, C. A., & Knight, R. A. (2014). Relating sexual sadism and psychopathy to one another, non-sexual violence, and sexual crime behaviors. *Aggressive Behavior, 40*(1), 12–23. https://doi.org/10.1002/ab.21505

Ruscio, J., Haslam, N., & Ruscio, A. M. (2006). *Introduction to the taxometric method: A practical guide.* Lawrence Erlbaum.

Ruscio, J., & Ruscio, A. M. (2004). Clarifying boundary issues in psychopathology: The role of taxometrics in a comprehensive program of structural research. *Journal of Abnormal Psychology, 113*(1), 24–38. https://doi.org10.1037/0021843X.113.1.24

Schooler, J. (2014). Metascience could rescue the replication crisis. *Nature, 515*(7525). https://doi.org/10.1038/515009a

Seto, M. C., Lalumière, M. L., Harris, G. T., & Chivers, M. L. (2012). The sexual responses of sexual sadists. *Journal of Abnormal Psychology, 121*(3), 739–753. https://doi.org/10.1037/a0028714

Stefanska, E. W., Nitschke, J., Carter, A. J., & Mokros, A. (2019). Sadism among sexual homicide offenders: Validation of the sexual sadism scale. *Psychological Assessment, 31*(1), 132–137. http://dx.doi.org/10.1037/pas0000653

Thornton, D. (2010). Evidence regarding the need for a diagnostic category for a coercive paraphilia. *Archives of Sexual Behavior, 39*(2), 411–418. https://doi.org/http://dx.doi.org/10.1007/s10508-009-9583-6

Walters, G. D., Knight, R. A., & Långström, N. (2011). Is hypersexuality dimensional? Evidence for the DSM-5 from general population and clinical samples. *Archives of Sexual Behavior, 40*(6), 1309–1321. https://doi.org/10.1007/s10508-010-9719-8

Warren, J. I., Hazelwood, R. R., & Dietz, P. E. (1996). The sexually sadistic serial killer. *Journal of Forensic Sciences, 41*(6), 970–974. https://doi.org/10.1520/JFS14033J

Zinik, G., & Padilla, J. (2016). Rape and paraphilic coercive disorders. In A. Phenix & H. M. Hoberman (Eds.), *Sexual offending: Predisposing antecedents, assessments and management* (pp. 45–66). Springer Science + Business Media.

14

Online Sexual Deviance and Pedophilia

Ethel Quayle

University of Edinburgh, UK

Introduction: Online Sexual Deviance

It is difficult to separate online sexual deviance and pedophilia from online sexual offending, as the majority of studies in this area have used forensic or clinical samples rather than community samples (e.g., Beier et al., 2015). Behaviors associated with online sexual deviance toward children often involve force or enticement to take part in sexual activities. These include the production, preparation, consumption, sharing, dissemination or possession of child exploitation material (CSEM) and the solicitation of children for sexual purposes (sometimes called "grooming"), whether or not it results, or is intended to result, in a contact offense (ECPAT International, 2016; May-Chahal & Palmer, 2018; Quayle, 2016). These activities can exist whether or not a child has access to the internet (May-Chahal et al., 2014). This chapter considers the role of the internet in CSEM-related crimes and the ways that the products of these crimes (images or text) may provide useful evidence of sexual interest and risk of future offending. Online sexual deviance expressed through violent sexual pornographies provides a useful context for considering the role of sexually explicit media (SEM) in both sexually normative behavior as well as sexual violence.

Scale of the Problem

Meaningful prevalence estimates of activities reflecting online sexual deviance involving children are highly problematic (Wager et al., 2018). Overall it appears that these activities are increasing, but it is unclear whether this may reflect police activity resulting in more convictions (Wolak et al., 2011). However, a meta-analysis of the prevalence of online solicitation amongst youth indicated that prevalence rates have decreased over time (Madigan et al., 2018).

Data related to online CSEM comes from the UK Internet Watch Foundation (IWF, 2018) using public reports and active searches. In 2018, 105,047 URLs were confirmed as containing CSEM, having links to images, or advertising it (15% increase from the previous year). Since 2014 there was a drop in children assessed as under 10 years-old, but these images were likely to include more serious forms of abuse, including sexual torture. There was an increase in images of 11–15-year-olds involving "self-produced" content using webcams or smart phones and shared online. A recent collaborative report from IT industry and child protection agencies (Google, NCMEC and Thorn) indicated a growth of detected CSEM, an expanding international scope of abuse, and the evolution of technologies and mediums used to create and distribute CSEM online. This study used anonymized metadata associated with the 23,494,983

Sexual Deviance: Understanding and Managing Deviant Sexual Interests and Paraphilic Disorders,
First Edition. Edited by Leam A. Craig and Ross M. Bartels.
© 2021 John Wiley & Sons, Ltd. Published 2021 by John Wiley & Sons, Ltd.

NCMEC (U.S. National Center for Missing and Exploited Children) reports related to suspected CSEM that were received from 1998 until 2017 (Bursztein et al., 2019). While there are limitations with this database which may bias the results, the study does provide a good indicator of the how CSEM reports have evolved. As I will go on to discuss, in terms of sexual deviance, these images and their content are potentially the best indicator that we have of online sexual deviance related to children.

Pornography, Deviance, and Violence

With almost universal access to the internet in high-income countries and the proliferation of smartphone technology, pornography appears to be more accessible, anonymous and diverse than ever before (Davis et al., 2018; Klein & Cooper, 2019). Data from Porn Hub (2019), which claims to be the world's largest free pornography site (images and videos), reported in 2019 over 42 billion visits, with a year-on-year increase in searches, downloads and content uploaded to their site. While not illegal, they host SEM which may be considered atypical rather than non-normative. A general interest in paraphilia is not uncommon, with nearly 50% of non-offending adults expressing an interest in at least one paraphilic category and approximately one-third having experience with such a practice at least once. Interests in voyeurism, fetishism, frotteurism, and masochism are most common (Joyal & Carpentier, 2017), between 22% and 44% of men and women admitting to at least one paraphilic interest (Mundy & Cioe, 2019), with highest rates associated with fetishism (24%) and voyeurism (18%; Ahlers et al., 2009). Frequently used search terms on Porn Hub include hentai (overtly sexualized manga), anal, teen, public, and gangbang. One of the most popular categories of SEM is POV (Point of View pornography), where someone holds the camera themselves and photographs their genitals during any sexual act (Brodesco, 2016). The effect of POV gives the viewer the sense that they are experiencing the sexual acts. In 2019 hentai remained the second most popular category of pornography for people aged between 18 and 24 and 25 and 34 years.

Clearly not all SEM are equal and some (for example, "teen" images and videos) may be bordering on illegal or created to give the impression that they really are of minors rather than adults (e.g., Peters et al., 2014). An online study from Australia asking how frequently heterosexual people aged 15–29 saw a range of pornographic media over the previous 12 months reported that a significantly higher proportion of respondents indicated seeing violence rather than romance/affection when they watched pornography (Davis et al., 2018). The violence was largely directed toward women. Pornography use associated with deviance and violence is not new. Barron and Kimmel (2000) measured the level of sexually violent content, the amount of consensual and non-consensual activity, and the gender of what they described as victim and victimizer in magazines, videos and Newsnet (internet newsgroups). There was a consistent increase in the amount of violence from one medium to the next. In both magazines and videos sampled, violence was portrayed as consensual, whereas in Usenet it appeared to be largely non-consensual and being inflicted by men. This study is not without its limitations (the Usenet group was largely made up of text) but it does suggest that SEM may have changed across each technical development which may be associated with attitudes and behaviors that support some forms of violence. More recently, Vogels and Sullivan (2019) in a general population survey looked at exposure to "rough sex" in SEM and its relationship with a desire for, or participation, in the same. Their definition of "rough sex" included hair pulling, spanking, scratching, biting, bondage, fisting, and double penetration. While their survey could not examine causality or directionality, exposure to this content in SEM was associated with a desire for and participation in "rough sex."

Concerns about the impact of violent SEM on sexual behavior, led to a new criminal offense in the UK of possessing extreme pornography (Criminal Justice and Immigration Act 2008) and later amended to include rape pornography. Under this act an extreme pornographic image is defined as one that: (a) "portrays, in an explicit and realistic way;" (b) acts which are life-threatening, or result, or are likely to result, in serious injury to a person's anus, breasts or genitals, or portray rape or other forms of non-consensual sexual penetration, as well as images of bestiality and necrophilia; and the images must be (c) "grossly offensive, disgusting, or otherwise of an obscene character." McGlynn and Bows (2019) used freedom of information requests to look at the characteristics of those charged under this act, as well as types of pornography used (591 cases). Importantly, to meet the criteria for extreme pornography the images must *appear* to be real. Of 366 cases, 85% related to bestiality. The majority of men charged were 20 to 50 years-old but included 21 people under 16 and 11 people over the age of 70. For over half of 125 cases where data was available, an additional offense was recorded most of which were sexual, although it was unclear from police data whether these were CSEM offenses.

The relationships between SEM, sexually violent media (SVM) and behavior is inconclusive, although a recent critical review of 43 studies using adolescent and young adult samples did find that exposure to SEM and SVM is associated with more accepting attitudes to dating and sexual violence (Rodenhizer & Edwards, 2019) and positively related to actual and anticipated dating and sexual violence victimization, perpetration, and bystander non-intervention. Of importance to this chapter, pre-existing attitudes to dating and sexual violence, and media preferences, moderated these relationships. A meta-analysis of the relationship between pornography consumption and acts of sexual aggression in general population studies (Wright et al., 2016) indicated that SEM was associated with sexual aggression (verbal and physical) in both males and females, and in cross-sectional and longitudinal studies. They concluded that violent content may be an exacerbating factor in sexual violence as opposed to a causal factor. An earlier review by Seto et al. (2001) noted the difficulties in operationally defining what constitutes pornography but argued that people who are already predisposed to sexually offend are the most likely to show an effect of pornography exposure and are the most likely to show the strongest effects. In a similar vein, Malamuth (2018), when considering existing studies that had examined the effect of exposure to non-consenting adult pornography and child pornography (CSEM), found converging evidence that pornography use may add to the risk of sexual aggression but only for those men already predisposed to being sexually aggressive due to more primary causes than pornography use.

Online Deviance and Pedophilic Interests

Online sexual deviance may relate to individuals or groups. Early work by Durkin et al. (2006) posited the idea that "pathological communities, once largely suppressed by time, space, and societal restraints, can now create and use virtual communities" (p. 595). Such communities reinforce rule violation and allow the expansion of deviant interests, including sexual engagement with children. There have been few supporting studies outside of research on peer2peer networks as "communities of CSEM-users" (Bissias et al., 2016; Steel, 2009; Wolak et al., 2014). However, Dalins et al. (2018) examined dark web activity (TOR: a web browser that anonymizes web traffic using the *Tor* network) and found that while the majority of activity on TOR related to commerce (narcotics and illegal financial services), less frequent, victim-based activities such as child exploitation and illicit/illegal pornography was identified within the network and presented unanticipated motivations. About one quarter of the domains were forums—discussions by "self-confessed" pedophiles regarding predatory behavior and the collecting or sharing of CSEM. Three domains (5%) provided education and training materials for child exploitation, with particular reference to grooming vulnerable children. In the context of online sexual grooming of children, opportunities afforded by internet platforms not only allow access to young people but facilitate rapid acquisition of expertise (Quayle et al., 2014).

Online child sexual materials and activities are, across most jurisdictions, illegal and associated with pedophilia and hebephilia (Seto, 2008; Seto et al., 2006). Much of what we know is drawn from forensic samples but general population studies have examined the prevalence and correlates of CSEM activities. Seto et al. (2015) used a population-representative sample of 1,978 young Swedish men (aged 17–20) and indicated that 4.2% of their sample had viewed CSEM. Using a multivariate logistic regression analysis, 7 of 15 tested factors independently predicted CSEM viewing and explained 42% of the variance. These included: ever had sex with a male, likely to have sex with a child aged 12–14, likely to have sex with a child aged 12 or less, a perception of children as seductive, having friends who have watched child pornography (CSEM), frequent pornography use, and ever having viewed violent pornography. A further study by Dombert et al. (2016) using an online survey of 8,718 German men found that 4.1% reported sexual fantasies involving prepubescent children, 3.2% reported sexual offending against prepubescent children, and 0.1% reported a pedophilic sexual preference. Sexual fantasies of prepubescent children were also positively associated with sexual offending against children (most frequently CSEM-use). However, as noted by Seto (2010), not all persons admitting sexual interest in children would meet the necessary Diagnostic and Statistical Manual of Mental Disorders-Fifth Edition (DSM-5; APA, 2013) diagnostic criteria for pedophilic disorder in terms of symptom intensity and persistence and only 20–50% of people who commit sexual offenses against children can be classified as pedophilic (Gerwinn et al., 2018; Schmidt et al., 2013). It is also the case that many men who self-identify as having pedophilic interests (sometimes called minor-attracted persons) do not engage in sexual activity with children or CSEM use (Cohen et al., 2018) and evidence higher inhibition (Kargel et al., 2016). Seto (2010) argued for the relevance of CSEM use and internet solicitation when considering a diagnosis of pedophilia. Seto et al. (2006) examined whether being charged with a CSEM offense is a valid diagnostic indicator of pedophilia as represented by an index of phallometrically assessed sexual arousal to children in 685 people referred for a sexological assessment of sexual interests and behavior. CSEM offenders showed greater sexual arousal to children than adults and differed from groups who committed contact sexual offenses against children, sex offenses against adults, and general sexology patients. They concluded that CSEM offending is a stronger indicator of pedophilia than contact sex offending against a child. Sexual stimuli included both images (slides) and audiotaped narratives in the phallometric test. One explanation for these findings is that some non-pedophilic men sexually victimize children because of antisocial tendencies, where pubescent females are used for sexual gratification. People are likely to choose pornography that corresponds with their sexual interests; therefore men who are not pedophilic are more likely to choose adult pornography, given ease of access over CSEM. This study, which has been profoundly influential, has not to my knowledge been replicated. The authors noted that their CSEM population was not a representative sample, and it may also be the case that men who display high rates of masturbatory behavior in relation to images may be likely to show higher sexual responsivity when exposed to slides. Nonetheless these findings are important and, as suggested, should be replicated with non-forensic, non-clinical samples. McPhail et al. (2019) provide an important review of the validity of phallometric testing for sexual interests in children.

CSEM as Evidence of Specific Sexual Interests

Glasgow (2010) noted the importance of downloaded CSEM (alongside other sexual material) to analyze unequivocal evidence of sexual deviance, alongside personality deviance known to be associated with risk. He used a series of case studies to demonstrate that digital evidence of sexual images saved on devices provides insights into preferred material used to generate augmented sexual and interpersonal fantasies, which may evolve over time and change the types of images sought. This can reflect changing sexual interests, an escalation of instrumental behavior and indications of growing compulsivity. CSEM also provides an accurate record of what the offender accessed which can be compared with self-reports. Polygraph studies indicate accounts often differ in relation to the age of the children in the images, the level of sexual victimization and acknowledgment of previous contact offenses (Bourke et al., 2015; Buschman et al., 2010). This issue may be critical in understanding pedophilic deviance in this population and what Seto (2009) described as a "seeming paradox" that this group (largely men) are likely to be pedophiles, yet few of them go on to have a detected contact sexual offense against a child, especially where there is no prior history of offending.

Of the few studies that have examined seized CSEM, most have focused on the relationship between CSEM collections and contact victimization. For example, Long et al. (2013) analyzed data from a subset of 60 offenders: 30 convicted of CSEM and contact offenses against children (dual offenders) and 30 with only known CSEM offenses. The two groups differed in previous convictions, access to children and the number, proportion, and type of CSEM viewed. Using the 5-point scale from UK Sentencing Guidelines Council (2007), dual offenders possessed a higher proportion of Level 3 and 4 images compared to CSEM-only offenders, of children with a smaller age range, and most dual offenders possessed CSEM that matched the gender and age of their contact victims. The SAP levels were: Level 1—images depicting erotic posing with no sexual activity; Level 2—non-penetrative sexual activity between children or solo masturbation by a child; Level 3—non-penetrative sexual activity between adults and children; Level 4—penetrative sexual activity involving a child or children, or both children and adults and Level 5—sadism of, or by, an animal. Long et al. (2013) suggested a potential homology between CSEM possession, victim selection and offending behavior. A further study by Smid et al. (2015) using 150 police files explored differences between CSEM-only suspects and dual offenders as well as variables related to direct victimization among CSEM-only suspects. A representative sample of identified CSEM for each offender was analyzed using a modified version of the COPINE scale (Taylor et al., 2001). The last five items of this scale correspond to those in the SAP Guidelines (used by Long et al., 2013). CSEM-only suspects, where further investigation revealed direct victimization, were more likely to have images containing victims below 5 years than CSEM-only suspects and more likely to have content depicting severe forms of victimization. The sample sizes were small so the results should be interpreted with some caution. The authors concluded that whether their results suggest that possession of extreme CSEM truly reflects greater sexual deviance, as compared to those who possess less extreme material but have committed a contact offense against children, raises complex issues, and may reflect how deviance is both operationalized and measured.

A final unpublished study by Eke and Seto (2017) also examined similarities between CSEM collection characteristics and child victims. They used an existing sample of 372 cases of men convicted of CSEM offenses between 1995 and 2009 which included men who had pre-, index, post-, or historical contact sexual offenses against a child. Of the 372, 81 had committed a contact sexual offense, 39 had attempted online contact with a child (20 overlapping with the contact offenders). Nine of the CSEM group were excluded as their collection was only of images of their victim. The sample also included offenders who had CSEM they produced and collected (72 in total), which in the main was part related to either a previous, or the index, offense. Their results indicated that the average age of contact victims was significantly related to age preferences in CSEM collections. For example, the older the age of the victim, the greater the likelihood that the collection of CSEM focused on pubescent content. CSEM content was also congruent with the gender of contact victims.

Seigfried-Spellar and Rogers (2013) addressed whether deviant pornography use follows a Guttman-like progression in that preferred image content may change over time. In this study 630 respondents from a survey sampling panel completed a questionnaire which assessed adult-only pornography, bestiality images, and CSEM consumption. Respondents' age at which they commenced viewing adult pornography was used to determine whether those who engaged in adult pornography at a younger age were more likely to transition into deviant pornography use (bestiality and CSEM). Their results indicated that 254 respondents reported using non-deviant adult pornography, 54 used bestiality (sexual activity between an adult and/or child with an animal), and 32 used CSEM. Importantly, of the 32 CSEM consumers, 60% ($n = 19$) also collected both non-deviant adult and animal pornography, 34% ($n = 11$) consumed only non-deviant adult pornography, and only 6% ($n = 2$) had just bestiality content. An earlier study by Endrass et al. (2009) of 231 Swiss men, who were charged with consumption of CSEM found that 40% of the sample were only in possession of CSEM, while the rest possessed other types of deviant content such as bestiality, sexual use of excrement or brutality. One in three participants possessed at least three types of illegal pornography. Seigfried-Spellar and Rogers (2013) demonstrated that deviant pornography use followed a Guttman-like progression in that people who started using pornography at a younger age were also more likely to engage in deviant (bestiality or child) images compared to people who had a later age of onset for pornography use. These studies are not without their limitations, but they raise interesting questions about exclusivity of, and changing patterns of, CSEM use.

Temporal patterns of CSEM consumption were examined by Fortin and Proulx (2019) through images and metadata extracted from the hard drives of 40 people convicted of CSEM possession. A sample of 61,244 images was categorized by the age of the children in the images and the severity of the victimization using the COPINE 10-point scale (Taylor et al., 2001), which ranges from 1 = non-erotic and non-sexualized pictures to 10 = sadistic/bestiality images involving children. Collecting CSEM followed four patterns. The first was a "Degenerating Spiral" (37.5% of the collections), which depicted a decrease in the age of the children over time and an increase in severity of victimization. In 20% of the sample, a "Sexualized Adolescent" pattern was characterized by an increase in victimization alongside an increase in the age of the children over the 24 months studied. The third pattern, "Boy/Girl-Love" (20% of the sample), indicated a decrease in victimization and a decrease in the age of the children. In the final pattern, "De-escalation" (22.5%), the severity of the images decreased over time and the victims became older. Case examples illustrate these different patterns. These cases indicated small numbers of very young children, a peak in children approximating 10 years-old and a gradual tail to 17 year-olds. Preference for children under six years was atypical: the most popular age was 6–12 years. Approximately 61% of the sample demonstrated exclusive age interests but for 16.9% the predominant age category collected was adults. The authors posit a variety of explanations for their results, which includes: CSEM collections are an indicator of sexual interests; that collectors become habituated to low-severity sexual content over time (congruent with patterns 1, 2 and 3 of the study) and seek out more egregious content; that collecting may be determined by the availability of content; and that CSEM behavior goes through a process of trial and error, discovery, and experimentation.

The fact that many of those who are identified or self-identify as using CSEM do not engage exclusively with this content is of interest but largely unexplored. Seto and Eke (2017) investigated correlates of sexual interest in children (CASIC) among convicted CSEM offenders focusing on information routinely available and which could not be faked. The goal was the development of a proxy variable for self-reported sexual interest in children. They were also interested in the amount of CSEM seized compared to the amount of adult pornography, which proved difficult because of missing data. Results indicated that six variables (scored absent or present) significantly predicted admission/diagnosis of sexual interest in children: (a) never married, (b) CSEM content included videos, (c) CSEM content included sex stories involving children, (d) evidence of interest in CSEM spanned two years or more, (e) volunteered in a role with high access to children, and (f) engaged in online sexual communication with a minor or officer posing as a minor. Within this sample, where data allowed, 90% also had adult pornography, and 87% had pornography depicting paraphilic themes (sadism, masochism, or bestiality). Parallel research (but not related specifically to online sexual activity) has evidenced that exclusivity of pedophilic interest (using DSM-IV-TR criteria: APA, 2000) has a strong relationship with sexual recidivism (Eher et al., 2015). In a study of a non-clinical sample of pedophilic men recruited from the Virtuous Pedophiles website, exclusivity of pedophilic interest was associated with having committed a sexual offense (self-reported and including arrest as well as conviction for sexual contact with a child aged 14 or young or for viewing CSEM). However, Kuhle et al. (2017) in a sample of 190 undetected, self-identified pedo- and/or hebephiles found that exclusivity of pedo/hebephilia and offense-supportive attitudes did not show any significant relation with offending behavior. It is unclear whether exclusivity in online sexual preferences expressed through possession of CSEM is the same as exclusivity of sexual interest, and in both national and supranational legislation "child" is defined as someone under the age of 18, meaning that CSEM will include children who have reached sexual maturity. Lykins et al. (2010) used self-report, offense history and phallometric assessment with gynephilic men exposed to slides and audiotaped narratives of interactions with prepubescent, pubescent adult males and females (as well as neutral activities). The highest levels of sexual arousal was shown to adult women with systematically decreasing arousal as female stimuli became younger and virtually no arousal to any male stimuli. Arousal to pubescent and pre-pubescent girls was higher than neutral stimuli.

Psychological and Demographic Characteristics of CSEM-Users

Elliott et al. (2019) and Henshaw et al. (2017) provide useful overviews of the psychological and demographic characteristics of CSEM offenders. Summarizing rather than reproducing these results, overall demographic data suggest that they are likely to be male (although Bickart et al. (2019) present an interesting study of female CSEM offenders), Caucasian and younger displaying typically higher IQ levels and academic achievements than contact offenders. Psychologically they are more likely to lack satisfactory intimate relationships, have been diagnosed with mood disorders (although less likely to access services), can be impulsive and sensation seeking but have fewer antisocial personality traits than contact offenders. Psychosexually they show higher sexual preoccupation and clinically paraphilic arousal to children. They are likely to also present with pro-offending rationalizations for accessing images, which is evidenced across many publications, particularly qualitative studies of CSEM offenders (Howitt & Sheldon, 2007; Rimer, 2019; Seto et al., 2010; Winder & Gough, 2010). However, as noted by Elliott et al. (2019) few studies have reported CSEM users endorsing beliefs that condone sexual contact between adults and children. In relation to this, Paquette et al. (2019) examined eight cognitive themes—uncontrollability, nature of harm, child as sexual being, child as partner, dangerous world, entitlement, virtual is not real, and internet is uncontrollable—and used bivariate analyses to determine whether they were linked to three indicators of criminal behaviors in a sample of 60 police interviews with men accused of CSEM offenses. They concluded that online sexual offense-supportive cognitions may not be criminogenic. A recent systematic review also found that overall endorsement by CSEM offenders of cognitive distortions traditionally associated with contact sex offenders was low, and that existing sex offender instruments are ineffective tools for use with CSEM offenders (Steel et al., 2020). Newer assessment instruments developed specifically for CSEM offenders show overall moderate endorsements present in tools such as the Cognitions on Internet Sexual Offending scale (Paquette & Cortoni, 2019).

Motivations for CSEM Use

Research in this area has attempted to understand what motivates online sexual offending against children (a recent overview is provided by Babchishin et al., 2018). Elliott and Beech (2009) developed an four-level offender typology: (1) periodically prurient (access impulsively and sporadically as part of a larger interest in pornography); (2) fantasy only (those who access/trade images to fuel a sexual interest in children and who have no known history of sexual offending); (3) direct victimization (who utilize online technologies as part of a larger pattern of contact and non-contact sexual offending); and (4) commercial exploitation, consisting of the criminally minded who produce or trade images to make money. A similar account classified offenders into subgroups, defined by the function of the images, the underlying motivation and the level of social networking in the behavior (Merdian et al., 2014). Both typologies focus on whether the motivation is to enable fantasy or direct contact victimization. This distinction has also been noted in online grooming offenders. Briggs et al. (2011) divided their sample into two subgroups: those driven by the motivation to commit an offline contact offense with an adolescent and a group driven by fantasy, who wish for cybersex only. However, in their sample of 51 men, 68.6% sent sexual images of themselves to the person they believed to be a minor and 31.3% created sexual content of themselves through a webcam.

Others research suggested that online offenders lie on a "deviance continuum" (Houtepen et al., 2014) related to the importance of fantasy as the motivation for offending. However, Broome et al. (2018) in their systematic review found that this contact and fantasy distinction was ambiguous, given that across studies both groups engage in online behaviors that provide them with online sexual gratification that can also lead to offline contact. In addition, they argued that no clear pattern of behavior was found to define contact and fantasy individuals. Seto (2019) described a motivation-facilitation model of sex offending, which examined relationships between paraphilic traits (predispositions), state factors (which facilitate acting on these predispositions), and situational factors (access and presence of a capable guardian). In the context of CSEM offenders, he concluded that many are motivated to engage sexually with children as they have pedophilic or hebephilic sexual interests but demonstrate high levels of self-control (or low in facilitation factors). This leaves them less likely to commit a contact offense but this, in the context of internet access, is insufficient to inhibit acting on the opportunity to commit CSEM offenses. These offenders have also been found to have greater access to technology but less access to children than contact offenders (Babchishin et al., 2015).

A final study of relevance is the use of script theory to examine the episodes and obstacles that moves an online offender to offline offending (Fortin et al., 2018). Script theory breaks down criminal acts into a series of steps and was used in an analysis of CSEM studies (as opposed to offender accounts) to examine how CSEM offenses could be understood dynamically. They outlined an offending path from adult pornography to consumption of CSEM, to distribution, to child luring, and, finally, to child sexual abuse and production of CSEM. For an offender to advance to the next episode, they must overcome certain obstacles (which mirror Finkelhor's (1984) model of sexual aggression). This study does suggest, as does forensic analysis of image-related data, that CSEM-related activities are not static but dynamic, and movement through different stages in the process may be influenced by individual variables as well as situationally specific ones (Quayle & Taylor, 2003). Specifically, use of adult pornography as an access route to CSEM has been identified in other studies (e.g., Winder et al., 2014).

CSEM and Contact Offending

The relationship between CSEM and contact offending has dominated this research agenda and has resulted in a critical evaluation of risk and its measurement (Hirschtritt et al., 2019). Online sexual offenders evidence high levels of paraphilic sexual interests, but show lower antisocial tendencies and have lower rates of reconviction than contact offenders (Faust et al., 2015; Goller et al., 2016; Seto & Eke, 2015). Higher recidivism rates are evidenced in offenders who have committed both online and offline sexual offenses against children (Eke et al., 2019; Goller et al., 2016)., However, much of this data relies on detected offenses. Elliott et al. (2019) examined the reoffending rates of 584 CSEM only (84.6%) and 106 mixed CSEM contact (15.4%) offenders from a UK community intervention program. After a 13-year average follow-up, proven reoffending rates were 24.8% for any reconviction and 12.6% for sexual reconvictions. However, the mixed group was twice as likely to receive any reconviction and three times more likely to receive a sexual reconviction. Only 2.7% of the CSEM only group was convicted of a subsequent contact offense. A move toward more sensitive risk assessment tools for CSEM populations has led to the development of the Child Pornography Offender Risk Tool (CPORT; Seto & Eke, 2015), alongside the CASIC (Seto & Eke, 2017). In the CPORT development study, case files of 266 men convicted of CSEM offenses (the majority of these for possession of images but 37% for distribution and 23% for production) were examined for candidate factors (based on existing studies) for risk. Twenty percent of these had committed a contact offense. This was compared to recidivism data for a five-year follow up period. During this time, 29% of the sample committed any new offenses, with 11% committing a new sexual offense (3% against a minor and 9% a new CSEM offense). Seven variables were identified that were associated with a greater likelihood of any sexual recidivism, whether contact, non-contact, or involving CSEM. These were: age at the time of the index investigation, 35 or younger; any prior criminal history; any failure on conditional release; any contact sexual offending; indication (admission or diagnosis) of sexual interest in prepubescent or pubescent children; more boy than girl content in CSEM; and more boy than girl content in other child-related materials. CPORT significantly predicted any sexual recidivism for CSEM recidivism specifically. A subsequent validation study (Eke et al., 2019) of 80 men convicted of CSEM offenses showed comparable results. Combining the two samples, CPORT predicted any sexual recidivism (AUC = .72) and CSEM recidivism specifically (AUC = .74), with similar accuracies. CPORT was also significantly predictive of these outcomes for the CSEM offenders who had no known contact offenses. However, the authors note that there are barriers for many practitioners in obtaining the relevant information needed for more accurate risk assessment in this population and these barriers are similar to those that relate to further research.

Conclusions

While there are challenges in defining sexual deviance, the online environment provides a window into the actual behavior of individuals through an evidence trail of text and images. This is of particular relevance in relation to crimes involving child sexual abuse images (CSEM). Online activities involving CSEM are illegal in most jurisdictions and have been clearly associated with pedophilia and hebephilia in forensic, clinical, and community samples (Dombert et al., 2016; Seto, 2008; Seto et al., 2015). Early research established that being charged with CSEM possession is a stronger indicator of pedophilia than contact sex offending against a child. CSEM collections on individual hard drives and remote storage may also provide evidence of specific sexual interests which may have greater validity than self-reports (Seto et al., 2006). This may be of relevance in predicting the likelihood of past contact offenses against a child and risk of future offending. There is also a limited body of evidence to suggest a homology between possession of types of CSEM images and the commission of contact offenses (Eke & Seto, 2017; Long et al., 2013; Smid et al., 2015). It is of importance that engagement with CSEM is likely to be nonexclusive and to follow a temporal pattern (Endrass et al., 2009; Fortin & Proulx, 2019; Seigfried-Spellar & Rogers, 2013). CSEM collections have also been used as a proxy variable for self-reported sexual interest in children and have led to the development of the CASIC scale (Seto & Eke, 2017). The relationship between CSEM and contact offending has led to a critical evaluation of risk and its measurement, as CSEM offenders evidence high levels of paraphilic sexual interests but show lower antisocial tendencies and have lower reconviction rates than contact offenders (Elliott et al., 2019; Henshaw et al., 2017). High recidivism rates are seen in people who have committed both online and offline detected sexual offenses against children (Eke et al., 2019). Moves toward more sensitive risk assessment tools for CSEM populations has led to the development of CPORT which has moderate predictive accuracy but shows promise in the risk assessment of adult male CSEM offenders but there is a need for further cross-validation studies (Eke et al., 2019).

References

American Psychiatric Association. (2000). *Diagnostic and statistical manual of mental disorders: DSM-IV-TR*. Author.

American Psychiatric Association. (2013). *Diagnostic and statistical manual of mental disorders* (5th ed.). Author.

Ahlers, C., Schaefer, G., Mundt, I., Roll, S., Eglert, H., Willich, S. & Beier, K. (2009). How unusual are the contents of paraphilias? Paraphilia-associated sexual arousal patterns in a community-based sample of men. *Journal of Sexual Medicine, 8*(5), 1362–1370. http://doi.org/10.1111/j.1743-6109.2009.01597.x

Babchishin, K., Merdian, H., Bartels, R., & Perkins, D. (2018). Child sexual exploitation materials offenders. *European Psychologist, 23*(2), 130–143. https://doi.org/10.1027/1016-9040/a000326

Babchishin, K.M., Hanson, R. K., & VanZuylen, H. (2014). Online child pornography offenders are different: A meta-analysis of the characteristics of online and offline sex offenders against children. *Archives of Sexual Behavior, 44*(1), 45–66. https://doi.org/10.1007/s10508-014–0270-x

Barron, M., & Kimmel, M. (2000). Sexual violence in three pornographic media: Toward a sociological explanation. *The Journal of Sex Research, 37*(2), 161–168. https://doi.org/10.1080/00224490009552033

Beier, K. M., Grundmann, D., Kuhle, L. F., Scherner, G., Konrad, A., & Amelung, T. (2015). The German Dunkelfeld Project: A pilot study to prevent child sexual abuse and the use of child abusive images. *The Journal of Sexual Medicine, 12*(2), 529–542. https://doi.org/10.1111/jsm.12785

Bickart, W., Mclearen, A., Grady, M., & Stoler, K. (2019). A descriptive study of psychosocial characteristics and offense patterns in females with online child pornography offenses. *Psychiatry, Psychology and Law, 26*(2), 295–311. https://doi.org/10.1080/13218719.2018.1506714

Bissias, G., Levine, B., Liberatore, M., Lynn, B., Moore, J., Wallach, H., Wolak, J. (2016). Characterization of contact offenders and child exploitation material trafficking on five peer-to-peer networks. *Child Abuse and Neglect, 52*, 185e199. https://doi.org/10.1016/j.chiabu.2015.10.022

Bourke, M. L., Fragomeli, L., Detar, P. J., Sullivan, M. A., Meyle, E., & O'Riordan, M. (2015). The use of tactical polygraph with sex offenders. *Journal of Sexual Aggression, 21*(3), 354–367. https://doi.org/10.1080/13552600.2014.886729

Briggs, P., Simon, W., & Simonsen, S. (2011). An exploratory study of internet-initiated sexual offenses and the chat room sex offender: Has the internet enabled a new typology of sex offender? *Sexual Abuse: A Journal of Research and Treatment, 23*(1), 72–91. https://doi.org/10.1177/1079063210384275

Brodesco, A. (2016). POV to the people: Online discourses about gonzo pornography. *Porn Studies, 3*(4), 362–372. https://doi.org/10.1080/23268743.2016.1241158

Broome, L., Izura, C., & Lorenzo-Dus, N. (2018). A systematic review of fantasy driven vs. contact driven internet-initiated sexual offences: Discrete or overlapping typologies? *Child Abuse & Neglect, 79*, 434. https://doi.org/10.1016/j.chiabu.2018.02.021

Bursztein, E., Bright, T., DeLaune, M., Elifff, D. M., Hsu, N., Olson, L. Shehan, J., Thakur, M., &Thomas, K. (2019). *Re-thinking the detection of child sexual abuse imagery on the Internet.* In *Proceedings of the 2019 World Wide Web Conference (WWW'19), May 13–17, 2019*, San Francisco, CA, USA.

Buschman, J., Bogaerts, S., Foulger, S., Wilcox, D., Sosnowski, D., & Cushman, B. (2010). Sexual history disclosure polygraph examinations with cybercrime offences: A first Dutch explorative study. *International Journal of Offender Therapy and Comparative Criminology, 54*(3), 395–411. https://doi.org/10.1177/0306624X09334942

Cohen, L., Ndukwe, N., Yaseen, Z., & Galynker, I. (2018). Comparison of self-identified minor-attracted persons who have and have not successfully refrained from sexual activity with children. *Journal of Sex & Marital Therapy, 44*(3), 217–230. https://doi.org/10.1080/0092623X.2017.1377129

Criminal Justice and Immigration Act. (2008). Legislation.Gov.Uk. https://www.legislation.gov.uk/ukpga/2008/4/part/5/crossheading/pornography-etc

Dalins, J., Wilson, C., & Carman, M. (2018). Criminal motivation on the dark web: A categorisation model for law enforcement. *Digital Investigation, 24*, 62–71. https://doi.org/10.1016/j.diin.2017.12.003

Davis, A., Carrotte, E., Hellard, M., & Lim, M. (2018). What behaviors do young heterosexual Australians see in pornography? A cross-sectional study. *The Journal of Sex Research, 55*(3), 310–319. https://doi.org/10.1080/00224499.2017.1417350

Dombert, B., Schmidt, A., Banse, R., Briken, P., Hoyer, J., Neutze, J., & Osterheider, M. (2016). How common is men's self-reported sexual interest in prepubescent children? *The Journal of Sex Research, 53*(2), 214–223. https://doi.org/10.1080/00224499.2015

Durkin, K., Forsyth, C., & Quinn, J. (2006). Pathological internet communities: A new direction for sexual deviance research in a post modern era. *Sociological Spectrum, 26*, 595–606. https://doi.org/10.1080/02732170600948857

ECPAT International. (2016). *Terminology guidelines for the protection of children from sexual exploitation and sexual abuse*. ECPAT.

Eher, R., Olver, M., Heurix, I., Schilling, F., & Rettenberger, M. (2015). Predicting reoffense in pedophilic child molesters by clinical diagnoses and risk assessment. *Law and Human Behavior, 39*(6), 571–580. http://dx.doi.org/10.1037/lhb0000144

Eke, A., Helmus, L., & Seto, M. (2019). A validation study of the Child Pornography Offender Risk Tool (CPORT). *Sexual Abuse: A Journal of Research and Treatment, 31*(4), 456–476. https://doi.org/10.1177/1079063218762434

Eke, A., & Seto, M. (2017). *Child pornography collection characteristics: Similarities with child victims*. ATSA. https://www.researchgate.net/project/Child-Pornography-Offedndr-Risk-Tool-CPORT

Elliott, I., & Beech, A. (2009). Understanding online child pornography use: Applying sexual offense theory to internet offenders. *Aggression and Violent Behavior, 14*(3), 180–193. https://doi.org/10.1016/j.avb.2009.03.002

Elliott, I., Mandeville-Norden, R., Rakestrow-Dickens, J., & Beech, A. (2019). Reoffending rates in a U.K. community sample of individuals with convictions for indecent images of children. *Law and Human Behavior, 43*(4), 369–382. https://doi.org/10.1037/lhb0000328

Endrass, J., Urbaniok, F., Hammermeister, L. C., Benz, C., Elbert, T., Laubacher, A., & Rossegger, A. (2009). The consumption of internet child pornography and violent and sex offending. *BMC Psychiatry, 9*, 43. https://doi-org.ezproxy.is.ed.ac.uk/10.1186/1471-244X-9-43

Faust, E., Bickart, W., Renaud, C., & Camp, S. (2015). Child pornography possessors and child contact sex offenders: A multilevel comparison of demographic characteristics and rates of recidivism. *Sexual Abuse: A Journal of Research and Treatment, 27*(5), 460–478. https://doi.org/10.1177/1079063214521469

Finkelhor, D. (1984). *Child sexual abuse: New research and theory*. Free Press.

Fortin, F., Paquette, S., & Dupont, B. (2018). From online to offline sexual offending: Episodes and obstacles. *Aggression and Violent Behavior, 39*, 33. https://doi.org/10.1016/j.avb.2018.01.003

Fortin, F., & Proulx, J. (2019). Sexual interests of child sexual exploitation material (CSEM) consumers—Four patterns of severity over time. *International Journal of Offender Therapy and Comparative Criminology, 63*(1), 55–76. https://doi.org/10.1177/0306624X18794135

Gerwinn, H., Weiß, S., Tenbergen, G., Amelung, T., Födisch, C., Pohl, A., et al. (2018). Clinical characteristics associated with paedophilia and child sex offending—Differentiating sexual preference from offence status. *European Psychiatry, 51*, 74–85. https://doi.org/10.1016/j.eurpsy.2018.02.002

Glasgow, D. (2010). The potential of digital evidence to contribute to risk assessment of internet offenders. *Journal of Sexual Aggression, 16*(1), 87–106. https://doi.org/10.1080/13552600903428839

Goller, A., Jones, R., Dittmann, V., Taylor, P., & Graf, M. (2016). Criminal recidivism of illegal pornography offenders in the overall population—A national cohort study of 4612 offenders in Switzerland. *Advances in Applied Sociology, 6*(2), 48–56. http://dx.doi.org/10.4236/aasoci.2016.62005

Henshaw, M., Ogloff, J.R.P., & Clough, J.A. (2015). Looking beyond the screen: A critical review of the literature on the online child pornography offender. *Sexual Abuse, 29*(5), 416–445. https://doi.org/10.1177/1079063215603690

Hirschtritt, M. E., Tucker, D., & Binder, R. L. (2019). Risk assessment of online child sexual exploitation offenders. *Journal of the American Academy of Psychiatry and the Law, 47*(2), 155–164. https://doi.org/10.29158/JAAPL.003830-19

Houtepen, J., Sijtsema, J., & Bogaerts, S. (2014). From child pornography offending to child sexual abuse: A review of child pornography offender characteristics and risks for cross-over. *Aggression and Violent Behavior, 19*(5), 466–473. https://doi.org/10.1016/j.avb.2014.07.011

Howitt, D., & Sheldon, K. (2007). The role of cognitive distortions in paedophilic offending: Internet and contact offenders compared. *Psychology, Crime & Law, 13*(5), 469–486. https://doi.org/10.1080/10683160601060564

Internet Watch Foundation. (2018). Annual Report. https://www.iwf.org.uk/sites/default/files/reports/2019-04/Once%20upon%20a%20year%20-%20IWF%20Annual%20Report%202018.pdf

Joyal, C., & Carpentier, J. (2017). The prevalence of paraphilic interests and behaviors in the general population: A provincial survey. *The Journal of Sex Research, 54*(2), 161–171. https://doi.org/10.1080/00224499.2016.1139034

Kärgel, C., Massau, C., Weiß, S., Walter, M., Borchardt, V., Krueger, T.H.C., Tenbergen, G., Kneer, J., Wittfoth, M., Pohl, A., Gerwinn, H., Ponseti, J., Amelung, T., Beier, K.M., Mohnke, S., Walter, H., & Schiffer, B. (2016). Evidence for superior neurobiological and behavioral inhibitory control abilities in non-offending as compared to offending pedophiles. *Human Brain Mapping, 38*(2), 1092–1104. https://doi-org.ezproxy.is.ed.ac.uk/10.1002/hbm.23443

Klein, J., & Cooper, D. (2019). Deviant cyber-sexual activities in young adults: Exploring prevalence and predictions using in-person sexual activities and social learning theory. *Archives of Sexual Behavior, 48*(2), 619–630. https://doi.org/10.1007/s10508-018-1251-2

Kuhle, L., Schlinzig, E., Kaiser, G., Amelung, T., Konrad, A., Röhle, R., & Beier, K. (2017). The association of sexual preference and dynamic risk factors with undetected child pornography offending. *Journal of Sexual Aggression, 23*(1), 3–18. https://doi.org/10.1080/13552600.2016.1201157

Long, M. L., Alison, L. A., & Mcmanus, M. A. (2013). Child pornography and likelihood of contact abuse: A comparison between contact child sexual offenders and noncontact offenders. *Sexual Abuse: A Journal of Research and Treatment, 25*(4), 370–395. https://doi.org/10.1177/1079063212464398

Lykins, A., Cantor, J., Kuban, M., Blak, T., Dickey, R., Klassen, P., & Blanchard, R. (2010). Sexual arousal to female children in gynephilic men. *Sexual Abuse: A Journal of Research and Treatment, 22*(3), 279–289. https://doi.org/10.1177/1079063210372141

Madigan, S., Villani, V., Azzopardi, C., Laut, D., Smith, T., Temple, J. R., Browne, D., & Dimitropoulos, G. (2018). The prevalence of unwanted online sexual exposure and solicitation among youth: A meta-analysis. *Journal of Adolescent Health, 63*(2), 133–141. https://doi.org/10.1016/j.jadohealth.2018.03.012

Malamuth, N. M. (2018). "Adding fuel to the fire"? Does exposure to non-consenting adult or to child pornography increase risk of sexual aggression? *Aggression and Violent Behavior, 41*, 74–89. https://doi.org/10.1016/j.avb.2018.02.013

May-Chahal, C., Mason, C., Rashid, A., Walkerdine, J., Rayson, P., & Greenwood, P. (2014). Safeguarding cyborg childhoods: Incorporating the on/offline behaviour of children into everyday social work practices. *British Journal of Social Work, 44*(3), 596–614. https://doi.org/10.1093/bjsw/bcs121

May-Chahal, C., & Palmer, E. (2018). *Rapid evidence assessment characteristics and vulnerabilities of victims of online-facilitated child sexual abuse and exploitation*. www.iicsa.org.uk.

McGlynn, C., & Bows, H. (2019). Possessing extreme pornography: Policing, prosecutions and the need for reform. *The Journal of Criminal Law, 83*(6), 473–488. https://doi.org/10.1177/0022018319877783

McPhail, I., Hermann, C., Fernane, S., Fernandez, Y., Nunes, K., & Cantor, J. (2019). Validity in phallometric testing for sexual interests in children- a meta-analytic review. *Assessment, 26*(3), 535–551. https://doi.org/10.1177/1073191117706139

Merdian, H., Curtis, C., Thakker, J., Wilson, N., & Boer, D. (2014). The endorsement of cognitive distortions: Comparing child pornography offenders and contact sex offenders. *Psychology, Crime & Law, 20*(10), 971–993. https://doi.org/10.1080/1068316X.2014.902454

Mundy, C., & Cioe, J. (2019). Exploring the relationship between paraphilic interests, sex, and sexual and life satisfaction in non-clinical samples. *The Canadian Journal of Human Sexuality, 28*(3), 304–316. https://link.gale.com/apps/doc/A611334169/AONE?u=ed_itw&sid=AONE&xid=338dcd43

Paquette, S., & Cortoni, F. (2019). The development and validation of the Cognitions of Internet Sexual Offending (C-ISO) Scale. *Sexual Abuse, 32*(8), 907–930. Advance online publication. https://doi.org/10:1079063219862281

Paquette, S., Longpré, N., & Cortoni, F. (2019). A billion distorted thoughts: An exploratory study of criminogenic cognitions among men who sexually exploit children over the internet. *International Journal of Offender Therapy and Comparative Criminology*. https://doi.org/10.1177/0306624X19873082

Peters, E. M., Morrison, T., McDermott, D. T., Bishop, C. J., & Kiss, M. (2014). Age is in the eye of the beholder: Examining the cues employed to construct the illusion of youth in teen pornography. *Sexuality & Culture, 18*, 527–546. https://doi.org/10.1007/s12119-013-9210-5

Porn Hub. (2019). *The 2019 year in review*. Retrieved January 6, 2019, from https://www.pornhub.com/insights/2019-year-in-review

Quayle, E., (2016) Researching online child sexual exploitation and abuse: Are there links between online and offline vulnerabilities? Global Kids Online. www.globalkidsonline.net/sexual-exploitation.

Quayle, E., Allegro, S., Hutton, L., Sheath, M., & Lööf, L. (2014). Rapid skill acquisition and online sexual grooming of children. *Computers in Human Behavior, 39*, 368–375. https://doi.org/10.1016/j.chb.2014.07.005

Quayle, E., & Newman, E. (2015). The role of sexual images in online and offline sexual behaviour with minors. *Current Psychiatry Reports, 17*(6), 1–6. https://doi.org/10.1007/s11920-015-0579-8

Quayle, E., & Taylor, M. (2004). *Child Pornography*. Taylor and Francis.

Rimer, J. (2019). "In the street they're real, in a picture they're not"—Constructions of children and childhood among users of online child sexual exploitation material. *Child Abuse & Neglect, 90*, 160–173. https://doi.org/10.1016/j.chiabu.2018.12.008

Rodenhizer, K. A., & Edwards, K. M. (2019). The impacts of sexual media exposure on adolescent and emerging adults' dating and sexual violence attitudes and behaviors: A critical review of the literature. *Trauma, Violence, & Abuse, 20*(4), 439–452. https://doi.org/10.1177/1524838017717745

Schmidt, A., Mokros, A., & Banse, R. (2013). Is pedophilic sexual preference continuous? A taxometric analysis based on direct and indirect measures. *Psychological Assessment, 25*(4), 1146–1153. https://doi.org/10.1037/a0033326

Seigfried-Spellar, K. C., & Rogers, M. K. (2013). Does deviant pornography use follow a Guttman-like progression? *Computers in Human Behavior, 29*(5), 1997–2003. https://doi.org/10.1016/j.chb.2013.04.018

Sentencing Guidelines Council. (2007). *Sexual Offences Act 2003: Definitive guideline*. Sentencing Council: London.

Seto, M. (2010). Child pornography use and internet solicitation in the diagnosis of pedophilia. *Archives of Sexual Behavior, 39*(3), 591–593. https://doi.org/10.1007/s10508-010-9603-6

Seto, M. (2019). The motivation-facilitation model of sexual offending. *Sexual Abuse: A Journal of Research and Treatment, 31*(1), 3–24. https://doi.org/10.1177/1079063217720919

Seto, M., & Eke, A. (2015). Predicting recidivism among adult male child pornography offenders: Development of the Child Pornography Offender Risk Tool (CPORT). *Law and Human Behavior, 39*(4), 416–429. http://dx.doi.org.ezproxy.is.ed.ac.uk/10.1037/lhb0000128

Seto, M., & Eke, A. (2017). Correlates of admitted sexual interest in children among individuals convicted of child pornography offenses. *Law and Human Behavior, 41*(3), 305–313. https://doi.org/10.1037/lhb0000240

Seto, M., Reeves, L., & Jung, S. (2010). Explanations given by child pornography offenders for their crimes. *Journal of Sexual Aggression, 16*(2), 169–180. https://doi.org/10.1080/13552600903572396

Seto, M. C. (2009). Pedophilia. *Annual Review of Clinical Psychology, 5*(1), 391–407. https://doi.org/10.1146/annurev.clinpsy.032408.153618

Seto, M. C. (2008). *Pedophilia and sexual offending against children: Theory, assessment, and intervention*. American Psychological Association. https://doi.org/10.1037/11639-000

Seto, M. C., Cantor, J. M., & Blanchard, R. (2006). Child pornography offenses are a valid diagnostic indicator of pedophilia. *Journal of Abnormal Psychology, 115*(3), 610–615. https://doi.org/10.1037/0021-843X.115.3.610

Seto, M. C., Hermann, C. A., Kjellgren, C., Priebe, G., Svedin, C. G., & Långström, N. (2015). Viewing child pornography: Prevalence and correlates in a representative community sample of young Swedish men. *Archives of Sexual Behavior, 44*, 67–79. https://doi.org/http://dx.doi.org/10.1007/s10508-013-0244-4

Seto, M. C., Maric, A., & Barbaree, H. E. (2001). The role of pornography in the etiology of sexual aggression. *Aggression and Violent Behavior, 6*(1), 35–53. https://doi.org/10.1016/S1359-1789(99)00007-5

Smid, W., Schepers, K., Kamphuis, J., Van Linden, S., & Bartling, S. (2015). Prioritizing child pornography notifications: Predicting direct victimization. *Sexual Abuse: A Journal of Research and Treatment, 27*(4), 398–413. https://doi.org/10.1177/1079063213514453

Steel, C., Newman, E., O'Rourke, S., & Quayle, E. (2020). A systematic review of cognitive distortions in online child sexual exploitation material offenders. *Aggression & Violent Behavior, 51*. https://doi.org/10.1016/j.avb.2020.101375

Steel, C. M. S. (2009). Child pornography in peer-to-peer networks. *Child Abuse & Neglect, 33*, 560–568. https://doi.org/10.1016/j.chiabu.2008.12.011

Taylor, M., Holland, G., & Quayle, E. (2001). Typology of paedophile picture collections. *The Police Journal: Theory, Practice and Principles, 74*(2), 97–107. https://doi.org/10.1177/0032258X0107400202

Vogels, E. A., & Sullivan, L. F. (2019). The relationship among online sexually explicit material exposure to, desire for, and participation in rough sex. *Archives of Sexual Behavior, 48*(2), 653–665. https://doi.org/10.1007/s10508-018-1290-8

Wager, N., Armitage, R., Christmann, K., Gallagher, B., Ioannou, M., Parkinson, S. et al (2018). Rapid evidence assessment: Quantifying the extent of online-facilitated child sexual abuse: Report for the Independent Inquiry into Child Sexual Abuse. http://cdn.basw.co.uk/upload/basw_103534-9.pdf.

Winder, B., & Gough, B. (2010). "I never touched anybody-that's my defence": A qualitative analysis of internet sex offender accounts. *Journal of Sexual Aggression, 16*(2), 125–141. https://doi.org/10.1007/s10508-014-0302-6

Winder, B., Gough, B., & Seymour-Smith, S. (2014). Stumbling into sexual crime: The passive perpetrator in accounts by male internet sex offenders. *Archives of Sexual Behavior, 44*(1), 167–180.

Wolak, J., Liberatore, M., Levine, B.N., 2014. Measuring a year of child pornography trafficking by U.S. computers on a peer-to-peer network. *Child Abuse and Neglect, 38*, 347–356. https://doi.org/10.1016/j.chiabu.2013.10.018

Wolak, J., Finkelhor, D., Mitchell, K. J. A., & Jones, L. M. (2011). Arrests for child pornography production- data at two time points from a national sample of U.S. law enforcement agencies. *Child Maltreatment, 16*(3), 184–195. http://dx.org/10.1016/j.chiabu.2013.10.018

Wright, P. J., Tokunaga, R. S., & Kraus, A. (2016). A meta-analysis of pornography consumption and actual acts of sexual aggression in general population studies. *Journal of Communication, 66*(1), 183–205. https://doi.org/10.1111/jcom.12201

Part V

Managing Sexual Deviance and Paraphilic Disorders

15

A Generalized Model for Identifying Risk-Related Change in Sexual Deviance

David Thornton

Introduction

The construct of *sexual deviance* plays a central role in research-based understandings of sexual offending. The phrase is a shorthand for "offense-related sexual deviance" since human sexuality is endlessly diverse and most variations from normative sexuality are harmless sources of pleasure and human connection (see DSM-5; APA, 2013, pp. 685–686), while only some are linked to antisocial sexual behavior. This chapter is primarily concerned with *sexual deviance* as an empirical construct and with ways of understanding it and identifying changes that signal a reduction in the risk associated with sexual deviance. Following the DSM-5's distinction between a paraphilia and a paraphilic disorder, relevant change is understood to include both changes in sexual deviance itself and change in the link between deviance and behavior. The goal here is the pragmatic one of providing useful advice to professionals who are asked to assess the degree to which someone with a history of sexual deviance continues to present an undiminished risk.

Empirical Foundations of the *Sexual Deviance* Construct

Empirical research into risk for sexual recidivism first became coherent when researchers collated and categorized studies relating ascertainable features of individuals convicted for sexual offenses to records of future arrests, charges, or convictions for sexual offending (Beech et al., 2003; Fisher & Thornton, 1993; Hanson & Bussière, 1998; Hanson & Morton-Bourgon, 2005). Given the many correlates of sexual recidivism, it was natural to organize them into categories and these empirical reviews consistently identified aspects of prior sexual offending and sexual deviancy as robust predictors of sexual recidivism.

Empirical research moved from identifying individual risk factors to exploring the properties of scales that combined risk factors to create a risk score. Well established scales of this kind include Static-99R and Static-2002R (Helmus et al., 2012) and Risk Matrix 2000 (Thornton et al., 2003). Factor analyses of these scales (Allen & Pflugradt, 2014; Brouillette-Alarie et al., 2016; Roberts et al., 2002) have consistently identified a factor reflecting antisocial traits and either one or two factors reflecting *sexual deviancy*. The most consistent *sexual deviancy* factor has usefully been labeled paraphilia/persistence and has loaded items that reflect persistence and rate of sexual reoffending as well as items reflecting paraphilic indicators such as non-contact sexual offenses or offenses against young, unrelated children. The third factor

Sexual Deviance: Understanding and Managing Deviant Sexual Interests and Paraphilic Disorders,
First Edition. Edited by Leam A. Craig and Ross M. Bartels.
© 2021 John Wiley & Sons, Ltd. Published 2021 by John Wiley & Sons, Ltd.

occurring in these analyses involves items depicting stranger aggression carried out by young, unmarried men. This has been variously interpreted as reflecting age, as reflecting a fusion of sexual sadism and hostility to women, or as reflecting the form that criminal sexual deviancy takes in young men (e.g., see Brouillette-Alarie et al., 2016). Despite uncertainty in interpretation of this third factor, these factor analyses clearly show that *sexual deviance* plays a central role in actuarial risk instruments.

Sexual deviance has also been clearly identified in research focused on psychological correlates of sexual recidivism. Research into psychological correlates can be organized and understood in terms of the Structured Risk Assessment (SRA) framework (Thornton, 2002, 2016; Thornton & Knight, 2015). This classifies enduring psychological factors related to sexual offending into four domains comprising Sexual Interests, Distorted Attitudes, Relational Style, and Self-Management. Although it was developed in the late 1990s, research has continued to support this framework. Thornton (2016) showed that the psychological factors identified as

Table 15.1 SRA need framework.

Domains	Subdomains	Examples of Specific Factors
Sexual interests	Offense-related sexual interests	Sexual interest in children Sexualized violence
	Poor sexual self-regulation (hypersexuality/sexual preoccupation)	Sexualized coping Sex disproportionately valued High rates of sexual activity High rates of sexual thoughts Impulsive sexual behavior Diverse sexual outlets Impersonal sexuality
Distorted attitudes	Victim schema	Women as deceitful Children as sexual
	Rights Schema	Sexual entitlement General entitlement
	Means Schema	Machiavellianism Violent world
Relational style	Inadequate relational style	Dysfunctional self-esteem Emotional congruence with children
	Intimacy deficits	Difficulty or disinterest in forming and sustaining marital-type relationships Relationships marred by violence or infidelity
	Aggressive relational style	Callousness Grievance thinking Angry belligerence
Self-management	Social deviance	Lifestyle impulsiveness Resistance to rules and supervision
	Dysfunctional coping	Poor problem-solving Poor emotional control

empirically supported or empirically promising by Mann et al. (2010)'s meta-analyses fall neatly into the four domains (see Table 15.1). Similarly, the items from empirically supported measures of dynamic risk factors such as the Violence Risk Scale-Sex Offense Version (VRS-SO: Olver et al., 2007) or the STABLE-2007 (Hanson et al., 2007) also fall into the four SRA domains (see Thornton, 2016, Table 1). Of particular interest is a recent meta-analysis by Berg et al. (2018) which assessed the predictive properties of measures of dynamic risk for sexual recidivism. This found that dynamic instruments were robustly predictive of sexual recidivism (d = 0.71, based on n = 5,699) and incrementally predictive relative to static-actuarial scales. Of note is that the scales included in this meta-analysis were either explicit implementations of the SRA framework or scales like the VRS-SO, whose components and items map into the SRA framework.

The SRA framework for describing psychological risk factors is thus well validated empirically and therefore can afford a basis for examining *sexual deviance*. It is outlined in Table 15.1 which is based on Thornton and Knight (2015) and Thornton (2016). Within this framework *Sexual deviance* is understood as referring to two interrelated constructs central to SRA's depiction of long-term vulnerabilities that contribute to sexual offending from the sexual interest domain. These are offense-related sexual interests (ORSI) and poor sexual self-regulation.

The different ORSI are psychologically distinct and in some samples even appear negatively correlated. The two main examples are Sexual Interest in Children (SIC) and Sexualized Violence (SV). SIC refers to an intense sexual interest in, or sexual preference for, prepubescent or pubescent children, while SV refers to an intense sexual interest in, or sexual preference for, forcing sex on an unwilling recipient or sexual arousal to inflicting violence, pain, terror, humiliation, destruction, or to exercising abusive control over another person. In contrast, the different elements of poor sexual self-regulation tend to be mutually reinforcing and often co-occur, although some apparent differences in their expression may result from an interaction between focus of sexual interests and available opportunities. For example, someone who is sexually interested in children might spend more time in sexual fantasy because opportunities to be sexual with specific live children are more limited. In contrast, in someone attracted to adults, poor sexual self-regulation might be expressed in a very large number of casual sexual partners. Common elements of poor sexual self-regulation include sexualized coping, sex being disproportionately valued relative to other motivations, high rates of sexual activity, large amounts of time spent engaging in sexual thoughts or fantasies, diverse sexual outlets, and impersonal sexuality.

There are obvious overlaps between the SIC and SV factors and the constructs of pedophilia and sexual sadism as defined by the DSM. There are important differences, however. In both cases SRA defines the focus of the abnormal sexual interest more broadly, while placing more emphasis on its having been expressed in a persistent and generalized way. Thus, for example, a man who engaged in sexual activity with one 12 year-old child over a period of six months might be seen as meeting DSM criteria for Pedophilia, but unless he acted sexually in relation to multiple young children or otherwise communicated a generalized and persistent interest in young children, he would not be seen as showing the SRA SIC factor. Similarly, a man whose repeated rapes were supported by persistent rape fantasies and who expressed a long-standing sexual preference for coercion would be seen as displaying the SRA SV factor but would not normally be diagnosed with sexual sadism.

Although sexual deviance is described in Table 15.1 as an interest, it is important to recognize that it does not exist in a vacuum, disconnected from other aspects of the individual's psychological functioning and lifestyle. Rather, there will be internal and external triggers that activate the arousal pattern leading to urges and fantasies, and there will be both distal and proximate approach behaviors woven through their lifestyle that lead to opportunities to offend. Thus, fully developed sexual deviance will be pervasive in the individual's life and have become a primary source of reward through which multiple needs are satisfied.

Evidence for Risk-Related Change in Sexual Deviance

A common assumption is that, once established in adulthood, the foci of offense-related sexual interests remain stable throughout adult life. There is certainly evidence for some stability, but it is not as absolute as is sometimes supposed. To the contrary, there is evidence that offense-related interests can either decline in intensity or have less impact on behavior.

Seto (2018) has summarized the available evidence for the stability of sexual interest in children. He reports that these interests commonly emerge in the teenage years and become more clearly distinguishable in the later teenage years, as the individual continues an interest in young children while their peers gradually shift the focus of their interests to more mature individuals as they themselves age. These interests then remain fairly stable in the adult years, lasting over multiple decades. Nevertheless, this stability is not absolute. Grundmann et al. (2016) reported only moderate stability coefficients (varying between 0.5s and 0.7s) for sexual interest in males and females at different levels of physical maturity (prepubescent, pubescent, and adult) over a period of about two and a half years. These stability coefficients are no doubt limited by imperfect reliability of measurement, but they certainly leave room for a moderate degree of change.

Similarly, there is some evidence that sexual interest in coercion can be stable. As Lalumiere et al. (2003) documented, about half of men convicted for rape show a sexual preference for coercion when assessed years later when they are in secure settings. Since these men presumably had these interests when they were offending, this indicates that for these individuals this sexual interest had remained for at least a period of years. Nevertheless, we do not have true prospective long-term longitudinal studies of this sexual interest.

To set against this evidence of the stability of offense-related sexual interests there is also significant evidence for change. To begin with, there is strong evidence that change in other factors can modify the effect of sexual deviance. This comes from two kinds of study: studies of the statistical effect of age, and studies of the statistical effect of time free in the community without known offending.

Sexual recidivism rates decline as a function of the age at which a man is released to the community following a conviction for a sexual offense. Hanson (2002) helpfully broke this age trend down, separating those with extra-familial child victims, those with familial victims, and those with older victims. All three groups showed marked declines in sexual recidivism rates from age 40 onward, with rates becoming very low once men entered their 60s. Subsequent research has confirmed these basic findings and established that they still hold when other static risk factors are statistically controlled (e.g., Hanson, 2006; Helmus et al., 2012; Skelton & Vess, 2008). Men with extrafamilial child victims are particularly likely to have pedophilic sexual interests, so these results strongly suggest that these interests either wane with age or at least come to exercise less control over behavior.

An even more powerful effect is implied by research into changes in risk as men serving a sentence for sexual offending spend increasing amounts of time in the community after release without known sexual reoffending (Hanson et al., 2018; Thornton et al., 2019). In essence this research demonstrates that for each five years that these men spend in the community free from known sexual offending their risk for future offending halves. This effect holds regardless of whether their victims were children or adults and is marked for those at higher actuarial risk. Since offense-related sexual interests are particularly common in those at high actuarial risk, these results indicate that it is both possible, and indeed common, for these interests to either wane markedly over a decade or for continuing interests to have much reduced expression in behavior.

These results should be considered with studies of how sexual arousal patterns change when individuals who start with offense-related sexual arousal participate in behavioral treatment designed to target this (McPhail & Olver, 2019). Both pharmacological and behavioral interventions are associated with clinically meaningful reductions in sexual arousal to pedo-hebephilic stimuli, as measured by PPG. The behavioral techniques described by McPhail and Olver include masturbatory reconditioning, olfactory reconditioning, covert sensitization, and satiation. These effects were sustained after short-term follow-up. Long-term follow-up was not studied. It might be argued that this effect of treatment is only short term and that participants would simply relapse after treatment ended. However, studies with the VRS-SO in which degree of change during treatment is rated, find that reduction in sexual deviance during treatment is associated with reduced sexual recidivism after release (Olver et al., 2018).

In sum, while there is evidence for stability over periods of years in sexual deviance, there is also strong evidence that under some circumstances sexual deviance can either wane or reduce its effect on behavior. It is unclear from the research which of these two mechanisms of change applies, and it is possible that both are involved. For example, someone might experience some of the behavioral techniques as reducing an unwanted arousal pattern and learn how to reapply them when necessary. The motivation to do this might then be sustained if they developed ways of living a satisfying life that did not depend on offense-related arousal.

Assessing Response to Treatment

From the previous sections of this chapter it can be seen that change in sexual deviance, understood as reductions in the intensity or the effects of sexual deviance, is certainly possible. However, McPhail and Olver's work does not imply that all those involved in treatment will benefit. How should the practicing clinician distinguish those for whom a meaningful reduction in sexual deviance has occurred?

Undoubtedly the best empirically validated measure of recidivism-related change in institutional treatment targeting sexual deviance is the Change score from the VRS-SO. Effects appear clinically meaningful and have generalized across multiple samples. How can this be applied? Obviously the most straightforward way to do this is to apply the VRS-SO itself and, where practical, the writer would recommend this. However, relatively few clinicians are trained in the use of this instrument and scoring it can be quite laborious. Can these results inform a more general understanding changes in sexual deviance? It is possible to approach this by examining how the VRS-SO Change score is coded.

The Change score uses a modified version of the Stage of Change Model. Most of what is coded as Change in the VRS-SO studies will have consisted of moving from Pre-Contemplation or Contemplation to what the VRS-SO labels Preparation or Action. The key evidence for this shift consists of (a) the person recognizing that a risk factor constitutes a problem for them, (b) the person seeking to address the risk factor in an observable way, and (c) behavior related to the risk factor changing. The consistency and temporal stability of the changes determines whether Preparation or Action is coded (Wong et al., 2003), with Preparation being coded when there are more lapses or when improved functioning was only recently developed. This is coded separately for each dynamic risk factor identified as a treatment need for this individual at the point of entering treatment.

What constitutes seeking to address sexual deviance in an observable way and related behaviors changing, and how can these occur in an institutional setting where the individual's access to potential victims has deliberately been limited? Table 15.2 illustrates the kinds of change that can occur and that should be looked for in an institutional setting. Of course the richness of the information about these matters will depend on the nature of the therapeutic regime the individual is in and the quality of its recording practices!

Table 15.2 Change indicators occurring in institutional settings.

Deviant Arousal Patterns	*Easier to satisfy through illegal behavior*
	Behavior Therapy or Mindfulness skills developed and applied to mitigate deviant arousal Reduced frequency of deviant thoughts, able to interrupt them without masturbation; rapidly stopping masturbating if experiences intrusive deviant thoughts
Triggers	*Stimuli that trigger deviant fantasies and urges*
	Avoids media that triggers deviant arousal Learns how to cope differently with interactions that used to trigger deviant arousal Develops healthier ways of functioning to replace thoughts and feelings that used to trigger deviant arousal
Victim Access Behaviors	*Behaviors that connect deviant arousal to offense opportunities*
	Identifies distal and proximate access behaviors embedded in lifestyle and notices expressions of those behaviors in institutional behavior. Learns to interrupt or avoid these behaviors Plans community lifestyle that excludes these behaviors; alternate lifestyle should include personally meaningful sources of reward; takes active steps to prepares for this alternate lifestyle and practices available elements of this lifestyle in the institution.

VRS-SO pre-treatment dynamic risk factors have been found to express three factors which are labeled sexual deviance, criminality, and treatment responsivity. The treatment responsivity factor combines a lack of insight into offense precursors, cognitive distortions, reluctance to engage in relevant treatment, and a propensity to return to situations where offense-precursors will operate. It will here be referred to as Distorted Attitudes, as the items can be seen as cognitive and behavioral expressions of an underlying positive attitude toward offending and this phrase places it appropriately within the SRA framework.

These results are nicely integrated in logistic regression models which allow five- and 10-year sexual recidivism rates to be predicted from a weighted combination of Static-99R, Pre-Treatment Dynamic Risk, and Change (Olver et al., 2018). The application of these models to individual cases has been helpfully operationalized through Excel spreadsheets that are available online (https://psynergy.ca/vrs-so). In what follows, some general principles for assessing change are tested by applying them to the VRS-SO items and then using the VRS-SO logistic equations to determine how much difference given patterns of change would produce in expected recidivism rates.

A useful way to approach this is define a threshold level of meaningful change for a dynamic risk factor and then to examine the effect of different patterns and degrees of change. This can then be examined for different initial risk presentations. Here meaningful change is defined, following the VRS-SO, as requiring (a) the person recognizing that a risk factor constitutes a problem for them, (b) the person seeking to address the risk factor in an observable way, and (c) behavior related to the risk factor changing so that lapses are unusual over the last six months and generally mild in intensity.

Four levels of change are then considered: (i) Rejection, where the person has been resistant to treatment influences and has not shown meaningful change for any of their risk factors; (ii) Limited Response, where meaningful change has occurred for about one-third of the person's risk factors; (iii) Broad Response, where meaningful change has occurred for two-thirds of the person's risk factors; and (iv) Comprehensive Response, where meaningful change has occurred for all applicable risk factors. Across the Limited, Broad and Comprehensive Response patterns we can then also ask how risk would change if meaningful responses had been sustained for two years (a duration that would normally be regarded as meeting the criteria for "action" in VRS-SO scoring).

This framework is intended for use with individuals who, prior to treatment, present a substantial risk. Three prototypical presentations will be considered. The first of these combines high levels of sexual deviance without supporting distorted attitudes or antisociality. The second combines high levels of sexual deviance and distorted attitudes with some, more minor, antisociality. The third combines high levels of sexual deviance with general antisociality and some, more minor pro-offending attitudes. To make these prototypes more clinically intelligible, a case study corresponding to each is sketched below.

Corresponding to the first prototype is what can be labeled Ego Dystonic Preferential Pedophilia. The individual has a strong, and preferential, sexual interest in young children, but they see acting on this as repugnant and seek to control themselves. However, they tend to over-react to life stress and this weakens their capacity for self-control, especially as they then drink to excess. Additionally, although they exercise conscious self-control, their attraction to children sometimes leads to a succession of seemingly irrelevant decisions that place them in situations where offending against children would be relatively easy. When this coincides with weakened self-control a process of cognitive deconstruction ensues leading to offending. They have also sometimes downloaded sexualized images of children from the internet, seeing these as a way to avoid offending against "real children." Their struggles with their paraphilia have left them increasingly isolated from social support and they have limited experience of adult romantic relationships. They have been convicted for sexual offenses on two occasions and are known to have committed contact offenses against three victims. The current sentencing occasion included both a contact sex offense and illegal images of children on their computer. Their psychometric profile is a Static-99 R score of 6 and a VRS-SO Initial Dynamic Risk score of 22 with points coming almost exclusively from sexual deviance.

Corresponding to the second prototype is what can be labeled Ego Syntonic Preferential Pedophilia. The individual has a strong, and preferential sexual interest in young children which is supported by seeing children as naturally sexual and sexual contact between adults and children as harmless. They have generally groomed potential victims but have occasionally offended opportunistically without using physical violence. Although not generally criminal, they are inclined to seek out situations where there is an opportunity to sexually offend against children and have been resistant to both prior treatment and community supervision. They have been convicted on two occasions for offenses against children, having five known victims of contact sex offenses and also having been found with illegal images of children on their computer. They have never married, and lack prosocial community supports, though they have been able to hold down steady employment. Their psychometric profile is a Static-99 R score of 6 with a VRS-SO Initial Dynamic Risk score of 30 with points coming mainly from sexual deviance but also substantially from Distorted Attitudes.

Corresponding to the third prototype is what can be labeled Antisocial Sadism. The individual has a strong attraction to violent rapes in which the victim is humiliated, terrified and brutalized. They have a history of going out hunting for potential victims but have also impulsively sexually assaulted a woman when feeling affronted by her. They take pride in their ability to manipulate potential victims using a mixture of charm and intimidation. They express hostile and adversarial attitudes towards women but do not minimize the women's distress. This is the second occasion they have been convicted for sexual assault and they have three officially known victims, one of whom was previously known to them. They also have a history of non-sexual crime including non-sexual violence and burglary. Their psychometric profile is a Static-99 R score of 6 with a VRS-SO Initial Dynamic Risk score of 33, with points coming in equal parts from sexual deviance and antisociality but also to some degree from Distorted Attitudes.

Table 15.3 shows 10-year sexual recidivism rates projected from the VRS-SO logistic regression equations for persons with the psychometric scores corresponding to the three prototypes. For each prototype the recidivism rates associated with the treatment response profiles corresponding to Resistance, Limited Change, Broad Change and Comprehensive Change are shown. These are based on assigning corresponding Change scores assuming Preparation stage or, for sustained change, the Action stage, as this is defined by the VRS-SO.

Since recidivism base rates can vary depending on arbitrary features, such as the efficiency of the criminal justice system in detecting offenses, it may be helpful express the risk associated with a more positive response to the risk associated with Resistance (see Table 15.4). Note that "sustained" here refers to the Change Profile having been sustained for two years. Thus, for example, for someone showing a Broad pattern of change over less than two years, the

Table 15.3 Ten-year sexual recidivism rates by need and change profile.

Need Profile	Ego Dystonic Preferential Pedophilia	Ego Syntonic Preferential Pedophilia	Antisocial Sadism
Static-99 R	6	6	6
VRS-SO Pre-Treatment Dynamic Risk	22	31	33
Number of Treatment Needs	9	12	15
Change Profile			
Rejection	29%	39%	43%
Limited Response	25%	35%	36%
Broad Response	21%	29%	29%
Comprehensive Response	18%	24%	22%
Sustained Limited Response	21%	29%	29%
Sustained Broad Response	16%	18%	17%
Sustained Comprehensive Response	11%	13%	10%

Table 15.4 Proportion of risk associated with resistance retained after positive responses.

Change Profile	Developing	Sustained
Limited	Close to 90%	About 70%
Broad	About 70%	About Half
Comprehensive	About 60%	About a Third

associated risk could be described as about 70% of the risk they would have presented if they had made no efforts at change (Resistance). In contrast, if a Broad pattern of change had been shown for at least two years, then the associated risk could be described as about half the risk they would have presented if they had made no efforts at change (Resistance).

Some general principles can be extracted from the above analysis.

(1) *Breadth of change matters.* The proportion of the individual's dynamic risk factors that they are regulating makes a big difference. Where sexual deviance is a substantial part of the individual's need profile, changing non-sexual risk factors can help but will not be sufficient to produce a substantial reduction in risk. But equally, if both sexual and non-sexual risk factors are a substantial part of the individual's need profile, then change in both general areas will be required.
(2) *Duration of change matters.* All change profiles are associated with materially greater reduction in risk where the change is sustained for at least two years.
(3) *Perfection is not required.* Although greater reduction in risk is associated with regulation of all identified dynamic risk factors, regulating even two-thirds of them in a sustained way is sufficient to produce a substantial reduction in risk.

Applying the Change Framework

Since the evidence base for the above framework comes from work with the VRS-SO, professionals seeking to evaluate the significance of change will do well to use that instrument. Nevertheless, when, for whatever reason, other instruments or forms of structured clinical judgment are used, it is possible to apply the general principles described above.

As an example, consider need assessment with the SRA-FV (Thornton & Knight, 2015). This identifies up to 10 criminogenic needs as long-term vulnerabilities, with each factor scored on a 0 to 2 range, with scores of 1.5 or higher indicating the presence of a long-term vulnerability. Suppose that, for a given individual, six of the long-term vulnerabilities were identified based on their history, then if after being offered treatment services they demonstrated management of at least four of these, sustained for over two years, then they would meet the criteria for a sustained broad change profile and their assessed risk could be abated accordingly. Note that, as indicated earlier, "managing" a long-term vulnerability here means (a) the person recognizing that the long-term vulnerability constitutes a problem for them, (b) the person is working to address the risk factor in an observable way, and (c) behavior related to the risk factor has changed so that lapses are rare.

Similarly, a professional might be using a checklist of psychological risk factors based on Mann et al. (2010)'s identification of psychologically meaningful risk factors. They might identify nine of these factors as having been applicable to the individual. If the individual showed management of six of these factors, sustained over two years, then they would meet the criteria for a sustained broad change profile.

In the above examples, emphasis has been placed on meeting the criteria for a sustained broad change profile because, in the writer's experience, this is a target that is achievable for the majority of individuals with sexual deviancy who are assessed as presenting a well above average risk for sexual recidivism. Further, the proportionate reduction in risk would be sufficient to bringing the individual down one Risk Matrix 2000 level (Lehmann et al., 2016; Thornton et al., 2003) or one standardized risk category for Static-99 R or other instruments that have been calibrated against these standards.

This threshold for substantial risk reduction may also usefully apply in a number of forensic contexts where individuals' liberties are restricted because they are deemed to pose a danger to others as a result of mental disorder. Once such a status has been assigned, a small dip below the technically required risk threshold is seldom enough to persuade courts to allow the person to be released. Rather, in practice, courts need to be persuaded both that a legally defined risk threshold is no longer met and that risk to the public has substantially reduced. Meeting the criteria for a sustained broad change profile will typically justify both these claims.

Conclusions

Sexual deviance, understood as hypersexuality or sexual preoccupation combined with offense-related sexual interests, is an important predisposing factor for sexual offending. Research with the VRS-SO has demonstrated that the degree to which it predisposes can be mitigated when specifiable kinds of change are made during treatment. This chapter has described these changes in a sufficiently abstract and generalized way that they could be applied in combination with any credible measure of sexual deviance. The degree of change required to produce a clinically meaningful degree of risk reduction is also described.

References

Allen, B. P., & Pflugradt, D. M. (2014). An exploration of the latent constructs of the Static-99. *International Journal of Offender Therapy and Comparative Criminology, 58*(11), 1376–1388. https://doi.org/10.1177/0306624X13496046

American Psychiatric Association. (2013). *Diagnostic and statistical manual of mental disorders* (5th ed.). https://doi.org/10.1176/appi.books.9780890425596

Beech, A. R., Fisher, D. D., & Thornton, D. (2003). Risk assessment of sex offenders. *Professional Psychology: Research and Practice, 34*(4), 339–352. https://doi.org/10.1037/0735-7028.34.4.339

Brouillette-Alarie, S., Babchishin, K. M., Hanson, R. K., & Helmus, L.-M. (2016). Latent constructs of the Static-99R and Static-2002R: A three-factor solution. *Assessment, 23*(1), 96–111. https://doi.org/10.1177/1073191114568114

Fisher, D., & Thornton, D. (1993). Assessing risk of re-offending in sexual offenders. *Journal of Mental Health, 2*(2), 105–117. https://doi.org/10.3109/09638239309018395

Grundmann, D., Krupp, J., Scherner, G., Amelung, T., & Beier, K. M. (2016). Stability of self-reported arousal to sexual fantasies involving children in a clinical samples of pedophiles and hebephiles. *Archives of Sexual Behavior, 45*(5), 1153–1162. https://doi.org/10.1007/s10508-016-0729-z

Hanson, R. K. (2002). Recidivism and age: Follow-up data from 4,673 sexual offenders. *Journal of Interpersonal Violence, 17*(10), 1046–1062. https://doi.org/10.1177/08862605-0201710-02

Hanson, R. K. (2006). Does Static-99 predict recidivism among older sexual offenders? *Sexual Abuse: A Journal of Research and Treatment, 18*(4), 343–355. https://doi.org/10.1007/s11194-006-9027-y

Hanson, R. K., & Bussière, M. T. (1998). Predicting relapse: A meta-analysis of sexual offender recidivism studies. *Journal of Consulting and Clinical Psychology, 66*(2), 348–362. https://doi.org/10.1037/0022-006X.66.2.348

Hanson, R. K., Harris, A. J. R., Letourneau, E., Helmus, L. M., & Thornton, D. (2018). Reductions in risk based on time offense free in the community: Once a sex offender, not always a sex offender. *Psychology, Public Policy, and Law, 24*(1), 48–63. http://dx.doi.org/10.1037/law0000135

Hanson, R. K., Harris, A. J. R., Scott, T. L., & Helmus, L. (2007). Assessing the risk of sexual offenders on community supervision: The Dynamic Supervision Project. User Report, Corrections Research, Ottawa. Public Safety Canada.

Hanson, R. K., & Morton-Bourgon, K. E. (2005). The characteristics of persistent sexual offenders: A meta-analysis of recidivism studies. *Journal of Consulting and Clinical Psychology, 73*(6), 1154–1163. https://doi.org/10.1037/0022-006X.73.6.1154

Helmus, L, Thornton, D, Hanson, R. K., & Babchishin, K. M. (2012). Improving the predictive accuracy of Static-99 and Static-2002 with older sex offenders: Revised age weights. *Sexual Abuse, 24*(1), 64–101. https://doi.org/10.1177/1079063211409951

Lalumière, M. L., Quinsey, V., Harris, G., Rice, M., & Trautrimas, C. (2003). Are rapists differentially aroused by coercive sex in phallometric assessments? In R. Prentky, E. Janus, & M. C. Seto (Eds.), *Sexually coercive behavior*. Annals of the New York Academy of Sciences.

Lehmann, R. J. B., Thornton, D., Helmus, L. M., & Hanson, R. K. (2016). Developing nonarbitrary metrics for risk communication: Norms for the risk matrix 2000. *Theory, Culture & Society, 43*(12), 97–122. https://doi.org/10.1177/026327697014004005

Mann, R. E., Hanson, R. K., & Thornton, D. (2010). Assessing risk for sexual recidivism: Some proposals on the nature of psychologically meaningful risk factors. *Sexual Abuse: A Journal of Research and Treatment, 22*(2), 191–217. https://doi.org/10.1177/1079063210366039

McPhail, I. V., & Olver, M. E. (2019). *Interventions of pedohebephilic arousal in men convicted for sexual offenses against children: A meta-analytic review*. Unpublished manuscript.

Olver, M. E., Mundt, J. C., Thornton, D., Beggs Christofferson, S. M., Kingston, D. A., Sowden, J. N., Nicholaichuk, T. P., Gordon, A., & Wong, S. C. P. (2018). Using the Violence Risk Scale-Sexual Offense version in sexual violence risk assessments: Updated risk categories and recidivism estimates from a multisite sample of treated sexual offenders. *Psychological Assessment, 30*(7), 941–955. https://doi.org/10.1037/pas0000538

Olver, M. E., Wong, S. C. P., Nicholaichuk, T. P., & Gordon, A. (2007). The validity and reliability of the Violence Risk Scale-Sex Offender version: Assessing sex offender risk and evaluating therapeutic change. *Psychological Assessment, 19*(3), 318–329. https://doi.org/10.1037/1040-3590.19.3.318

Roberts, C. F., Doren, D. M., & Thornton, D. (2002). Dimensions associated with assessments of sex offender recidivism risk. *Criminal Justice and Behavior, 29*(5), 569–589. https://doi.org/10.1177/009385402236733

Seto, M. C. (2018). *Pedophilia and sexual offending against children*. American Psychological Association.

Skelton, A., & Vess, J. (2008). Risk of sexual recidivism as a function of age and actuarial risk. *Journal of Sexual Aggression, 14*(3), 199–209. https://doi.org/10.1080/13552600802267098

Thornton, D. (2002). Constructing and testing a framework for dynamic risk assessment. *Sexual Abuse: A Journal of Research and Treatment, 14*(2), 137–151. https://doi.org/10.1177/107906320201400205. PMID: 11961888.

Thornton, D. (2016). Structured risk assessment. In A. Phenix & H. M. Hoberman (Eds.), *Sexual offending: Predisposing antecedents, assessments and management*. Springer.

Thornton, D., Hanson, R. K., Kelley, S. M., & Mundt, J. C. (2019). Estimating lifetime and residual risk for individuals who remain sexual offense free in the community. *Sexual Abuse*. online publication ahead of print. https://doi.org/10.1177/1079063219871573

Thornton, D., & Knight, R. A. (2015). Construction and validation of SRA-FV need assessment. *Sexual Abuse: A Journal of Research and Treatment, 27*(4), 360–375. https://doi.org/10.1177/1079063213511120

Thornton, D., Mann, R., Webster, S., Blud, L., Travers, R., Friendship, C., & Erickson, M. (2003). Distinguishing and combining risks for sexual and violent recidivism. In R. Prentky, E. Janus, &

M. Seto (Eds.), *Understanding and managing sexually coercive behavior*. Annals of the New York Academy of Sciences.

Van den Berge, J. W., Wineke, S., Schepers, K., Wever, E., van Beek, D., Janssen, E., & Gijs, L. (2018). The predictive properties of dynamic sex offender risk assessment instruments: A meta-analysis. *Psychological Assessment, 30*(2), 179–191. https://doi.org/10.1037/pas0000454.

Wong, S., Olver, M. E., Nicholaichuk, T. P., & Gordon, A. (2003). The Violence Risk Scale: Sexual Offender version (VRS-SO). *Regional Psychiatric Centre and University of Saskatchewan.*

16

Psychological Treatments for Paraphilias and Compulsive Sexual Behavior

Michael H. Miner[1] *and Rosemary Munns*[2]

[1,2] *University of Minnesota, USA*

Psychological Treatment of Paraphilias and Compulsive Sexual Behavior

The treatment of paraphilias and compulsive sexual behavior (CSB) are two separate areas of investigation, although there appear to be overlapping concepts between the models proposed for the intervention of each issue. Central to both issues are definitions of the constructs. Paraphilias have been the topic of writing and theorizing for centuries, with the most complete description of unconventional sexual behavior being Krafft-Ebing's *Psychopathia Sexualis* in 1886. Money (1999) identified and named over 136 different types of paraphilias, while Aggrawal (2009) estimates that there are probably at least 547 different categories of paraphilia. However, until publication of the *Diagnostic and Statistical Manual of Mental Disorders, Fifth Edition* (*DSM-5*; American Psychiatric Association, 2013), there has been no clearly articulated definition of paraphilias, although they have been described as sexual arousal to objects, situations, or non-consenting individuals, which are outside the range of usual sexual interests (Beech & Harkins, 2012). Problematic in this definition is to articulate what is "outside the range of usual sexual interests." There are certainly some sexual interests that clearly fit this conceptualization, but others are less clear. Until 1973, homosexuality was defined as a paraphilia, but that is no longer the case, although one could argue that the prevalence data currently available would still indicate that same sex sexual interest is not "usual," being reported by 5.8% of males and 1.5% of females in a recent U.S. survey of adult sexual behavior (Herbenick et al., 2017). The contemporary definition from the *DSM-5* is "any intense and persistent sexual interest other than sexual interest in genital stimulation or preparatory fondling with phenotypically normal, physically mature, consenting human partners" (American Psychiatric Association, 2013, p. 685).

CSB presents even more definitional problems. It is characterized by intense, distressing, and recurrent sexual urges and fantasies that significantly interfere with a person's daily functioning (e.g., with personal, interpersonal, and occupational responsibilities). CSB is widely disputed with regard to conceptualization, etiology, and nomenclature, and has been dubbed with such terms as "sexual addiction" (Carnes, 1983), "compulsive sexual behavior" (Coleman, 1991), "paraphilia related disorder" (Kafka & Hennen, 1999), "hypersexual disorder" (Kafka, 2010), and "out of control sexual behavior" (Braun-Harvey & Vigorito, 2015). Despite such disagreement, one of the hallmarks of all conceptualizations of hypersexuality, which we will use interchangeably with CSB due to lack of general agreement in

Sexual Deviance: Understanding and Managing Deviant Sexual Interests and Paraphilic Disorders,
First Edition. Edited by Leam A. Craig and Ross M. Bartels.
© 2021 John Wiley & Sons, Ltd. Published 2021 by John Wiley & Sons, Ltd.

nomenclature (Carnes, 1983, 1991; Coleman, 1991; Coleman et al., 2003; Kafka, 1997, 2010), is distress resulting from obsessive, compulsive, impulsive, and/or out of control sexual behavior (Black et al., 1997; Coleman et al., 2010; Dickenson et al., 2018). Moreover, several theoretical models of hypersexual behavior indicate that engaging in sexual behavior functions as a strategy to cope with, escape from, or avoid unwanted emotions (Kafka, 2010; Reid & Kafka, 2014). There are those that argue that CSB does not exist, but that the concept represents an effort to pathologize high sexual drive (Ley et al., 2014) and impose moral standards of acceptable levels of sexual behavior (Moser, 2013). In our recent work, we have found that CSB is related to two broad personality factors: Negative Emotionality and Constraint (Miner et al., 2016). These factors indicate that CSB is characterized by difficulties regulating and coping with negative affect and a tendency toward impulsivity, risk taking, and non-traditional values. We further found that those who met criteria for CSB responded differently to fluctuations in daily affect than those who did not. Specifically, negative affect interacted with positive activation to motivate sexual behavior in those with CSB, while no such interaction existed in non-CSB individuals. In the non-CSB sample, negative affect attenuated the probability of engaging in sexual behavior, while it failed to do so in those with CSB (Miner et al., 2019).

Treatment of men who have committed sexual crimes has focused attention on both the sexual arousal (paraphilias) and the ability to control one's sexual behavior (CSB). The remainder of this chapter will focus on methods that have been used to modify and address paraphilic sexual attractions and to help individuals to gain control over their sexual behavior.

Treatment of Paraphilias

While psychological treatment of paraphilias was initially the domain of psychoanalysis (Laws & Marshall, 2003), these methods were not shown to be particularly effective. With the move toward conditioning explanations of behavior, and the application of behavior theory to therapeutic interventions, most of the work on treating paraphilias comes out of a behavioral perspective, particularly classical conditioning and other contiguity paradigms. The research exploring the treatment of paraphilias has been conducted mainly with sexual offending samples, with the aim of affecting sexual arousal to children, sexual arousal to violent or sadistic themes, and sexual arousal to consensual sexual behavior. These interventions have applied aversive, reconditioning, or satiation paradigms.

Behavioral Interventions

Covert Sensitization

Covert Sensitization involves pairing the imagined deviant fantasy with an imagined unpleasant outcome. The unpleasant image is sometimes augmented with a noxious odor. Covert sensitization also takes on a more complex process, where the individual does not just focus on the sexual activity itself, but imagines the entire offending process. After completing the sexual act, either molesting a child, raping a woman, exposing, they continue the fantasy and imagine negative outcomes, such as being arrested, facing loss of family, humiliation, or being beaten up. While covert sensitization is a popular technique (Beech & Harkins, 2012; McGrath et al., 2010), there is little evidence of efficacy (Beech & Harkins, 2012; Marshall et al., 1999).

Olfactory Aversion

Olfactory aversion procedures involve the presentation of a noxious odor along with the presentation of some type of deviant sexual material. The purpose of the presentation is to establish a connection between induced physical discomfort and sexually explicit material that the individual found erotic (Adams et al., 1981). These procedures have usually taken two forms. In the first, a classical conditioning paradigm is used by pairing the presentation of a noxious stimulus with the presentation of either a fantasy or an image of the preferred deviant target. The classical counter-conditioning paradigm (Rimm & Masters, 1979) is thought to bring about inhibition of deviant sexual arousal by associating unpleasant physical sensations with the presentation of inappropriate sexual material, in place of the previously experienced pleasant sensation of sexual arousal. It has also been used successfully to change individual arousal patterns. This form of olfactory aversion has been used effectively to inhibit the sexual arousal of previously exhibitionist patients to imagery and photographs of exhibitionistic behavior (Maletzky, 1977) and to inhibit arousal to sadistic material of an individual with previously high involvement in sexually sadistic fantasies and activities (Laws et al., 1978).

In the second form, a noxious odor (i.e., dilute ammonia sulfide, aromatic ammonia, butyric acid, or valeric acid) has been used to augment the aversive imagery during covert sensitization (Levin et al., 1977). In this procedure the individuals are led through a fantasy that brings them to the point where they would perform an inappropriate sex act. At this point, the patient is directed to imagine extremely noxious stimuli (e.g., vomiting, parasites entering their mouth, etc.) and these images are augmented by the presentation of a noxious odor. Olfactory aversion as an augmentation of covert sensitization (often called assisted covert sensitization) has been successfully used in the treatment of various paraphilias, including exhibitionism (Maletzky, 1974) and pedophilia (Levin et al., 1977). In these cases, the authors found that the addition of a noxious odorous substance to the standard covert sensitization procedure led to a decrease in the individual's arousal to the target sexual object or, in the case of exhibitionism, to a decrease in sexual gratification to images of that activity.

Apparently, both forms of olfactory aversion have shown promise as means for eliminating sexual arousal to paraphilic content. In a more recently published case study, Marshall (2006a) again showed successful use of the counter-conditioning form of olfactory aversion in decreasing paraphilic arousal. The classical counter-conditioning paradigm seems more appealing due to the increased control that the therapist can exert over the pairing of negative reinforcement and sexual material, and to the decreased reliance on visualization, which is a skill that individuals may perform with varying degrees of success.

Orgasmic Reconditioning

Orgasmic reconditioning, also referred to as masturbatory conditioning, attempts to increase sexual arousal to adult, consenting sex through pairing stimuli with elicited sexual arousal. The value of this procedure derives from the assumption that various stimuli acquire erotic arousal properties by virtue of their association with orgasmic pleasure (McGuire et al., 1964). As originally practiced, orgasmic reconditioning involved having the individual initiate arousal to a fantasy involving their particular paraphilia. Approximately five seconds prior to ejaculation, they are asked to switch to fantasy content of a non-paraphilic nature. The point at which the individual changes fantasy content is slowly moved forward in time until, ultimately, they use only fantasies involving mutually consenting sexual behavior with an adult partner. It is important in this procedure that the individual never ejaculates while fantasizing about a paraphilic act, since the pairing of ejaculation and fantasy content is hypothesized to be the mechanism by which new sexual arousal patterns are to be established (Marquis, 1970).

While initial reports of this procedure were positive (LoPiccolo et al., 1972; Marquis, 1970), Conrad and Wincze (1976) found no evidence that orgasmic reconditioning had any effect on physiologic or behavioral arousal. This conflicting result was attributed to the reliance on self-reported measures in previous work. Conrad and Wincze (1976) found that their subjects were able to reach orgasm when using alternative fantasies and that such subjects were likely to report an increased attraction to material compatible with such fantasies. However, their relative physiologic responses were unchanged. Orgasmic reconditioning is contingent on the ability of the individual to change fantasy themes at the point of orgasm and to experience orgasm only when fantasizing to themes with non-paraphilic content. Thus, primary control of the treatment rests with the participant. It may be that the findings of Conrad and Wincze (1976) can be explained, in part, by failure of participants to consistently alter fantasy content at the appropriate time.

A procedure that allows for more control of the stimulus content of fantasies is the use of fantasy alternation. In this procedure the patient used fantasy with a deviant content for a prescribed block of time, and then in the next block uses fantasy with non-deviant content. These fantasies are alternated until termination of treatment (Abel et al., 1975). Laws and his colleagues (Foote & Laws, 1981; Laws & O'Neill, 1981; VanDeventer & Laws, 1978) have found orgasmic conditioning to effectively reduce arousal to paraphilic material and increase arousal to appropriate depictions of nude adults or descriptions involving mutually consenting sexual behavior among adults. They found a pattern in which paraphilic arousal decreases and non-paraphilic arousal increases, with a crossover occurring about the fourth week of treatment. This pattern was the same, regardless of whether fantasy content was alternated on a weekly basis (VanDeventer & Laws, 1978) or a daily basis (Foote & Laws, 1981).

The fantasy alternation procedure requires a reassessment of the theorized mechanism of action for orgasmic reconditioning. The studies by Laws and his colleagues have found a consistent pattern of change in the relative responding from a primacy of paraphilic stimuli to a primacy of non-paraphilic stimuli (Laws, 1985). These investigators have hypothesized that the opportunity to compare the fantasy content and to experience, perhaps for the first time in their lives, sexual arousal to "normal" sexual content, leads individuals to reassess their perceptions of themselves and their sexual behavior. It is this reassessment of themselves as something other than "sick perverts" and their behavior as something which can be controlled, that leads the individual to a change in arousal patterns (Laws & O'Neill, 1981; VanDeventer & Laws, 1978).

It has been suggested that the magnitudes and directions of changes in arousal patterns are unpredictable using fantasy alternation (Leonard & Hayes, 1983). Law's work would appear to confirm that fantasy alternation would not be useful with patients who show no clear preference for any class of sexually explicit stimuli, and appears to predict that the best candidates for orgasmic reconditioning are individuals who initially show high arousal to paraphilic material and minimal arousal to non-paraphilic stimuli (Laws, 1985; Laws & O'Neill, 1981).

The major problem with the fantasy alternation approach to orgasmic reconditioning is that the decrease in sexual arousal to paraphilic content is difficult to explain. Using Laws's cognitive restructuring explanation (Laws, 1985; Laws & O'Neill, 1981; VanDeventer & Laws, 1978), it would appear that the same resultant changes might be obtained by eliminating the paraphilic portion of the procedure. In fact, it has been found that orgasmic reconditioning, involving only socially acceptable fantasies, resulted in the same outcomes as using fantasy alternation (Kremsdorf et al., 1980). Not only was the pattern of results the same, but the length of treatment needed to bring pedophilic responses to 0% was the same as that found for previous cases using fantasy alternation.

In conclusion, orgasmic reconditioning has been used effectively with a wide range of paraphilias. The most promising form appears to be that in which no paraphilic themes are used in treatment sessions. This procedure is appealing since it does not result in the compliance problems associated with the original technique (Marquis, 1970) and provides the same information and advantages as the fantasy alternation approach, without its theoretic confusion.

Masturbatory Satiation

Masturbatory satiation requires prolonged, continuous masturbation while verbalizing aloud every variation the individual can think of on the theme of his paraphilic interest. Through this procedure stimulus satiation occurs, since the paraphilic fantasy is presented continuously until it becomes tedious, thus losing its motivation potential (Hull, 1943). Additionally, the repeated performance of self-manipulation results in fatigue and thus becomes aversive rather than reinforcing (Hull, 1943).

Marshall, in a series of single case experiments, found that masturbatory satiation is effective in reducing sexual arousal to paraphilic stimuli in sexually assaultive subjects (Marshall & Lippens, 1977) and in subjects whose sexual behavior was predominantly pedophilic (Marshall, 1979). The individual was required to continuously verbalize fantasy material based on his primary paraphilic interest (e.g., rape scenes or sex with a child) and was prompted during any prolonged silence. Sessions lasted from one to one and a half hours. In all cases, individuals showed a decay in their arousal to paraphilic stimuli and a maintenance of this lowered arousal at follow-up physiological assessments up to 10 months after treatment (Marshall, 1979). The effectiveness of masturbatory satiation was confirmed in a report of a multi-method treatment program (Rouleau et al., 1986). The authors also found that the masturbatory satiation component was more effective in decreasing individuals' faulty cognitions than was cognitive therapy. In a more recent case study, Marshall (2006b) again found this form of directed masturbation effectively decreased sexual interest in paraphilic content.

Verbal Satiation

Verbal satiation works through the process of stimulus satiation. That is, the individual fantasizes about their paraphilic theme, with no masturbatory manipulation, for at least 30 minutes each treatment session. This continuous repetition of the sexual stimuli continues until the attractiveness of the paraphilic fantasies has been reduced. This is thought to happen because the individual is repeatedly presented with the sexual material with no reinforcement. Therefore, the paraphilic fantasies and arousal to paraphilic material should extinguish (Hull, 1943; Rimm & Masters, 1979).

This procedure makes sense from a learning theory perspective. Satiation should be a good way to decrease the attractiveness of stimuli, such as sexually explicit depictions of children. This could be due to either of two well-established behavioral concepts, habituation and extinction. Habituation occurs when repeated applications of a particular stimulus results in decreased response (Rankin et al., 2009). In this case the same sexual fantasies have a reduced sexual arousal response. Indeed, there is evidence that people tire of repetitive sexual behaviors (Masters & Johnson, 1970) and that sexual fantasies elicited by pornography lose their attractiveness over time (Kutschinsky, 1970). The other possible mechanism is extinction, which differs from habituation in that extinction is thought to be related, not to the loss of the ability of the stimulus to elicit the response, but to the loss of the reinforcement characteristics of the stimuli due to continued presentation without reinforcing pairings (Bouton, 2004).

Ceniti and Malamuth (1984) found that repeated exposure to sexually violent pornography resulted in satiation of sexual arousal to rape themes in those subjects who were initially classified as "force oriented," due to an initial arousal to rape depictions that were similar to their arousal to non-rape depictions. One could expect rapists to respond similarly to a satiation procedure, since the arousal patterns seen in "force oriented" subjects in the study were analogous to the arousal patterns seen in convicted rapists (Abel et al., 1977). The research, to date, on satiation procedures has not been designed to explicate the mechanism underlying these procedures.

Cognitive Behavior Interventions

As the reader will note, there has been little or no research on behavioral interventions since the late 1980s, other than the case studies looking at the effectiveness of olfactory aversion and directed masturbation (Marshall, 2006a, 2006b). In general, the late 1980s and early 1990s brought a move away from strict behavioral techniques with the expansion toward cognitive aspects of therapy. An initial movement away from the strict behavior techniques was Relapse Prevention (RP; Marlatt & Gordon, 1985). This model discussed treatment of paraphilias and sexual arousal in two ways. First, rather than discarding the behavioral procedures, they were incorporated into the treatment programs for those who showed paraphilic sexual arousal (J. K. Marques et al., 1989; Nelson et al., 1989). At the same time, RP acknowledged that paraphilias were unlikely to change and that sexual fantasies and urges were likely to continue. These fantasies and urges were described as lapses, and patients were encouraged to realize that they would happen, and interventions were designed to help them cope with their emotional responses to them and to determine where they came from (Russell et al., 1989). With this addition, treatment providers describe the behavioral interventions as providing methods to control sexual urges and fantasies, rather than methods that would change the individual's arousal pattern themselves.

Paraphilic interest has long been addressed by those interested in sexual health and human sexuality. In general, these traditions have explored paraphilias within the same behavioral paradigms described above, but have been less concerned about changing sexual interest and more interested in understanding how they fit within the sexual scripts and repertoires of individuals. Our group at the Program in Human Sexuality developed an intervention program based on the Sexual Health Model (Robinson et al., 2002). A complete description of this program is available in Berg et al. (2017). The program diverges from other programs designed to treat individuals who have committed sexual offenses in that sexual fantasies are viewed, not as targets for change, but as targets for discussion. The underlying assumption is that paraphilias are unlikely to change and that individuals will continue to think about things they find sexually arousing. Further, it is assumed that keeping these interests secret adds to their salience and may also foster guilt and shame. Intervention is aimed at helping individuals understand that thoughts themselves are not problematic, but behaviors are, and the aim is to have individuals discuss their fantasies and determine their place within the individual's offending cycle (Berg et al., 2017). This technique for intervention with sexual fantasies has not been tested and a recent meta-analysis indicates that those sex offender treatment programs that include some form of arousal reconditioning resulted in larger treatment effects than those without this component (Gannon et al., 2019). However, preliminary analyses from California's Sex Offender Treatment and Evaluation Project (SOTEP) showed significant decreases in sexual arousal to paraphilic stimuli across their treatment sample, regardless of whether they received behavioral treatment or not, indicating that a multi-component cognitive behavioral intervention appears to influence arousal to paraphilic content, independent of whether or not the arousal was directly targeted by behavioral techniques (J. Marques et al., 1994). This would be consistent with Laws's (1985) argument that the change in arousal patterns seen with masturbatory reconditioning is due to changes in cognition, which is the explicit target of the J. Marques et al.

(1994) intervention. However, it was overall decrease in sexual arousal within a phallometric procedure, and not arousal to paraphilic content per se, that predicted decreased sexual offending upon release (J. Marques et al., 1994).

In summary, the psychological treatment of paraphilias has primarily been based in classical conditioning paradigms. Most of the work was done in the late 1970s and early 1980s and showed short-term effectiveness of these paradigm in decreasing arousal to the paraphilic content and, in some cases, increasing arousal to non-paraphilic content. However, there have been no large scale, long-term efficacy or effectiveness studies that show that these gains in the laboratory either generalize to the community or are maintained over time. More recent studies have focused less on individuals with paraphilias and more on those identified as sexual offenders, some proportion of whom also have paraphilic interests. These studies have explored multi-faceted programs, some of which include focus on paraphilic interest using the established behavioral procedures and others that have addressed paraphilic interest from a more sexual health and social cognitive perspective. While Gannon et al. (2019) indicated that those programs that included behavior techniques for addressing paraphilic arousal were more effective than those that did not, it is far from clear, at this point, whether classical conditioning paradigms are superior to cognitive interventions that focus on helping individuals accept their paraphilic interests and develop self-management strategies that help them avoid acting on those fantasies which harm others and/or are illegal.

Treatment of Compulsive Sexual Behavior

There are many different terms used to define non-paraphilic sex problems and each has implications for the therapeutic methods applied and targets addressed. Carnes (1983) uses the term sexual addiction where the sexual behaviors are viewed as a disease and a 12-step model of addiction is used as a guideline for treatment. Coleman et al. (2018) use the term Impulsive/Compulsive Sexual Behavior (ICSB) framing the sexual behavior problems in an integrated biopsychosocial and sex positive model. Braun-Harvey and Vigorito (2015) define these sexual behaviors as out-of-control sexual behaviors. The sexual behaviors are sociocultural in nature and arise from inter- and intra-personal conflicts regarding sexual values. Sexual value conflicts are impacted by biological, social, and psychological experiences. Marty Kafka's (2000) model of CSB emphasizes neurobiological factors contributing to these sexual behaviors. Kafka's model does incorporate psychological factors into treatment, although it often focuses primarily on medication for treatment (Kafka, 2000).

The sexual addiction model is based on the disease model of Alcoholics Anonymous (Alcoholics Anonymous, 1976, 2001). According to this model, sexual addiction is viewed as a chronic disease that is outside the control of the person (Carnes, 1983; Sex Addicts Anonymous, 2005). The sexual addiction disease continues to progress within the person and, as with alcoholism (Jellinek, 1960), results in insanity or death. Treatment uses the 12-step program guidelines with the goal of remission from the disease, as there is no cure. Carnes (1983) argues that there is something in the brain that is different from non-addicts Research has focused on trying to identify these Central Nervous System (CNS) dysfunctions, with some finding disruptions in the areas of the brain consistent with addiction (Gola et al., 2015, 2017; Voon et al., 2014), while others have failed to find such CNS disruptions (Miner et al., 2009; Prause et al., 2015). The treatment focus of an addictions model uses the 12 steps of Sex Addicts Anonymous (SAA) (Sex Addicts Anonymous, 2005). The typical treatment model focuses on getting clients through the first five steps during an inpatient or outpatient treatment phase and then having clients complete the rest of the 12 steps with assistance from a sponsor and a 12-step community support group.

The basic assumptions of the sexual addiction according to (Carnes, 1991) is that sexual preoccupation and sexual behaviors have a medication effect for various emotions and family and life problems. Birchard (2015) defines sexual addiction as a pattern of sexual behaviors containing four main components: "(1) It is experienced as out of control and preoccupying. (2) People try to stop, but they cannot remain stopped. (3) The sexual behavior brings about harmful consequences. (4) It is primarily used to anaesthetize some negative feeling state." These behaviors are not only consistent with the addictions model, but are common across all of the conceptualizations of CSB and form the core components of the proposed DSM-5 hypersexual behavior disorder (Kafka, 2010) and the current ICD-11 Compulsive Sexual Behavior Disorder (World Health Organization, 2018).

Sexual Addictions Treatment

Central to treatment from an addictions perspective is accepting powerlessness over the sexual behaviors and that these behaviors have caused your life to be unmanageable. This is an abstinence model focusing on eliminating the sexual behaviors that are addictive. Unlike alcohol or illicit drugs, sex is a primary drive and, thus, total abstinence from any type of sexual behavior is likely an unattainable goal. This treatment model defines clients' sexual behavior within three concentric circles. The inner circle lists the sexual behaviors that are the most shameful, hurtful, and problematic. These sexual behaviors are the ones from which clients abstain. The middle circle contains risky sexual behaviors, sexual behaviors that could lead to engaging in the sexual behaviors identified in the inner circle. The outer circle involves a range of healthy behaviors that are sexual and non-sexual. These behaviors are viewed as healthy behaviors that assist with coping and/or are the rewards of sobriety (Sex Addicts Anonymous, 2005). Treatment focuses on assisting clients in understanding and applying the steps to their particular behaviors.

The basic assumptions of treatment are that an addict needs to work through the 12 steps to obtain and remain in remission from sexual addiction. While initial parts of treatment may be within a structured, professionally facilitated inpatient or outpatient program, the 12-step model puts emphasis on working with a sponsor, someone who also has a sexual addiction that has completed the steps or is further along in completing the steps, and attending meetings. Thus, central to treatment from the addictions approach is an inability to control one's sexual behavior and the use of peer social supports. There appears to be no research that has tested the effectiveness of these methods. However, there is evidence from alcoholism and other areas of addiction that peer and social supports are important factors in maintaining abstinence from addictive substances (Stein & Carnes, 2018).

Cognitive Behavior Therapy

Cognitive Behavior Therapy (CBT) is commonly used as a treatment intervention for a variety of behavioral addictions and mental health issues. CBT is a combination of changing behaviors and cognitions. Beck—the founder of cognitive therapy—recognized how thoughts played a significant role in mood disorders. Feelings emerge from thoughts. CBT focuses on changing behaviors and behavior patterns by changing the meaning or interpretation of events. In sexual compulsive behavior, the focus of CBT is developing an understanding of the function of problematic sexual behaviors. Treatment focuses on developing a diagrammatic explanation of the history and function of problematic sexual behaviors that can assist the client and therapist in simplifying the complex problem. It is important to identify precipitants, vulnerability factors, triggers, and modifiers (Birchard, 2015) of the problematic sexual behaviors. Precipitants are circumstances, factors, or events in the client's history that precede engaging in the problematic sexual behavior. Triggers are the circumstances, events and/or emotional states that lead someone to engage in the sexual behavior in the present. The emotional states could include depression, anxiety, shame, loneliness, low self-esteem, etc. The problematic sexual behaviors are often self-soothing and used to manage or cope with these emotional states and vulnerability factors, despite the harmful consequences experienced because of these behaviors. While there have been few studies specifically looking at the effect of CBT on sexual compulsive behavior, as noted earlier in this chapter, CBT has been applied to sexual offending behavior and there are some data to support its use with paraphilic and sexual offending behavior. Since such behaviors are also thought to be related to self-regulation, it would seem likely that CBT would have similar effects as a treatment for CSB.

In a randomized outcome study of a seven-week CBT treatment program for individuals meeting criteria for hypersexual behavior disorder (Kafka, 2010), Hallberg et al. (2019) found indications of effectiveness in reducing sexual behaviors, indications of CSB and mental health symptoms. In a small study which also used random assignment to treatment or a waitlist control group, Crosby and Twohig (2016) found significant improvement in men who were concerned about their pornography use after being exposed to Acceptance and Commitment Therapy—a particular form of CBT.

The Mentalization-Based Therapy for Sexual Addiction (MBT-SA) is another form of CBT and is described as a straightforward model focusing on understanding behaviors, thoughts, and feelings of the self and others (Berry & Berry, 2014). In this model the subjective behaviors, cognitions, and emotional impact as experienced by the client is the focus of treatment. Treatment focuses on the client understanding the sexual behaviors in a contextual model, with a basis in social constructionism. Clients focus on critically deconstructing their beliefs regarding what "normal" sexual behavior should be and developing an understanding of sexual behaviors in the context of their sociocultural experiences and relationships (Berry & Berry, 2014). Mentalizing is the process of understanding the dynamic nature of thoughts and feelings, in the context of intentionality and changeability. The core objective of treatment is to assist clients in developing or restoring reflexive functioning to increase intentional control over mental states and problematic sexual behaviors. MBT holds that effective mentalization is a core element of psychological health and wellbeing and underlies a wide variety of psychopathologies (Bateman & Fonagy, 2012; Luyten et al., 2012).

Integrated Biopsychosocial and Sex Positive Model

The integrated biopsychosocial and sex positive model defines ICSB as a clinical syndrome characterized by intense, distressing, and recurrent sexual urges and fantasies that significantly interfere with a person's daily functioning. "Impulsive" refers to sexual behaviors that a person finds difficult to resist, whereas "compulsive" is defined as sexual behaviors that a person may experience an overwhelming urge to engage in. Thus, ICSB incorporates both impulsive and compulsive behaviors. Persons struggling with this disorder can have both or either to varying degrees. The basic assumptions of this model is that there are a multitude of underlying mechanisms that come together to create this problem. Thus, treatment requires a thorough assessment of the individual to determine the biological, psychological, and sociocultural factors that have contributed to the development and maintenance of ICSB (Coleman et al., 2018).

This integrated model is conceptualized as a modified biopsychosocial approach to treatment. Biological, psychological, and sociocultural influences are integrated and embedded into one another. ICSB occurs in an interplay of physiological, genetic, social, cognitive, emotional, and cultural influences over time. Psychological influences are the result of the interactions between biological and environmental influences. ICSB assumes that latent biological factors are manifest behaviorally under specific environmental, cultural, and social pressures. In this perspective, sexual behaviors are adaptive in one context and maladaptive in another context. The focus of treatment is for the therapist to maintain a sex positive therapeutic approach while working with clients to understand the underlying mechanisms supporting the sexual behaviors without judgment. Further, persons with ICSB are viewed as having identity and intimacy impairments resulting from psychosexual development, which have been influenced by family of origin interpersonal dysfunction, attachment issues, ongoing interpersonal interactions, and social learning and conflicts related to cultural norms regarding sexual behavior. Psychological interventions focus on identifying and repairing intimacy and identity deficits. Therapy addresses intrapsychic, interpersonal dysfunction and works to resolve socio-cultural conflicts with the individual's values. The therapy process uses interventions from family systems, social learning, attachment, and interpersonal theories. As with the other intervention strategies, while there is support for the targets and processes, there has been no direct investigation of the efficacy of this particular intervention (Coleman et al., 2018).

In summary, there are some common assumptions regarding the symptoms and treatment processes across the various conceptualizations of hypersexuality, sexual addiction, out of control sexual behavior, and ICSB. These sexual behaviors are considered maladaptive and used as a way of soothing or coping with various emotions and life events. Treatment focuses on stopping the problematic sexual behaviors, identifying behavior and thought patterns that reinforce the sexual behaviors, developing skills for intervening in these patterns, and developing a support system. These common elements are also consistent with current models of sexual offender treatment (Berg et al., 2017; Gannon et al., 2019) and may be useful within a self-regulation model that addresses control of maladaptive sexual behaviors, be they paraphilic or non-paraphilic.

Conclusions

The common issue in both the treatment of paraphilia and CSB is that research is limited and provides little evidence of long-term effectiveness. Paraphilias are not always harmful, and when both partners consent to paraphilic behaviors, or when the behaviors do not negatively impact the individual or others, there is little reason to intervene. However, when such behaviors are upsetting to the individual, cause significant dysfunction, or harm others, there is a need for intervention. The research has predominantly explored behavioral interventions that were designed to eliminate the sexual interest. In more modern programs, providers have acknowledged that paraphilic interests are unlikely to change. Thus, interventions must focus on controlling, regulating, or avoiding behavior.

The reformulated concepts of treating paraphilic behavior are consistent with the treatments of CSB, which seek to identify the purpose that the behaviors serve, identify the precursors and motivators of such behaviors, and help the individual to develop new ways of coping with the precursors, and offer new strategies to meet the needs that motivate the unwanted and maladaptive sexual behaviors. As such, treating paraphilias and CSB both draw upon self-regulation models. In the case of paraphilias, it is likely that the sexual interests and arousal are not changeable, so the individual must learn to control their behavior. With CSBs, regardless of the conceptualization guiding treatment, self-regulation may be particularly aimed at learning to regulate negative affect, as this has been hypothesized to be a driver of these behaviors

(Coleman et al., 2018) and has been found to be associated with CSB (Miner et al., 2016, 2019). The major need in treating maladaptive sexual behaviors, be they paraphilias or CSBs, is for well-constructed empirical studies to explore the efficacy of the various models and methods described in this chapter. These studies should explore the mechanisms by which change occurs, both short-term outcomes and long-term outcomes. Such studies will need to overcome a number of measurement issues, including defining appropriate outcome variables and how to measure those variables. The two studies of CBT provide a good start, but until more studies are conducted, we can only conclude that there are some promising models for treatment of paraphilias and CSB. We have little evidence to choose between the various models and procedures at present. Additionally, while there is some evidence that sex offender treatment programs that include behavioral procedures are more effective than those that do not include such procedures (Gannon et al., 2019), the evidence is weak and the mechanism by which these procedures affect long-term outcome (i.e., sexual reoffending) is unclear.

References

Abel, G. G., Barlow, D. H., Blanchard, E. B., & Guild, D. (1977). The components of rapists' sexual arousal. *Archives of General Psychiatry, 34*(8), 895–903. https://doi.org/10.1001/archpsyc.1977.01770200033002

Abel, G. G., Blanchard, E. B., Barlow, D. H., & Flanagan, B. (1975, December). *A case report of the behavioral treatment of a sadistic rapist.* Paper presented at the meeting of the Association for Advancement of Behavior Therapy, San Francisco, CA.

Adams, H. E., Tollison, C. D., & Carson, T. P. (1981). Behavior therapy with sexual deviations. In S. M. Turner, K. S. Calhoun, & H. E. Adams (Eds.), *Handbook of clinical behavior therapy* (pp. 318–346). John Wiley.

Aggrawal, A. (2009). *Forensic and medico-legal aspects of sexual crimes and unusual sexual practices.* Taylor and Francis.

Alcoholics Anonymous. (1976). *Alcoholics anonymous: The story of how many thousands of men and women have recovered from alcoholism* (3rd ed.). A.A. World Services.

Alcoholics Anonymous. (2001). *Alcoholics anonymous: The story of how many thousands of men and women have recovered from alcoholism* (4th ed.). A.A. World Services.

American Psychiatric Association. (2013). *Diagnostic and statistical manual of mental disorders* (5th ed.). Author.

Bateman, A. W., & Fonagy, P. (Eds.). (2012). *Handbook of mentalizing in mental health practice.* American Psychiatric Publishing.

Beech, A. R., & Harkins, L. (2012). DSM-IV paraphilia: Descriptions, demographics and treatment interventions. *Aggression and Violent Behavior, 17*(6), 527–539. https://doi.org/10.1016/j.avb.2012.07.008

Berg, D., Munns, R., & Miner, M. (2017). Treating sexual offending. In Z. D. Peterson (Ed.), *The Wiley handbook of sex therapy* (pp. 129–142). John Wiley & Sons.

Berry, M. D., & Berry, P. D. (2014). Mentalization-based therapy for sexual addiction: Foundations for a clinical model. *Sexual and Relationship Therapy, 29*(2), 245–260. https://doi.org/10.1080/14681994.2013.856516

Birchard, T. (2015). *CBT for Compulsive Sexual Behavior: A guide for professionals.* Routledge.

Black, D. W., Kehrberg, L. L., Flumerfelt, D. L., & Schlosser, S. S. (1997). Characteristics of 36 subjects reporting compulsive sexual behavior. *The American Journal of Psychiatry, 154*(2), 243–249. https://doi.org/10.1176/ajp.154.2.243

Bouton, M. E. (2004). Context and behavioral processes in extinction. *Learning and Memory, 11*, 485–494. http://learnmem.cship.org/content/11/5/485.full.html#ref-list-1

Braun-Harvey, D., & Vigorito, M. (2015). *Treating out of control sexual behavior: Rethinking sex addiction*. Springer Publishing Company, LLC.

Carnes, P. (1983). *The sexual addiction*. CompCare.

Carnes, P. (1991). *Don't call it love*. Bantam Books.

Ceniti, J., & Malamuth, N. M. (1984). Effects of repeated exposure to sexually violent or nonviolent stimuli on sexual arousal to rape and nonrape depictions. *Behaviour Research and Therapy, 22*(5), 535–548. https://doi.org/10.1016/0005-7967(84)90056-1

Coleman, E. (1991). Compulsive sexual behavior: New concepts and treatments. *Journal of Psychology and Human Sexuality, 4*(2), 37–52. https://doi.org/10.1300/J056v04n02_04

Coleman, E., Dickenson, J. A., Girard, A., Rider, G. N., Candelario-Perez, L. E., Becker-Warner, R., Kovic, A.G., & Munns, R. A. (2018). An integrative biopsychosocial and sex positive model of understanding and treatment of impulsive/compulsive sexual behavior. *Sexual Addiction & Compulsivity, 25*(2–3), 125–152. https://doi.org/10.1080/10720162.2018.1515050

Coleman, E., Horvath, K., Miner, M., Ross, M. W., Oakes, M., & Rosser, B. R. S., & Men's INTernet Sex (MINTS-II) Team. (2010). Compulsive sexual behavior and risk for unsafe sex among internet using men who have sex with men. *Archives of Sexual Behavior, 39*(5), 1045–1053. https://doi.org/10.1007/s10508-009-9507-5

Coleman, E., Raymond, N., & McBean, A. (2003). Assessment and treatment of compulsive sexual behavior. *Minnesota Medicine, 86*(7), 42–47. www.MMAonline.net

Conrad, S. R., & Wincze, J. P. (1976). Orgasmic reconditioning: A controlled study of its effects upon the sexual arousal and behavior of adult male homosexuals. *Behavior Therapy, 7*(2), 155–166. https://doi.org/10.1016/S0005-7894(76)80271-7

Crosby, J. M., & Twohig, M. P. (2016). Acceptance and commitment therapy for problematic Internet pornography use: A randomized trial. *Behavior Therapy, 26*(3), 355–366. https://doi.org/10.1016/j.beth.2016.02.001

Dickenson, J. A., Gleason, N., Coleman, E., & Miner, M. H. (2018). Prevalence of distress associated with difficulty controlling sexual urges, feelings, and behaviors in the United States. *JAMA Network Open, 1*(7), e184468–e184468. https://doi.org/10.1001/jamanetworkopen.2018.4468

Foote, W. E., & Laws, D. R. (1981). A daily alternation procedure for orgasmic reconditioning with a pedophile. *Journal of Behavior Therapy and Experimental Psychiatry, 12*(3), 267–273. https://doi.org/10.1016/0005-7916(81)90057-4

Gannon, T. A., Olver, M. E., Mallion, J. S., & James, M. (2019). Does specialized psychological treatment for offending reduce recidivism? A meta-analysis examining staff and program variables as predictors of treatment effectiveness. *Clinical Psychology Review, 73*, Article no. 101752.

Gola, M., Wordecha, M., Sescousse, G., Kossowski, B., & Marchewka, A. (2015). Increased sensitivity to erotic reward cues in subjects with compulsive sexual behaviors. *Journal of Behavioral Addictions, 4*(S1), 16–17. https://doi.org/10.1556/JBA.4.2015.Suppl.1

Gola, M., Wordecha, M., Sescousse, G., Lew-Starowicz, M., Kossowski, B., Wypych, M., Makeig, S., Potenza, M.N., & Marcheska, A. (2017). Can pornography be addictive? An fMRI study of men seeking treatment for problematic pornography use. *Neuropsychopharmacology, 42*(5), 2021–2031. https://doi.org/10.1038/npp.2017.78

Hallberg, J., Kaldo, V., Arver, S., Dhejne, C., Jokinen, J., & Öberg, K. G. (2019). A randomized controlled study of group-administered cognitive behavior therapy for hypersexual disorder in men. *Journal of Sexual Medicine, 16*(5), 733–745. https://doi.org/10.1016/j.jsxm.2019.03.005

Herbenick, D., Bowling, J., Fu, T.-C., Dodge, B., Guerra-Reyes, L., & Sanders, S. (2017). Sexual diversity in the United States: Results from a nationally representative probability sample of adult women and men. *PLoS ONE, 12*(7), e0181198. https://doi.org/10.1371.journal.pone0181198

Hull, C. L. (1943). *Principles of behavior*. Appleton.

Jellinek, E. M. (1960). *The disease concept of alcoholism*. Hillhouse Press.

Kafka, M. P. (1997). Hypersexual desire in males: An operational definition and clinical implications for men with paraphilias and paraphilia-related disorders. *Archives of Sexual Behavior, 26*(5), 505–526. https://doi.org/10.1023/A:1024507922470

Kafka, M. P. (2000). The paraphilia-related disorders: Nonparaphilic hypersexuality and sexual compulsivity/addiction. In S. R. Leiblum & R. C. Rosen (Eds.), *Principles and practice of sex therapy* (3rd ed., pp. 471–503). Guilford Press.

Kafka, M. P. (2010). Hypersexual disorder: A proposed diagnosis for DSM-V. *Archives of Sexual Behavior, 39*(2), 377–400. https://doi.org/10.1007/s10508-009-9574-7

Kafka, M. P., & Hennen, J. (1999). The paraphilia-related disorders: An empirical investigation of nonparaphilic hypersexual disorders in 206 outpatient males. *Journal of Sex and Marital Therapy, 25*(4), 305–319. https://doi.org/10.1080/00926239908404008

Krafft-Ebing, R. (1886). *Psychopathis sexualis*. Fredinand Enke.

Kremsdorf, R. B., Holmen, M. L., & Laws, D. R. (1980). Orgasmic reconditioning without deviant imagery: A case report with a pedophile. *Behavior Research and Therapy, 18*(3), 203–207. https://doi.org/10.1016/0005-7967(80)90037-6

Kutschinsky, B. (1970). *Studies on pornography and sex crimes in Denmark*. New Social Science Monographs.

Laws, D. R. (1985). Sexual fantasy alternation: Procedural considerations. *Journal of Behavior Therapy and Experimental Psychiatry, 16*(1), 39–44. https://doi.org/10.1016/0005-7916(85)90028-X

Laws, D. R., & Marshall, W. L. (2003). A brief history of behavioral and cognitive behavioral approaches to sexual offenders: Part 1. Early developments. *Sexual Abuse, 15*(2), 75–92. https://doi.org/10.1023/A:1022325231175

Laws, D. R., Meyer, J., & Holmen, M. L. (1978). Reduction of sadistic arousal by olfactory aversion: A case study. *Behaviour Research and Therapy, 16*(4), 281–285. https://doi.org/10.1016/0005-7967(78)90026-8

Laws, D. R., & O'Neill, J. A. (1981). Variations on masturbatory conditioning. *Behavioural and Cognitive Psychotherapy, 9*(2), 111–136. https://doi.org/10.1017/S014134730000731X

Leonard, S. R., & Hayes, S. C. (1983). Sexual fantasy alternation. *Journal of Behavior Therapy and Experimental Psychiatry, 14*(3), 241–249. https://doi.org/10.1016/0005-7916(83)90055-1

Levin, S. M., Barry, S. M., Gambaro, S., Wolfinsohn, L., & Smith, A. (1977). Variations of covert sensitization in the treatment of pedophilic behavior: A case study. *Journal of Consulting and Clinical Psychology, 45*(5), 896–907. https://doi.org/10.1037/0022-006X.45.5.896

Ley, D., Prause, N., & Finn, P. (2014). The emperor has no clothes: A review of the "pornography addiction" model. *Current Sexual Health Reports, 6*(2), 94–105. https://doi.org/10.1007/s11930-014-0016-8

LoPiccolo, J., Stewart, R., & Watkins, B. (1972). Treatment of erectile failure and ejaculatory incompetence of homosexual etiology. *Journal of Behavior Therapy and Experimental Psychiatry, 3*(3), 233–236. https://doi.org/10.1016/0005-7916(72)90082-1

Luyten, P., Fonagy, P., Lowyck, B., & Vermote, R. (2012). Assessment of mentalization. In A. W. Bateman & P. Fonagy (Eds.), *Handbook of mentalizing in mental health practice* (pp. 43–65). American Psychiatric Publishing, Inc.

Maletzky, B. M. (1974). "Assisted" covert sensitization in the treatment of exhibitionism. *Journal of Consulting and Clinical Psychology, 42*(1), 34–40. https://doi.org/10.1037/h0036060
Maletzky, B. M. (1977). "Booster" sessions in aversion therapy: The permanency of treatment. *Behavior Therapy, 8*(3), 460–463. https://doi.org/10.1016/S0005-7894(77)80082-8
Marlatt, G., & Gordon, J. R. (1985). *Relapse prevention*. Guilford Press.
Marques, J., Nelson, C., West, M. A., & Day, D. M. (1994). The relationship between treatment goals and recidivism among child molesters. *Behaviour Research and Therapy, 32*(5), 577–588. https://doi.org/10.1016/0005-7967(94)90148-1
Marques, J. K., Day, D. M., Nelson, C., & Miner, M. H. (1989). The Sex Offender Treatment and Evaluation Project: California's relapse prevention program. In D. R. Laws (Ed.), *Relapse prevention with sex offenders* (pp. 247–267). Guilford Press.
Marquis, J. N. (1970). Orgasmic reconditioning: Changing sexual object choice through controlling masturbation fantasies. *Journal of Behavior Therapy and Experimental Psychiatry, 1*(4), 263–271. https://doi.org/10.1016/0005-7916(70)90050-9
Marshall, W. L. (1979). Satiation therapy: A procedure for reducing deviant arousal. *Journal of Applied Behavior Analysis, 12*(3), 377–389. https://doi.org/10.1901/jaba.1979.12-377
Marshall, W. L. (2006a). Ammonia aversion with an exhibitionist: A case study. *Clinical Case Studies, 5*(1), 15–24. https://doi.org/10.1177/1534650103259755
Marshall, W. L. (2006b). Olfactory aversion and directed masturbation in the modification of deviant preferences: A case study of a child molester. *Clinical Case Studies, 5*(1), 3–14. https://doi.org/10.1177/1534650103259754
Marshall, W. L., Anderson, D., & Fernandez, Y. (1999). *Cognitive behavioural treatment of sexual offenders*. Chichester.
Marshall, W. L., & Lippens, K. (1977). The clinical value of boredom: A procedure for reducing inappropriate sexual interests. *The Journal of Nervous and Mental Disease, 165*(4), 283–287. https://doi.org/10.1097/00005053-197710000-00009
Masters, W., & Johnson, V. E. (1970). *Human sexual inadequacy*. Little, Brown.
McGrath, R. J., Cumming, G. F., Burchard, B. L., Zeoli, S., & Ellerby, L. (2010). *Current practices and emerging trends in sexual abuser management*. Safer Society Press.
McGuire, R. J., Carlisle, J. M., & Young, B. G. (1964). Sexual deviations as conditioned behavior: A hypothesis. *Behaviour Research and Therapy, 2*(2–4), 185–190. https://doi.org/10.1016/0005-7967(64)90014-2
Miner, M. H., Dickenson, J., & Coleman, E. (2019). Effects of emotions on sexual behavior in men with and without hypersexuality. *Sexual Addiction & Compulsivity, 26*(1–2), 24–41. https://doi.org/10.1080/10720162.2018.1564408
Miner, M. H., Raymond, N., Mueller, B. A., Lloyd, M., & Lim, K. O. (2009). Preliminary investigation of the impulsive and neuroanatomical characteristics of compulsive sexual behavior. *Psychiatry Research, 174*(2), 146–151. https://doi.org/10.1016/j.pscychresns.2009.04.008
Miner, M. H., Swinburne Romine, R., Raymond, N., Janssen, E., MacDonald, A., III, & Coleman, E. (2016). Understanding the personality and behavioral mechanisms defining hypersexuality in men who have sex with men. *Journal of Sexual Medicine, 13*(9), 1323–1331. https://doi.org/10.1016/j.jsxm.2016.06.015
Money, J. (1999). *The lovemap guidebook: A definitive statement*. Continuum International Publishing Group.
Moser, C. (2013). Hypersexual disorder: Searching for clarity. *Sexual Addiction & Compulsivity, 20*(1), 48–58. https://doi.org/10.1080/10720162.2013.775631

Nelson, C., Miner, M., Marques, J., Russell, K., & Achterkirchen, J. (1989). Relapse prevention: A cognitive-behavioral model for treatment of the rapist and child molester. *Journal of Social Work & Human Sexuality, 7*(2), 125–143. https://doi.org/10.1300/J291v07n02_07

Prause, N., Steele, V. R., Staley, C., Sabatinelli, D., & Hajcak, G. (2015). Modulation of late positive potentials by sexual images in problems users and controls inconsistent with "porn addiction". *Biological Psychology, 109*(1), 192–199. https://doi.org/10.1016/j.biopsycho.2015.06.005

Rankin, C. H., Abrams, T., Barry, R. J., Bhatnagar, S., Clayton, D., Colombo, J., Coppola, D.L., Geyer, M.A., Glanzman, Marsland, S., McSweeney, F.K., Wilson, D.G., Wu, C.F., & Thompson, R. F. (2009). Habituation revised: An updated and revised description of the behavioral characteristics of habituation. *Neurobiology of Learning and Memory, 92*(2), 13–138. https://doi.org/10.1016/j.nlm.2008.09.012

Reid, R. C., & Kafka, M. P. (2014). Controversies about hypersexual disorder and the DSM-5. *Current Sexual Health Reports, 6*(4), 259–264. https://doi.org/10.1007/s11930-014-0031-9

Rimm, D. C., & Masters, J. C. (1979). *Behavior therapy: Techniques and empirical findings* (2nd ed.). Academic Press.

Robinson, B. E., Bockting, W. O., Rosser, B. R. S., Miner, M., & Coleman, E. (2002). The Sexual Health Model: Application of a sexological approach to HIV prevention. *Health Education Research: Theory & Practice, 17*(1), 43–57. https://doi.org/10.1093/her/17.1.43

Rouleau, J. L., Abel, G. G., Mittelman, M. S., Becker, J. V., & Cunningham-Rathner, J. (1986, February). *Effectiveness of each component of a treatment program for non-incarcerated pedophiles. Paper presented at NIMH Conference on Sex Offenders*, Tampa, FL.

Russell, K., Sturgeon, V. H., Miner, M. H., & Nelson, C. (1989). Determinants of the abstinence violation effect in sexual fantasies. In D. R. Laws (Ed.), *Relapse prevention with sex offenders* (pp. 247–267). Guilford Press.

Sex Addicts Anonymous. (2005). *Sex addicts anonymous.* International Service Organization of SAA.

Stein, T. D., & Carnes, P. (2018). Sex addiction, the 12 steps and therapy. In T. Birchard & J. Benfield (Eds.), *The Routledge international handbook of sexual addiction* (pp. 203–211). Routledge.

VanDeventer, A. D., & Laws, D. R. (1978). Orgasmic reconditioning to redirect sexual arousal in pedophiles. *Behavior Therapy, 9*(5), 748–765. https://doi.org/10.1016/S0005-7894(78)80006-9

Voon, V., Mole, T. B., Banca, P., Porter, L., Morris, L., Mitchell, S., Lapa, T.R., Karr, J., Harrison, N.A., Potenza, M.N., & Irvine, M. (2014). Neural correlates of sexual cue reactivity in individuals with and without compulsive sexual behaviours. *PLoS One, 9*(7), e102419. https://doi.org/10.1371/journal.pone.0102419

World Health Organization (2018). *ICD-11 for mortality and morbidity statistics.* https://icd.who.int/browse11/l-m/en#/http%3a%2f%2fid.who.int%2ficd%2fentity%2f1630268048. Author.

17

Managing Paraphilic Interests in the Community

An International Perspective

Klaus M. Beier

Institute of Sexology and Sexual Medicine, Charité –Universitätsmedizin Berlin, Germany

Introduction: Problematic Sexual Interests, Paraphilias, and Paraphilic Disorders

Principally, mate choice in humans appears to be less dependent on innate sexually salient stimuli than in non-human animals (e.g., rodents). Following the model of "exotic becomes erotic" (Bem & Daryl, 1996), features of potential mates are determined by differential behavioral tendencies in prepubescence based on prenatal organizational effects of sex hormones on the brain. If this model holds true, such developmentally determined mechanisms for developing mate choice may explain the greater variability of outcomes (i.e., the potential idiosyncrasy of sexually salient stimuli) to be found in humans than in species depending on innate salience.

According to clinical knowledge in sexology, human sexual preference shows a multidimensional structure organized along three basic axes: (1) the preferred gender of the sex partner (male and/or female), (2) the preferred (body development) age of the sex partner (body scheme of children, adolescents, adults, elderly persons), and (3) the preferred kind and modus of sexual activity with and without sex partner(s) (i.e., type, object, method, etc.; Beier et al., 2005; Beier & Loewit, 2013; see also Seto, 2017).

The final manifestation of sexual preference structure takes place during youth and remains a constituent in its basic features for life (for pedophilia and hebephilia, see Grundmann et al., 2016). This includes even particular sexual inclinations (e.g., fetishism or masochism), which also manifest from youth on and which partly or completely characterize the sexual structure of the person involved. Precisely these forms of individual manifestation on the three axes determine which stimuli sexually attract the individual, and this alone yields a huge spectrum of possibilities in principle. The important point, however, is that the greatest intensity of pleasure is attained by the personal arousal pattern, and that this pattern therefore essentially governs the sexual experience of each individual. But this also means that sexually stimulating signals that deviate from the personal arousal pattern do not tend to yield a comparable intensity of pleasure—even when eagerly desired. A male who is sexually oriented to females (axis 1), then to the adult development shape (axis 2), and in sexual interaction to female feet (axis 3), will hardly experience the same intensity of pleasure during coital intimacy with a woman as he would in giving attention to her feet, which could (considerably) differ from the sexual preference pattern of the real (female) partner.

From a sexological point of view, cases are only diagnosed as disorders of sexual preference (ICD-10: WHO, 1992) or as paraphilic disorders (DSM-5: APA, 2013; ICD-11; 2018, cf.

Sexual Deviance: Understanding and Managing Deviant Sexual Interests and Paraphilic Disorders,
First Edition. Edited by Leam A. Craig and Ross M. Bartels.
© 2021 John Wiley & Sons, Ltd. Published 2021 by John Wiley & Sons, Ltd.

Table 17.1) if they cause distress by virtue of their divergent sexual impulses. As such, persons who have such inclinations but do not suffer on account of them are not considered disturbed, ill, or in need of treatment, so long as they do not impair or endanger others or themselves by acting upon their sexual needs.

Initial epidemiological data shows that the prevalence of paraphilia-related sexual arousal patterns is higher than assumed (Ahlers et al., 2011; Joyal & Charpentier, 2017; Langström & Zucker, 2005). This is true for German-speaking countries based on data from the Berlin Male Study (BMS) in which the prevalence of erectile dysfunction, its age dependency, and its relation to general health variables and general quality of life measures were determined in 6,000 men aged 40–79. In the first phase of this study, 1,915 men took part (Schäfer et al., 2003). These men were then invited to take part in a further comprehensive sexological study by responding to an extensive questionnaire on sexual experiences and behaviors, including that of their (female) partners (later also examined). The outcome was a sample of 373 men, of whom 63 were single and 310 were involved in a relationship. In addition, 108 female partners were interviewed in person. The data provided an indication of possible paraphilia-related

Table 17.1 Disorders of sexual preference according to ICD-10/paraphilic disorders according to DSM-5 and ICD-11.

ICD-10	Disorders of Sexual Preference	DSM-5	Paraphilic Disorders	ICD-11	Paraphilic Disorders
F65.0	Fetishism	302.81	Fetishistic disorder	6D36	Paraphilic disorder involving solitary behavior or consenting individuals
F65.1	Transvestic fetishism	302.3	Transvestic-fetishistic disorder		
F65.2	Exhibitionism	302.4	Exhibitionistic disorder	6D30	Exhibitionistic disorder
F65.3	Voyeurism	302.82	Voyeuristic disorder	6D31	Voyeuristic disorder
F65.4	Pedophilia	302.2	Pedophilic disorder	6D32	Pedophilic disorder
F65.5	Sadomasochism	302.83	Sexual masochistic disorder	6D36	Paraphilic disorder involving solitary behavior or consenting individuals
		302.84	Sexual sadistic disorder	6D33	Coercive sexual sadism disorder
		302.89	Frotteuristic disorder	6D34	Frotteuristic disorder
F65.6	Multiple disorders of sexual preference				
F65.8	Other disorders of sexual preference			6D35	Other paraphilic disorder involving non-consenting individuals
F65.9	Sexual disorders not otherwise specified	302.9	Not otherwise specified paraphilic disorder	6D3Z	Paraphilic disorder, unspecified

tendencies within the general population based on arousal patterns characterized by frequency of occurrence in sexual fantasies, during masturbation (as fantasy content), and during actual practice (Ahlers et al., 2011).

A total of 57.6% of the men questioned acknowledged one of these arousal patterns as part of their fantasies, 46.9% used them for arousal enhancement during masturbation, and 43.9% acted out these patterns on the behavioral level (see Table 17.2). The percentages were far smaller in females: 27.8% of the women acknowledged one of the questioned arousal patterns as part of their fantasies, 23.1% used them for arousal enhancement during masturbation, and also 23.1% acted out these patterns on the behavioral level (see Table 17.3). Even though the virtually unavoidable, indeed obligatory, selection effects do not allow assumptions to the general population, these figures are nevertheless a relevant indication of presumptive distribution, which explains the extent and diversity of offers from the pornography industry.

It is to be assumed, however, that the most "deviant" sexual impulses are rooted in the "normal" sexual response and only turn into pathological disorders by their isolation or generalization. The DSM-5 (APA, 2013) and subsequently the ICD-11 (WHO, 2018) takes this into account by coding a diagnosis only if the person in question claims to suffer on account of the paraphilic inclination, if it restricts significant social or vocational life functions, or if it potentially endangers others above and beyond the person himself as a result of being acted upon. In this case, the DSM-5 and ICD-11 use the term "paraphilic disorder" and distinguish it from paraphilia (without significant distress or danger to others). This is true for pedophilia as well, which—according to the DSM-5—is now primarily seen as a sexual orientation/sexual interest and not as a disorder. Only if significant distress and/or impaired social functioning is connected with a pedophilic inclination (which is difficult to separate from the impact of stigmatization of people with pedophilia; see Jahnke et al., 2015) and/or sexual offenses are committed against children, will it be diagnosed as a pedophilic disorder.

Table 17.2 Prevalence of PASAPs in males.

	Level of Experience		
PASAP	**Sexual Fantasy (%)**	**Masturbation Fantasy (%)**	**Sociosexual Behavior (%)**
Fetishism	29.5	26.0	241
Transvestic fetishism	4.8	5.6	2.7
Masochism	15.5	13.4	12.1
Sadism	21.4	19.6	15.3
Voyeurism	34.3	24.1	17.7
Exhibitionism	3.5	3.2	2.1
Frotteurism	13.1	7.0	6.4
Pedophilia	9.4	5.9	3.8
Others	6.2	6.2	4.6
Presence of at least one PASAP	**57.6**	**46.9**	**43.7**

Note: Prevalence of paraphilia-associated sexual arousal patterns (PASAP) on different experience levels in men between 40 and 79 years (population-based sample); results of the Berlin Male Study II (BMS; Responses for different arousal patterns were prompted on a 5-step rating scale with gradings from "none" to "very strong." All answers from "few" to "very strong" were rated as a response to a sexual arousal pattern ($N = 373$).

Table 17.3 Prevalence of PASAPs in females.

	Level of Experience		
PASAP	**Sexual Fantasy (%)**	**Masturbation Fantasy (%)**	**Sociosexual Behavior (%)**
Fetishism	13.9	13.0	12.0
Transvestic fetishism	0.0	0.0	0.0
Masochism	17.6	15.7	16.7
Sadism	7.4	5.6	6.5
Voyeurism	9.3	9.3	0.9
Exhibitionism	1.9	1.9	0.9
Frotteurism	2.8	2.8	2.8
Pedophilia	1.9	2.8	0.9
Others	2.8	1.9	0.0
Presence of at least one PASAP	**27.8**	**23.1**	**23.1**

Note: Prevalence of paraphilia-associated sexual arousal patterns (PASAP) on different experience levels in female partners of male participants between 40 and 79 years (population-based sample); results of the Berlin Male Study (BMS) II (Responses for different arousal patterns were prompted on a 5-step rating scale with gradings from "none" to "very strong." All answers from "few" to "very strong" were rated as a response to a sexual arousal pattern ($N = 108$).

Concerning pedophilia and hebephilia, Grundmann and colleagues (2016) presented evidence of the retrospective, as well as prospective, stability of sexual arousability to different gender and age categories. Similarities in behavioral expressions have been shown by Seto (2012). Moreover, functional magnetic resonance imaging has, thus far, shown similar brain areas to be involved in the processing of teleiophilic and pedophilic visual sexual stimuli (Polisois-Keating & Joyal, 2013). More such data are urgently needed in a debate that often appears to reflect wishful thinking based on teleio-heteronormativity.

Given these findings, it is quite remarkable that a significant number (nearly one-third) of the men questioned in the BMS II regarded paraphilia-related sexual arousal patterns as inadequate, and voluntarily declined to act upon them—even if they do not harm or endanger others (e.g., fetishistic impulses). Nonetheless, another remarkable number of participants revealed a potential to violate the sexual autonomy of others (e.g., exhibitionism, voyeurism, frotteurism) or had already done so (e.g., child sexual abuse) in the past. It is not infrequent for different paraphilias to occur side by side; a great number of exceptional inclinations are known about, which the international classification systems summarize as, "not otherwise specified paraphilias" or "other disorders of sexual preference."

However, the empirical data suggest that all kinds of paraphilic arousal patterns, both common and exceptional, are a domain of male sexuality and can therefore become relevant, especially during male puberty and adolescence. The same applies to a pedophilic inclination (sexual attraction to a prepubescent body scheme, i.e., before the growth of pubic hair and breasts, etc.). Hebephilia is an independent disorder of sexual preference (sexual attraction to an early pubescent body scheme with initial growth of pubic hair and breasts, etc., i.e., Tanner Stages 2 and 3) which is not yet specifically coded in the International Classification System of the World Health Organization (ICD-10 and ICD-11) or the American Psychiatric Association (DSM-5).

Problematic Sexual Behavior: The Concept of Dissexuality

Dissexuality covers all forms of sexual behavior by which the health and/or wellbeing of others is damaged or their sexual autonomy is impaired. Dissexuality is defined as the failure to conform to social norms—regardless of whether that failure has been prosecuted or not. It includes all harmful sexual conduct (physical or psychological violence) and is defined as irresponsible sexual behavior that disregards the individual rights of others (Beier, 1995). Attempts at or actual performance of sexual acts in front of, with, or by prepubescent or pubescent minors or other persons unable to give their consent also belong to the category of sexual behavior disorders (the so-called "pedo-sexual" acts; in criminal law: "child sexual abuse" or CSA). Some cases of dissexual behavior are due to acting out paraphilias; in other words, a paraphilic impulse pattern can be the root of disturbed sexual behavior, defined as acts of inclination. In other cases, dissexual behavior is related to a different primary problem, such as a personality disorder, intellectual disability, low sociosexual experience (as in some adolescents), or—presumably most important of all—boundary-violating family constellations that have generally unfavorable conditions for child development (including female offenders in such family settings). These cases of sexual abuse are motivationally understood (from the perspective of the offender) as substitute acts, compensating for the actually desired sexual interaction with an adult and consenting partner, which, for various reasons, is not obtainable in a socially acceptable manner. This means that disorders of sexual preference and sexual behavior must be clearly differentiated, not confused or conflated.

Figure 17.1 shows that much of the entire spectrum of paraphilias has nothing to do with harmful sexual contact (i.e., dissexuality). Conversely, dissexuality is usually not attributed to paraphilia. In simple terms, most men with disorders of sexual preference ("paraphilia") are not dissexual, and the large number of men with sexual behavior disorders ("dissexuality") are not paraphilic. CSA studies with legally registered cases (those covered by the German term "Hellfeld", which literally means "bright field") show that approximately 40% of violations can be assigned to pedophilically motivated offenders and 60% to substitute actions (see Beier, 1998; Seto, 2008). Moreover, only a small number of dissexual acts are known to the legal authorities ("Hellfeld"), meaning that the majority generally do not come to the attention of the authorities (those covered by the German term "Dunkelfeld", which means "dark field").

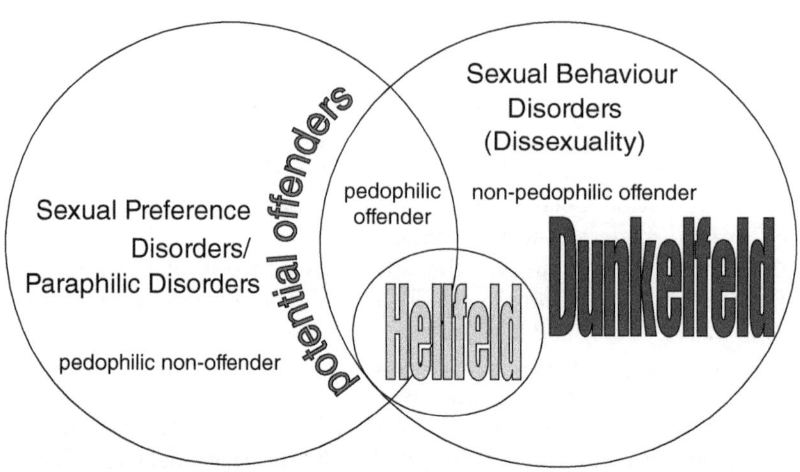

Figure 17.1 Disorders of sexual preferences and sexual behavior. Dunkelfeld: cases not officially registered; Hellfeld: officially known cases.

Clinical Aspects Concerning Assessment, Treatment and Prevention

Considering that—according to the epidemiological data—a significant proportion of men and a smaller, but still visible, proportion of women have sexual preference particularities, it makes sense to place targeted offers for treatment in the healthcare system. These should be preventively effective in two ways: (1) insofar as significant distress caused by the inclination must be avoided, and (2) whenever the case has the possibility of endangering others (e.g., if the paraphilia is associated with a risk due to the preference's particularity, such as sadism or pedophilia), the paraphilic inclination can be influenced in a way that does not lead to any harmful acting out. This requires the provision of appropriate skills in the healthcare system (which implies specific training on top of existing psychiatric and psychotherapeutic skills), where it is obvious that adequate tasks are completely lacking. This includes, for example, conducting the assessment of a sexual history with the exploration of the sexual preference structure, as well as knowledge and skills for the assessment and treatment of sexual preference disorders. Unfortunately, in the case of an impending risk of sexual offending (which is generally assumed with pedophilia), the therapists involved typically avoid taking on the necessary responsibility (see Jahnke et al., 2015).

Concerning the epidemiology of even more frequent sexual dysfunctions, the situation is by no means different, and there is also a major deficit with regards to sexological couple-related interventions (Hoyer, 2013). This can only be compensated by adjusting medical school learning content and by establishing appropriate training courses. Doing so would also help facilitate preventive measures for children at schools (e.g., educational modules could be run by students of medical school and students of psychology). In addition to that, the establishment of outpatient clinics or—in so far as a potential risk of sex offending is associated with a preference disorder—specialized centers would be most beneficial.

Due to the manifestation of paraphilic patterns during puberty and their immutability over the rest of the life-span, it is necessary for those affected to "come to terms" with these inner experiences and, thus, be more or less confronted with their own self-doubt. This, in the end, results from the concern that their partner might not accept the way they truly are (i.e., not love them anymore if their sexual fantasy content were out in the open—even if they have no intention of putting these fantasies into practice). This insecurity is so substantially affected by relationship experience ("Can I find true acceptance from my partner?") that a partnership is difficult to establish or is permanently at risk of ending if one already exists.

On the one hand, there might be anxiety about the course of a paraphilic inclination ("Will it pass, will it remain, or might it even grow stronger?"), while on the other hand, a long hide-and-seek situation is established (i.e., shielding the paraphilic pattern from the perception of the partner). The latter can lead to an irreparable loss of confidence when the inclination is revealed by other circumstances (e.g., discovering significant internet activities is increasingly common). However, if a relationship does exist and both partners have an authentic interest in a common perspective, couple-oriented interventions can improve satisfaction and contentment within the relationship. Four factors are crucial to planning treatment options (Beier, 2010):

1. The Proportion of the Paraphilic Pattern According to the Sexual Preference Structure in General

It makes a big difference whether the paraphilic pattern characterizes the entire sexual preference structure, or whether it exists in addition to a non-paraphilic pattern, possibly being able to integrate it on a partnership level. For example, in the case of an exclusive masochistic paraphilia, in which the person is sexually excitable solely in connection with fantasized scenarios of being mutilated by the partner, then there is no way to otherwise have sexually intense equivalent experiences. This, in turn, leads to potential sexual dysfunction (e.g., erectile disorder, see point 2). Subsequently, the partnership is significantly burdened, if the partner is kept in the dark about the paraphilia and the underlying issues that are the actual cause of the symptoms, making it impossible for the partner to understand the difficulties in their sexual communication.

2. The Additional Occurrence of Sexual Dysfunctions

Any sexual dysfunction may be a symptom of some other medical condition (e.g., orgasmic disorder in multiple sclerosis). In this context, it must be kept in mind that the cause of the dysfunction could be paraphilia-related. That is, the person with the paraphilic preference may not want to burden any sexual interactions with their paraphilic stimulus. This, in turn, makes them insecure during intimacy and afraid that revealing the paraphilic fantasy could disturb the desired closeness and intimacy with the partner. The dysfunction itself, however, as a symptom, is quite visible to the partner and cannot be hidden like the fantasy. If a couple in this situation asks for help, it might, for both partners, be an important step of the therapy to explain the connection between the dysfunction and the paraphilic pattern.

3. Valence of the Paraphilic Stimulus in the Inner Experience

The paraphilic stimulus (e.g., a fetish in case of a fetishist inclination) can sometimes substitute attachment. This is because experiencing the stimulus is not only sexually exciting but is also a psycho-emotionally stabilizing component (comparable to the attachment to another person). This implicates a huge risk for the partnership and the efficacy of therapeutic intervention, especially when the bond to the paraphilic stimulus (e.g., a fetish) has reached the same (or even a greater) relevance for the intrinsic value than the attachment to a real partner. Indeed, clinical experience shows that, particularly in fetishist preference patterns (such as diaper fetishism), the attachment to the fetish can be so strong that it overwhelms the significance of a real partner. Here, couple-related interventions do not stand much chance.

4. Ability of Self-Restriction

A limiting factor in therapeutic work is not only the significance of the paraphilic stimulus in terms of self-estimation (see introduction), but also—and therefore by no means congruent—the ability for self-restriction within the relationship. Even in the case of an exclusive paraphilic pattern (e.g., sadism with an arousing content associated with injury or mutilation of the partner), it might be a higher priority to maintain relationship contentment. This could be because the concerned person considers it an important resource for quality of life and, therefore, wants to live his life in a relationship situation. A most important motivational factor in this context is a sense of responsibility for any existing (or planned) children of their own.

Pedophilia, Hebephilia, and Sexual Offending Against Children

Paraphilic interests that would endanger others if acted upon need specific attention. This is particularly true in the case of CSA. It is well established that childhood adversity, including sexual abuse, dramatically increases the risk for developing a wide range of psychiatric disorders, as well as certain medical conditions, later in life (Leeb et al., 2011). Enduring effects of abuse on the developing brain and its regulatory outflow systems, the autonomic, endocrine, and immune systems are very likely to contribute to disease vulnerability (McCrory et al., 2011). Furthermore, the prevalence of sexual offending against children is high and has developed into a global health issue. A review of 38 prevalence studies in 21 countries resulted in prevalence rates of recalled childhood sexual victimization of approximately 20% for women and 10% for men (e.g., Pereda et al., 2009). Quite obviously, official statistics account for only a fraction of all CSA and the use of child sexual exploitation material (CSEM), inappropriately called "child pornography offenses." Cases not reported to the authorities constitute the largest part of sexual offending against children (as highlighted already in German, referred to as "Dunkelfeld"). For this reason, the healthcare system should focus more on assessment, treatment, and prevention within the community.

There are two possible approaches to prevent CSA. One way is to focus on potential victims, and the other is to focus on potential offenders. If it were somehow possible to reach those who are liable to cause CSA and influence their behavior, then that would be primary prevention at its best, as there would be no offense and no harm done to others. To achieve this goal, it is necessary to have specialized knowledge about the different kinds of offenders. For example, on one hand, there are those who show no sexual preference disorder, for whom the child serves as a surrogate for a sexual relationship with a consenting partner; and on the other hand, there are those who do show a sexual preference disorder, namely pedophilia and/or hebephilia.

As pointed out earlier, sexual preference in general manifests itself during adolescence and remains stable thereafter. All attempts to change sexual orientation have failed (Spitzer, 2012). Generally speaking, it is fate and not choice—in a holistic way of understanding—as a combination of biological and psychosocial circumstances. Therefore, it would be wrong to condemn the preference itself by moral standards. This is true for pedophilia and hebephilia, too. Both can be considered as being stable (Grundmann et al., 2016) and as a form of sexual orientation (DSM-5; APA, 2013; Martijn et al., 2020; Seto, 2017). Thus, people with pedophilia and hebephilia will always be at higher risk of offending and/or reoffending than those without a pedophilic/hebephilic inclination, mainly in the Dunkelfeld (i.e., the judicially unreported cases). Empirical data suggests that people with pedophilia and hebephilia have higher levels of comorbidity and distress due to the problems associated with their sexual preference. As a result, they are more likely than other sexual offenders to seek treatment (Konrad et al., 2017).

Furthermore, the prevalence of pedophilia is—conservatively estimated—about 1% of the male population (Ahlers et al., 2011) and this group accounts for approximately 40% of officially registered offenders (Seto, 2008). Calculating with 1% of the male population and the (increasing) accessibility of child abuse images on a worldwide scale (i.e., the internet), it can be calculated that there might be 23.5 million pedophilically-inclined persons (mostly men) based on 7.6 billion in world population. In the light of this calculation, in Europe with its 500 million inhabitants, there might be at least 1.5 million pedophilically-inclined men and potential users of child abuse images and other sexual exploitation material.

The Prevention Project Dunkelfeld

In spite of the potentially large prevalence of pedophilically-inclined individuals, community-based specialized diagnostic and therapeutic programs within the Dunkelfeld remain scarce. For that reason, the Institute of Sexology and Sexual Medicine in Berlin launched a prevention approach in 2005 called Prevention Project Dunkelfeld (PPD). This was done by generating a media campaign designed to encourage self-identified (but not officially registered) pedophiles and hebephiles to seek professional help in order to avoid committing CSA and the use of CSEM.

For that purpose, it was important to stress the difference between sexual preference and sexual behavior. That is, a pedophilic inclination in an individual does not mean that they will consequently act upon their fantasies. CSA (a behavior) on one hand and pedophilia (a preference disorder) on the other hand are two distinct phenomena investigated in forensic and sexological research. While an intuitive link between both exists, they can, and often do, occur independently. Quite obviously, pedophilia is an emotionally charged and controversial topic, which might be an explanation for not putting it into focus within the healthcare system, where it belongs.

The Dunkelfeld approach—addressing pedophilia as a diagnosis (according to the ICD-11 of the WHO) and not as a crime—was successful. Despite the fact that pedophilia is the most socially stigmatized disorder, pedophilically-inclined persons can be reached for preventive purposes. On average, 15–20 individuals per month contacted the research office in Berlin. From the beginning up to December 2018, there were 2,736 applications, 1,620 assessments, and treatment offers for 616 individuals. The help-seeking men are, on average, 37 years old. They came from all levels of society, most of them were single at the time of questioning, and one-third had children of their own. Half of them had already committed CSA and three-quarters admitted using CSEM in the Dunkelfeld (Beier et al., 2015). Currently, the PPD is being expanded. In addition to the one in Berlin, 10 further contact points in other German States have been successfully established. Furthermore, up to December 2019, there have been 12,077 applications, 3,613 assessments, and 2,007 treatment offers within the whole network known as "don't offend" (www.dont-offend.org).

In a specialized one-year treatment program (Beier 2021), participants learn to ensure impulse control by using cognitive behavioral techniques and sexological concepts (e.g., integrating the sexual preference into the personal sexual identity), as well as pharmaceutical options (mostly androgen deprivation therapy). In terms of the participants that approach the PPD for help, the data clearly show that nearly half have already offended against children within the Dunkelfeld, and nearly 80% have used child abuse images. Only a very small number had been detected by law enforcement institutions. Most of them are pedophilically- or hebephilically-inclined, with a very low risk of being caught by the police.

Advertising via Related Keywords

For that reason, the internet serves as a platform for advertising PPD in terms of a primary prevention approachfor pedophiles unknown to the justice system. This is achieved through a multi-level approach, addressing (potential) users of CSEM through co-operations with search engine providers (i.e. BING and Google) that show tailored messages to people searching for keywords related to CSEM. Users of CSEM are additionally addressed through a software developed by the Institute of Sexology and Sexual Medicine, that automatically shares files on deep and dark web filesharing platforms, which seemingly contain explicit material, but instead present messages that encourage seeking help. Additionally, a broader population is addressed through social media channels (Facebook, Instagram, YouTube etc.) through either sponsored advertisements or media-cooperations with channel providers (von Heyden, 2018).

The Prevention Project for Juveniles

Since 2014, the prevention work has been opened up in Berlin to reach adolescents with an erotic preference toward children's body scheme—initiating public relations activities tailor-made to catch the attention of adolescents by way of flyers, posters and the social media (Beier et al., 2016; see www.just-dreaming-of-them.org). Up to December 2019, there were 293 applications, 156 fully completed assessments, and treatment offers for 92 juveniles.

The average age of the interested adolescents was 15.4 years (only males). Up to 20% of the juveniles contacted the project themselves, while the others were introduced by parents, clinical professionals, guardians, or social workers.

From those juveniles with completed assessments, 80% already had sexually offended (15% use of CSEM, 51% CSA, 14% mixed), 83% had siblings, 37% were exclusively attracted toward children (33% non-exclusively attracted toward children; 25% attracted toward adults), and 73 were offered therapy, with 61 actually beginning therapy. Of those 93 juveniles with a non-/exclusive sexual preference toward children, 56% had at least one comorbid psychiatric disorder, mostly ADHD (21%), conduct disorders (38%), mental retardation (25%) or autism spectrum disorders (12%).

The results show that the project does prevent sexual offending against minors and the consumption of child abusive images. Until now, every adolescent involved has chosen to refrain from CSA behavior and/or the use of CSEM. The patients are grateful for the guidance and are willing to accept advice if they develop trust and do not feel judged or condemned because of their fantasies. Since the approach was successful and it has been possible to reach pedophiles from the community (and encourage them to change their habits of harming others and to stabilize their law-abiding behavior), the German Parliament voted (in November, 2016) for legislation to finance specialized anonymous treatment services for self-referred pedophilically-inclined individuals through the general health insurance system. The law has been in force since January 1, 2017. The aim is to help these individuals to achieve constant behavioral control and not act upon their impulses toward children. This will be evaluated in the next four years in preparation of the decision to maintain the concept.

The International Extension

Integration of this prevention work into the healthcare system is the right strategy and should be done an international scale. Pedophilia is a part of human sexuality and it is to be found in every culture and in every country. Also, the consumption of child abuse images is a topic of international concern because of the worldwide web and its global accessibility. Until now, only in Germany is such an on-site, face-to-face, and anonymous treatment offered. However, it is internationally visible, which would account for the fact that the project websites have received visits from 107 countries with countless personal requests. Examples of such requests are as follows (original texts were not modified):

> *Portugal: "Help Me!! I am a pedophile, but never abused any child. I did Sexual Abuse Risk Assessment (SARA) and had 39 points, but there is no explanation on that score. What does that mean? I look this kind of pornography, it makes me have an enormous weight on my conscience. Sometimes I get days, almost months without access. But always come back to fall into temptation. What can you do to help me?"*
>
> *USA: "I am a hebephile, but I don't know what to do. I am from America, but America does not provide access to help for this issue, nor do I have health insurance to pay for any preventative therapy. I just don't know what to do. I am afraid of my own impulses and afraid of what others would say about me. Please help."*

Global efforts have resulted in the promulgation of legal instruments such as the UN Convention of the Rights of the Child (UNICEF, 1989). Article 34 concerns protecting the child from all forms of sexual exploitation and sexual abuse and makes specific reference to preventing the exploitative use of children in pornographic performances and material. Apart from these global instruments, regional instruments have been developed to tackle the use of CSEM and to protect children (see Gillespie, 2012), but none of them deals with prevention measures that focus on the potential offenders. Furthermore, the enforceability of international law demonstrates tangible weaknesses, because it is a long stretch from signing treaties to the actual implementation of measures and being rewarded by seeing results. The European Parliament enacted a very clear legislative act on this issue, namely, the Directive 2011/92/EU of the European Parliament and of the European Council in December, 2011 on combatting sexual abuse and sexual exploitation of children and child pornography. The directive covers offenses concerning sexual abuse (Article 3), offenses concerning sexual exploitation ("causing or recruiting a child to participate in pornographic performances, or profiting from or otherwise exploiting a child for such purposes"; Article 4), offenses concerning child pornography (Article 5), and the solicitation of children for sexual purposes ("the proposal, by means of information and communication technology by an adult to meet a child who has not reached the age of sexual consent for the purpose of committing any of the offenses referred to in Article 3 to Article 5"; Article 6). Furthermore, "incitement, aiding and abetting, and attempt should be punished by all member states" (Article 7).

Of utmost interest is Article 22, which is a regulation concerning "preventive intervention programs or measures." It states: "Member states shall take necessary measures to ensure that persons who fear that they might commit any of the offenses referred to in Article 3 to 7 may have access where appropriate to effective intervention programs or measures designed to evaluate and prevent the risk of such offenses being committed." In Article 23 dealing with "prevention," member states "shall take appropriate measures, such as education and training to discourage and reduce the demand that fosters all forms of sexual exploitation of children," claiming to take "appropriate action, including through the internet, such as information and awareness-raising campaigns, research and education programs ...."

Interestingly, Article 24 deals with intervention programs or measures "on a voluntary basis in the course of or after criminal proceedings." It states: "member states shall take the necessary measures to ensure that effective intervention programs or measures are made available to prevent or minimize the risks of repeated offenses of a sexual nature against children. Such programs or measures shall be accessible at any time during the criminal proceedings, inside and outside prison, in accordance with national law."

Germany has no Mandatory Report Laws but countries which do (e.g., USA, Canada, India) could at least focus on pedophilically-inclined people who may potentially offend in the Dunkelfeld for preventive purposes. In the light of this, cooperation between the Berlin Institute and India began in 2015, offering treatment for pedophilically-inclined individuals who had not yet offended (cf. www.pppsv.org). For that purpose, the Berlin Institute of Sexology has initiated an online program to be used anonymously and free of charge for assessment and treatment (now available in English, German, Spanish, Portuguese, French, Marathi, Russian, Turkish and Hindi; further languages to follow; cf. www.troubled-desire.com). This digital tool makes it possible to differentiate between people who have the potential to offend and those who have already offended. This will provide the opportunity to refer law-abiding pedophiles to personal treatment and offer those that have offended at least something in their self-motivated search for desistance from CSA and/or the use of CSEM.

Within the first 18 months (25 October, 2017 to 25 April, 2019), the assessment module of Troubled Desire was started by 3,208 visitors from 78 countries, most of whom were from Germany, USA, India, UK, Switzerland, France, Netherlands, Canada, Austria, and Australia. Of these users, 90% confirmed a sexual preference for prepubescent body age (pedophilia) and/or a sexual preference for the early pubescent body age (hebephilia), very often in mixed (non-exclusive) form. Of these, 73.2% reported using CSEM, with 55.7% using it weekly or daily, and with 88.5% occurring within the Dunkelfeld. Also, 38% had committed CSA (which includes all sexually motivated physical contact behavior from touching to violent behavior), 86.1% of which took place in the Dunkelfeld (Beier, 2019).

Conclusions

Paraphilic interests are obviously a constituent part of human sexuality, or the other way around: there will never be human sexuality without paraphilias. According to epidemiological data, there is no doubt about a high prevalence of paraphilic patterns within the general population, with greater rates seen in men than in women. From a clinical point of view, there is strong evidence concerning the implications of an additional source of human sexuality: the attachment dimension, that is, the significance of intimacy in terms of acceptance, admiration, and trust within a relationship. The attachment dimension is endangered, even if the paraphilic inclination is not harmful to others when acted out.

Realizing the impact of sexual health and wellbeing in positive intimate relationships as a protective factor for the development of stress-related disorders (i.e., cardio-vascular diseases, diabetes, obesity, anxiety disorders or depression), it makes a lot of sense to enhance the capacity of the healthcare system regarding the assessment and treatment of paraphilic inclinations.

This is even more necessary in the case of paraphilias that can cause harm to others when acted out, such as pedophilia, sadism, frotteurism, and exhibitionism etc. Focusing on pedophilia and hebephilia, the German Dunkelfeld Project has proved that it is possible to manage these paraphilic inclinations within the community as a challenge for specialized healthcare professionals outside the legal system. In the near future, the comparatively riskless viewing of child abusive material through the countless offers on the internet will lead to a situation where, at an early stage (i.e., during adolescence), practically every pedophilically and/or hebephilically-inclined individual will have been exposed to the temptation of viewing these images and will become a more or less experienced consumer. This makes the consumption of child abusive material a crucial target for primary prevention and, in consequence, it will be necessary to mobilize the internet itself for relating these preventive measures.

Looking at the success of the PPD approach—including the one in India—it should not be an unrealistic call to address the whole spectrum of paraphilic inclinations in order to fulfil the demand of the WHO to enhance sexual health within the general population. Therefore, the transfer of knowledge to implement prevention and intervention strategies on the general level of society is a necessary and internationally relevant task that should be supplemented by a specialized institution in this regard. This would enable the establishment of online offers like Troubled Desire (www.troubled-desire.com) in several languages for diagnostics and treatment through public relations, particularly via social media, country by country. At the same time, it is important to establish a network of therapists in the various countries so that, in line with national legislation, direct and personal assessment and treatment of people with a pedophilic sexual preference who are willing to be treated can be carried out.

For this purpose, a policy is needed to affect the structural framework for the implementation of effective concepts concerning the prevention of CSA and the use of CSA images through lobbying in each country. In addition to that, the social discourse should be enhanced by the regular publication of scientific findings on the topic, including new challenges, such as the growing problem of grooming. In terms of future goals and perspectives, mechanisms for the management and coordination of prevention activities should combine efforts from different stakeholders (e.g., government ministries, hospitals, health insurance schemes, the pharmaceutical industry). These efforts will not succeed if stakeholders from the health sector are not aware of and do not understand the correlation between (and the serious impact of) paraphilic disorder and health in general, and the long-term consequences of CSA in particular.

References

Ahlers, C. J., Schaefer, G. A., Mundt, I. A., Roll, S., Englert, H., Willich, S., & Beier, K. M. (2011). How unusual are the contents of paraphilias—Prevalence of paraphilia-associated sexual arousal patterns (PASAPs) in a community–based sample of men. *Journal of Sexual Medicine, 8*, 1362–1370.

APA (American Psychiatric Association). (2013). *Diagnostic and statistical manual of mental disorders, fifth edition revised (DSM-5)*. APA Press.

Beier, K. M. (1995). *Dissexualität im Lebenslängsschnitt: Theoretische und empirische Untersuchungen zu Phänomenologie und Prognose begutachteter Sexualstraftäter*. Springer.

Beier, K. M. (1998). Differential typology and prognosis for dissexual behaviour: A follow-up study of previously expert-appraised child molesters. *International Journal of Legal Medicine, 111*, 133–141.

Beier, K. M. (2010). Sexuelle Präferenzstörungen und Bindungsprobleme. *Sexuologie, 17*, 24–31.

Beier, K. M. (2019). Proactive strategies to implement prevention programs for persons with sexual interest in children. IASR 45th Annual Meeting, Mexico City, July 24–27.

Beier, K.M. (2021). *Pedophilia, Hebephilia and Sexual Offending against Children*. The Berlin Dissexuality Therapy, Springer 2021.

Beier, K. M., Amelung, T., Kuhle, L., Grundmann, D., Scherner, G., & Neutze, J. (2015). Hebephilia as a sexual disorder. *Fortschritte der Neurologie – Psychiatrie, 83*, e1–e9.

Beier, K. M., Bosinski, H. A. G., & Loewit, K. (2005). *Sexualmedizin, München*. Elsevier, Urban & Fischer 2. Auflage.

Beier, K. M., & Loewit, K. (2013). *Sexual medicine in clinical practice*. Springer.

Beier, K. M., Oezdemir, U. C., Schlinzig, E., Groll, A., Hupp, E., & Hellenschmidt, T. (2016). "Just dreaming of them": The Berlin Project for Primary Prevention of Child Sexual Abuse by Juveniles (PPJ). *Child Abuse & Neglect, 52*, 1–10.

Bem, B., & Daryl, J. (1996). Exotic becomes erotic: A developmental theory of sexual orientation. *Psychological Review, 103*, 320–335.

Gillespie, A. A. (2012). Child Pornography in international law. In E. Quayle & K. N. Ribisl (Eds.), *Understanding and preventing online sexual exploitation of children* (pp. 60–76). Routledge.

Grundmann, D., Krupp, J., Scherner, G., Amelung, T., & Beier, K. M. (2016). Stability of self-reported arousal to sexual fantasies involving children in a clinical sample of pedophiles and hebephiles. *Archives of Sexual Behavior, 45*, 1153–1162.

Hoyer, J. (2013). Sexual dysfunctions and outpatient psychotherapy. *Psychotherapeut, 58*, 371–378.

Jahnke, S., Imhoff, R., & Hoyer, J. (2015). Stigmatization of people with pedophilia: Two comparative surveys. *Archives of Sexual Behavior, 44*, 21–34.

Joyal, C. C., & Carpentier, J. (2017). The prevalence of paraphilic interests and behaviors in the general population: A provincial survey. *Journal of Sex Research, 54*, 161–171.

Konrad, A., Haag, S., Scherner, G., Amelung, T., & Beier, K. M. (2017). Previous judicial detection and paedophilic sexual interest partially predict psychological distress in a non-forensic sample of help-seeking men feeling inclined to sexually offend against children. *Journal of Sexual Aggression, 23*, 266–277.

Langström, N., & Zucker, K. J. (2005). Transvestic fetishism in the general population: Prevalence and correlates. *Journal of Sex & Marital Therapy, 31*, 87–95.

Leeb, R. T., Lewis, T., & Zolotor, A. J. (2011). A review of physical and mental health consequences of child abuse and neglect and implications for practice. *American Journal of Lifestyle Medicine, 5*, 454–468.

Martijn, F. M., Babchishin, K. M., Pullman, L. E., & Seto, M. C. (2020). Sexual attraction and falling in love in persons with pedohebephilia. *Archives of Sexual Behavior,* Advanced online version. https://doi.org/10.1007/s10508-019-01579-9

McCrory, E., De Brito, S. A., & Viding, E. (2011). The impact of childhood maltreatment: A review of neurobiological and genetic factors. *Frontiers in Psychiatry, 2*, 48.

Pereda, N., Guilera, G., Forns, M., & Gómez-Benito, J. (2009). The prevalence of child sexual abuse in community and student samples: A meta-analysis. *Clinical Psychology Review, 29*, 328–338.

Polisois-Keating, A., & Joyal, C. C. (2013). Functional neuroimaging of sexual arousal: A preliminary meta-analysis comparing pedophilic to non-pedophilic men. *Archive of Sexual Behavior, 42*, 1111–1113.

Schäfer, G. A., Engert, H. S., Ahlers, C. J., Roll, S., Willich, S. N., & Beier, K. M. (2003). Erektionsstörungen und Lebensqualität: Erste Ergebnisse der Berliner Männer-Studie. *Sexuologie, 10*, 50–60.

Seto, M. C. (2008). *Pedophilia and sexual off ending against children: Theory, assessment, and intervention*. American Psychological Association.

Seto, M. C. (2012). Is pedophilia a sexual orientation? *Archives of Sexual Behavior, 41*, 231–236.

Seto, M. C. (2017). The puzzle of male chronophilias. *Archives of Sexual Behavior, 46*, 3–22.

Spitzer, R. L. (2012). Spitzer reassesses his 2003 study of reparative therapy of homosexuality. *Archives of Sexual Behavior, 41*, 757–757.

UNICEF. (1989). UN Convention of the Rights of the Child. https://www.unicef.org/child-rights-convention/convention-text

von Heyden, M. (2018). *Internet-based strategies for the cause-related prevention of child sexual abuse*. Conference Paper presented at the 9th EUSPR Conference, Lisbon (25 October, 2018).

World Health Organization. (1992). *International statistical classification of diseases and related health problems: ICD-10 (10th revision)*. Author.

World Health Organization. (2018). International Statistical Classification of Diseases and Related Health Problems: ICD-11 (11th revision). Author. https://www.who.int/classifications/icd/en

18

Pharmacological Treatments for Individuals with Paraphilic Disorders or at Risk for Sexual Offending

Daniel Turner[1] *and Peer Briken*[2]

[1] *Department of Psychiatry and Psychotherapy, University Medical Center Mainz, Germany*
[2] *Institute for Sex Research, Sexual Medicine and Forensic Psychiatry, University Medical Center Hamburg-Eppendorf, Germany*

Introduction

When reviewing the scientific literature one can find diverse reports about the use of pharmacological agents for the treatment of deviant sexual fantasies and/or behaviors. Most treatment studies were performed with persons convicted of sexual offenses (PCSOs) because they show a relatively high prevalence of paraphilic disorders (Eher et al., 2019). However, the findings of previous research as well as the recommendations given throughout the present chapter can mostly be generalized to persons without sexual convictions with paraphilic disorders. There are studies concerning the use of selective-serotonin-reuptake-inhibitors (SSRIs), tricyclic antidepressants, antipsychotics, lithium carbonate, anticonvulsants, and testosterone-lowering medications (TLM; Briken et al., 2001; Cesnik & Coleman, 1989; Corretti & Baldi, 2010; Greenberg et al., 1996; Kafka & Hennen, 2000; Nelson et al., 2001). However, currently only the use of SSRIs and TLM is recommended for the treatment of paraphilic disorders (as a clinically relevant diagnostic construct overlapping with sexual deviance), while all other pharmacological agents should only be applied if comorbid disorders call for their usage (Thibaut et al., 2010). This accounts especially for anti-psychotics because in clinical practice they seem to be employed quite frequently despite these recommendations (Turner et al., 2018; Turner et al., 2013b). An exceptionally important point that always has to be kept in mind is that none of these pharmacological agents directly influences the content of the deviant sexuality and all agents lead "only" to a general reduction of paraphilic but also non-paraphilic fantasies, urges and/or behaviors. In some cases, though, pharmacological treatment is needed in order to increase receptiveness for psychotherapeutic interventions (Briken & Kafka, 2007).

The following chapter will first give an overview of the existing empirical evidence concerning the efficacy of the currently recommended pharmacological agents, followed by a discussion of current treatment and management guidelines for adults and adolescents. Closing the chapter, we will discuss legal and ethical aspects related to the pharmacological treatment of paraphilic disorders.

Selective Serotonin Reuptake Inhibitors (SSRIs)

The neurotransmitter serotonin has various effects and functions within the human central nervous system, e.g., on affect regulation, on the sleep-wake cycle, appetite, pain, and, last but not least, sexuality (Turner et al., 2013a). By blocking serotonin transporters, SSRIs hamper the reuptake of serotonin into the presynaptic membrane, thereby leading to an increase of active

Sexual Deviance: Understanding and Managing Deviant Sexual Interests and Paraphilic Disorders,
First Edition. Edited by Leam A. Craig and Ross M. Bartels.
© 2021 John Wiley & Sons, Ltd. Published 2021 by John Wiley & Sons, Ltd.

serotonin within the central nervous system. SSRIs were primarily developed for the treatment of depression, anxiety disorders, and obsessive-compulsive disorders. However, it was observed that many patients complained about a reduction of their sexual desire and sexual functioning during SSRI therapy (Briken et al., 2011; Corona et al., 2009). Indeed, serotonin does have primarily inhibiting effects on sexual functioning and it leads to a delay in erection and ejaculation (Pfaus, 2009). Some studies have shown that this effect is also observable in patients or PCSOs with a paraphilic disorder, leading to a decrease in sexual fantasizing, sexual desire, and a lower masturbation frequency to paraphilic fantasies (e.g., Greenberg et al., 1996; Kraus et al., 2006). However, this effect is not specific to paraphilic fantasies, desires or behaviors and accounts for non-paraphilic sexual functioning as well. Besides reducing overall sexual functioning, SSRIs also lead to a decrease in obsessive-compulsive symptoms and an increase in impulse control, explaining why SSRIs seem to be especially useful in patients with intense sexual urges, an intense sexual preoccupation and/or comorbid hypersexual behaviors (Houts et al., 2011; Wainberg et al., 2006; Winder et al., 2018). Furthermore, it was suggested that SSRIs could also promote pro-social and affiliative behaviors in PCSOs (Beech & Mitchell, 2005).

Most treatment studies in PCSOs or persons without sexual convictions with paraphilic disorders assessed the efficacy of Fluoxetine (Prozac®) and Sertraline (Zoloft®; Adi et al., 2002); however, no differences concerning the effectiveness of different SSRIs in reducing paraphilic sexual fantasies and urges have been found so far (Greenberg et al., 1996). A recent meta-analysis found that the prevalence of sexual dysfunctions in general is highest under therapy with Sertraline (80%), Citalopram (79%), Paroxetine (71%), and Fluoxetine (70%; Serretti & Chiesa, 2009). It usually takes two to four weeks before reductions of paraphilic symptomatology can be observed under SSRI treatment (Hill et al., 2003). Adverse effects during SSRI treatment include nervousness, sleeping disorders, headache, dizziness, weight gain, nausea, hyponatremia, prolongation of the QT-interval and bleedings if combined with non-steroidal antirheumatics or anticoagulants (Garcia et al., 2013). However, due to their overall good tolerance SSRIs are suitable for treatment over several years and can be used in adolescents as well.

Testosterone-Lowering Medications

TLM that are used in the treatment of paraphilic disorders have in common that they lead to an intense reduction of serum testosterone concentrations. Depending on the individual dosage of the applied agent, testosterone levels are partly reduced below the so-called castration level (usually defined as serum testosterone concentrations < 20–50 ng/dL; Nishiyama, 2014). The production and secretion of testosterone is under the control of the hypothalamic-pituitary-gonadal axis and follows a negative feedback mechanism. Low serum testosterone levels stimulate the production and secretion of the gonadotropin-releasing hormone (GnRH or synonymously luteinizing hormone-releasing hormone, LHRH) in the hypothalamus. GnRH, in turn, binds to specific GnRH receptors in the pituitary gland, thereby leading to an increased production and secretion of luteinizing hormone (LH) and follicle-stimulating hormone (FSH). Finally, LH binds to specific receptors in the testes and stimulates the production of testosterone in the Leydig cells of the testes. High testosterone concentrations again impede this regulatory cycle.

After its secretion testosterone is usually transferred into its more active metabolite 5-alpha-dihydrotestosterone. Testosterone and 5-alpha-dihydrotestosterone promote the development and differentiation of the male primary and secondary sexual characteristics, the development of muscular and bone mass and induce the production of erythrocytes. Concerning sexuality, testosterone is involved in the emergence of erections and ejaculations and increases general sexual desire. Although it was shown that altered testosterone concentrations are not related to the occurrence of paraphilic sexual fantasies, behaviors or interests (Wong & Gravel, 2016), several studies have shown that reduced serum testosterone concentrations can lead to a considerable decrease in the frequency and intensity of paraphilic sexual fantasies and behaviors in PCSOs (Briken et al., 2001; Rösler & Witztum, 1998; Thibaut et al., 2010; Turner & Briken, 2018b), but non-paraphilic sexuality is affected as well.

Currently three different agents are subsumed under the term TLM and are regularly used in the treatment of paraphilic disorders: (1) cyproterone acetate (CPA), (2) medroxyprogesterone acetate (MPA), and (3) gonadotropin-releasing hormone (GnRH-) agonists.

Cyproterone Acetate (CPA, Androcur®)

CPA is a synthetic testosterone antagonist with antiandrogenic as well as progestogenic effects. At first, CPA binds to androgen receptors in the testes and/or different brain areas and competitively replaces testosterone and 5-alpha-dihydrotestosterone from these receptors, thereby inhibiting their effect on sexuality and other body functions and inhibits their synthesis via the above mentioned negative feedback mechanism. Through its progestational properties CPA also directly inhibits the production and secretion of LH in the pituitary gland, thereby leading to a further decrease of serum testosterone concentrations.

CPA is available in tablet form or as an injectable depot solution. So far, several studies have been published showing that CPA leads to a considerable decrease in paraphilic sexual urges, fantasies and behaviors (e.g., Cooper & Cernovovsky, 1992; Lippi & van Staden, 2017; Turner et al., 2013b). It has to be noted, though, that most previous studies were uncontrolled observation studies, included only small samples or are in the meantime quite outdated. Nevertheless, in clinical practice CPA is used quite frequently (Czerny et al., 2002; Turner et al., 2013b). There are five older double-blind studies which have found that CPA is slightly more effective in reducing sexual fantasies, urges and behaviors compared to ethinylestradiol (Bancroft et al., 1974) and placebo (Bradford & Pawlak, 1993; Cooper, 1981; Cooper, Cernovovsky et al., 1992) and shows no differences in its efficacy compared to medroxyprogesterone acetate (Cooper, Sandhu et al., 1992). The most recent study on the efficacy of CPA was conducted in South Africa and compared 13 PCSOs treated with CPA (150 mg to 300 mg i.m./month) and 63 PCSOs treated with other psychotropic medications; however, the precise agents were not mentioned. In that study, CPA treatment resulted in lower levels of sexual desire, a lower frequency of sexual activities and less pleasurable sexual activities than the other psychotropic agents (Lippi & van Staden, 2017). CPA treatment can be accompanied by diverse mild as well as severe side effects which are mainly caused by the reduced testosterone concentrations. Observed adverse effects are: weight gain, hot flushes, pain at the site of injection, lethargy and depression, gynecomastia, thromboembolic events as well as liver and kidney dysfunctions (Assumpcao et al., 2014). Most side effects are reversible once treatment has been terminated. More recently however, studies revealed that individuals with a history or current use of CPA had significantly more meningeomas and were significantly younger at the onset of menigeoma. Therefore, the use of CPA as first line medication to supress testosterone is now obsolete in some countries.

Medroxyprogesterone Acetate (MPA, DepoProvera®)

MPA is a synthetic gestagen which is mainly used as an ovulation inhibitor for contraception. Almost exclusively in the U.S. it is also used for the treatment of paraphilic disorders in PCSOs. MPA has mainly progestogenic effects and inhibits the production and secretion of GnRH and

LH via the negative feedback mechanism of the hypothalamic-pituitary-gonadal axis. Furthermore, MPA directly reduces testosterone serum concentrations by inducing the enzyme testosterone-alpha-reductase, which deactivates 5-alpha-dihydrotestosterone, and MPA increases the binding of testosterone to the testosterone hormone-binding globulin, thereby reducing the serum concentrations of free testosterone.

MPA is available as oral medication or as an injectable depot solution, and the depot preparation should be preferred due to its higher bioavailability. Comparably to CPA, several studies on the effectiveness of MPA have been published; however, nearly all studies were uncontrolled and were conducted in the 1980s and 1990s (e.g., Kravitz et al., 1996; Maletzky et al., 2006; Wincze et al., 1986). Only three older double-blind studies exist showing a superior efficacy of MPA compared to placebo in the reduction of paraphilic as well as non-paraphilic sexual urges, fantasies, and behaviors (Hucker et al., 1988; Kiersch, 1990; Wincze et al., 1986). To our knowledge, the most recent study assessing the usefulness of MPA was a retrospective file study conducted in the U.S. comparing 79 mainly pedophilic PCSOs treated with MPA and psychotherapy with 196 PCSOs treated psychotherapeutically without additional MPA treatment showing that MPA was superior in reducing deviant sexual behaviors (Maletzky et al., 2006). More recent studies are nevertheless, to our knowledge, lacking; at least in the U.S., MPA is used on a quite regular basis in certain PCSOs (McGrath et al., 2010; Turner et al., 2017).

Side effects observed during MPA treatment are comparable to those found during CPA treatment and include weight gain, hot flushes, pain at the site of injection, lethargy and depression, gynecomastia, thromboembolic events as well as liver and kidney dysfunctions. However, again, most side effects are reversible once treatment has been terminated (Maletzky & Field, 2003).

Gonadotropin-Releasing Hormone (GnRH-) Agonists and Antagonists

Among TLM, GnRH-agonists were introduced most recently to the treatment of paraphilic fantasies and behaviors in PCSOs. In recent years a notable increase in the use of GnRH-agonists in the treatment of paraphilic disorders in PCSOs has been observed (Czerny et al., 2002; Turner et al., 2013b). GnRH-agonists bind to GnRH receptors in the pituitary gland and lead to a permanent stimulation of these receptors. Permanent receptor binding initially leads to a rapid increase of LH secretion followed by an extensive upsurge of testosterone serum concentrations during the first two to four weeks of treatment (the so-called "flare-up effect"). After this period the permanent stimulation leads to a de-sensibilization and downregulation of GnRH receptors in the pituitary gland, resulting in a decrease in testosterone serum levels, usually below castration level.

So far, GnRH-agonists are available as an injectable depot solution only. In the meantime, three systematic reviews concerning the efficacy of GnRH-agonists have been published (Briken et al., 2003; Lewis et al., 2017; Turner & Briken, 2018b). These systematic reviews have suggested that GnRH-agonists seem to be more effective than CPA and MPA concerning the reduction of paraphilic sexual urges, fantasies and behaviors. At the same time, though, GnRH-agonists also lead to a complete decline of non-paraphilic sexual fantasies and behaviors, indicating that they are suitable for a small, particular group of PCSOs only (Briken et al., 2003; Turner & Briken, 2018b). So far, no double-blind studies assessing the effectiveness of GnRH-agonists in PCSOs have been conducted and thus the current state of research is almost exclusively based on case reports and cross-sectional studies (Briken et al., 2017). In one of our own study, which has not been included in any of the previously mentioned systematic reviews, we found in a group of 38 PCSOs from one forensic psychiatric hospital in Germany that after the start of GnRH-agonist treatment a considerable risk reduction measured with the Stable-2007 could be observed (Sauter et al., 2019). In particular, improvements in the Stable-2007 risk domains general and sexual self-regulation were observable in the group treated with GnRH-agonists. Before the start of GnRH-agonist treatment, the included PCSOs were treated with psychotherapy only for an average of seven years, suggesting that in a selected group of PCSOs GnRH-agonist treatment might be a necessary precondition to achieve therapeutic success. It must be taken into account that in German forensic psychiatric hospitals, particularly severely disturbed and dangerous offenders are treated until the danger caused by the disturbance no longer exists (Briken et al. 2019).

Adverse effects observed during the treatment with GnRH-agonists are mainly comparable to those seen under CPA or MPA treatment. Furthermore, a considerable loss of bone mineral density up to manifest osteoporosis has been found in some patients (Turner & Briken, 2018b). Therefore, bone mineral density should be monitored regularly and any deficiency, if present, should be treated accordingly. Only recently for the first time a GnRH antagonist has been evluated in an RCT. This trial found that degarelix reduced the risk score for committing child sexual abuse in men with pedophilic disorder 2 weeks after initial injection. It might be that this medication has the potential as a rapid-onset treatment option but further experiences and studies are needed.

Current Treatment Guidelines

While we have introduced the currently recommended agents for the treatment of paraphilic disorders in PCSOs in the early part of this chapter, the question remains, who should be treated with which pharmacological agents. In this context, one should refer to the guidelines about the biological treatment of paraphilias published by the World Federation of Societies of Biological Psychiatry (WFSBP) in 2010 for adults (updated in 2020) and 2016 for adolescents, which provide recommendations for the pharmacological treatment of adolescent and adult PCSOs with a paraphilic disorder (Thibaut et al., 2010, 2016, 2020). First, it has to be noted that pharmacological treatment should in all cases be used as an add-on to psychotherapeutic interventions only. Beyond that the WFSBP guidelines propose a risk-based approach, meaning that the selection of the most appropriate medication should be based on the individual's risk of exhibiting sexually violent behaviors, as well as on the intensity of the self-reported and observed paraphilic urges. Further factors that were recommended by persons with broad experience in treating patients with a paraphilic disorder are a history of previous treatment failures, sexual violations while under community supervision or while being placed in an institution, CNS dysfunction, and the use of force in sexual crimes (Turner et al., 2014). Table 18.1 presents the current guidelines for adults.

In adolescents convicted of sexual offences, psychotherapy should always be the first line treatment irrespective of the severity of the paraphilic symptomatology (Thibaut et al., 2016). Only in adolescent patients with a paraphilic disorder in whom psychotherapy has not been sufficiently successful after a reasonable period of time might one consider additionally using pharmacological agents. In patients with a low to medium risk for sexually violent behaviors one might consider applying SSRIs, while in patients with a high to very high risk one should refer to TLM in addition to psychotherapy and SSRIs. The guidelines do not distinguish between CPA/MPA and GnRH-agonists; however, they recommend using TLM always in the lowest possible dose and, if possible, for a maximum of six months before re-evaluating the usefulness of further using TLM. Only in adolescents convicted of sexual offences who are at least 16 years old and whose sexual characteristics are fully developed (at least Tanner stage V) could longer treatment periods be considered (Thibaut et al., 2016). Keeping the above

Table 18.1 Guidelines for the Biological Treatment of Paraphilias of the World Federation of Societies of Biological Psychiatry (WFSBP; adapted according to Thibaut et al., 2010, 2020).

Level 1	
• Aim: control of paraphilic sexual fantasies and behaviors without impact on non-paraphilic sexual functioning.	• Psychotherapy (preferentially cognitive-behavioral therapy)
Level 2	
• Aim: control of paraphilic sexual fantasies and behaviors with minor impact on non-paraphilic sexual functioning. • Appropriate for paraphilic disorders with low risk of sexual violence, i.e., exhibitionism, voyeurism.	• Psychotherapy (preferentially cognitive-behavioral therapy) • SSRIs: use same dosages as would be used in obsessive-compulsive disorders.
Level 3	
• Aim: control of paraphilic sexual fantasies and behaviors with substantial reduction of non-paraphilic sexual functioning. • Appropriate for paraphilic disorders with medium risk of sexual violence, for example, fondling without risk of penetration. • No satisfactory results at level 2 after 4–6 weeks of SSRIs at high dosages.	• Psychotherapy (preferentially cognitive-behavioral therapy) • Antiandrogen (CPA: oral, 50–300 mg/day or i.m. 200–400 mg once weekly or every 2 weeks) or MPA: 50–300 mg/day if CPA is not available. However, given the risk of meningeoma, in some contries CPA can be used only when other treatments are deemed inappropriate.
Level 4	
• Aim: control of paraphilic sexual fantasies and behaviors with almost complete reduction of non-paraphilic sexual functioning. • Appropriate for paraphilic disorders with medium to high risk of sexual violence, for example, pedophilic disorders. • No sexually sadistic fantasies and/or behaviors.	• Psychotherapy (preferentially cognitive-behavioral therapy) • Long-acting GnRH-agonists (i.e. leuprolide acetate 11.25 mg i.m. every 3 months). • To prevent the flare-up effect add CPA/MPA one week before and during the first four weeks of GnRH-agonist treatment.
Level 5	
• Aim: control of paraphilic sexual fantasies and behaviors with complete suppression of non-paraphilic sexual functioning. • High to very high risk of sexual violence, for example, sexually sadistic disorder or pedophilic disorder.	• Psychotherapy (preferentially cognitive-behavioral therapy) • Use full-dose CPA/MPA in addition to GnRH-agonists. • SSRIs may also be added.

mentioned risk for menigeoma in mind, CPA should not be used as first line therapy for adolescents anymore.

Close monitoring of adverse effects is a necessary requirement during pharmacological treatment, especially during TLM treatment. Assessing blood pressure and body weight on a weekly basis is recommended. At least every three months, blood analysis should be performed, including a full blood count as well as the determination of liver enzymes, fasting glucose levels, lipids and electrolytes. Especially when using GnRH-agonists, bone mineral density using osteodensitometry should be checked every two years or every year in case of a familial risk of osteoporosis or in patients over 50 years of age. Furthermore, psychiatric examinations should be performed on a regular basis in order to detect signs and symptoms of depression, emotional disturbances, or suicidality. If side effects occur, they should be treated or if they are too intense one should consider terminating treatment (Thibaut et al., 2010; Turner & Briken, 2018b).

Besides the monitoring of side effects, therapeutic success should also be checked closely. Testosterone serum concentrations should be assessed at least every three to six months in order to verify treatment compliance or to detect concealed testosterone supplementation. Furthermore, the nature, intensity, and frequency of paraphilic sexual fantasies and behaviors should be assessed monthly. The evaluation of deviant sexual fantasies and behaviors should mainly be based on the patient's self-report; however, it can also be supported by more indirect measures such as penile plethysmography, eye-tracking or other attention-based measures. The risk for future sexual violence should also be assessed regularly using a dynamic risk assessment instrument, like the Stable-2007 (Thibaut et al., 2010; Turner & Briken, 2018b).

Regular monitoring of the therapeutic success is an essential prerequisite to detect the most suitable time point to de-escalate or even terminate the current therapy regime. In particular, termination of therapy presents a problem that has so far not been sufficiently addressed by previous research efforts. The WFSBP guidelines recommend a minimal treatment duration of two years in patients with mild paraphilias and a duration of three to five years in patients with severe paraphilias and a high risk of sexual violence (Thibaut et al., 2010, 2020). In one study an abrupt rebound upsurge of serum testosterone concentrations in a group of PCSOs who had been treated with GnRH-agonists for three months was found, while a much smoother upsurge could be observed in PCSOs who had been treated for six months. Furthermore, a more rapid increase in paraphilic sexual fantasies and urges after treatment termination was observable in the group treated for only three months (Koo et al., 2014). Comparably, Voß et al. (2016) followed 11 PCSOs from Germany who were treated with TLM for an average of 78 months (range 14 to 148 months) before TLM treatment was terminated. The authors found that it took on average five months (range 2 to 18 months) until testosterone serum concentrations were in the normal range again, while sexual functioning reoccurred with some further delay. None of the patients reported an increase in (sexual) aggressive thoughts or behaviors (Voß et al., 2016). Thus, a minimal treatment duration of at least six months may be reasonable. Furthermore, it is suggested that treatment should never be terminated abruptly and termination should be closely monitored, including frequent measurements of serum testosterone concentrations as well as assessments of paraphilic sexual fantasies and behaviors.

We recently developed and validated the "Change or Stop Testosterone Lowering Medication (COSTLow)-Scale," which can be used to support the decision whether or not a pharmacological treatment should be changed or stopped in an individual PCSO (Briken, Turner et al., 2018). The COSTLow-Scale consists of 15 items which can be assigned to five different categories: age of the patient and duration of previous therapy, therapeutic alliance, psychopathology and risk factors, therapy motivation and compliance, and external control mechanisms (Briken, Turner et al., 2018). In any case, the decision to actually change or stop TLM treatment should always be made in close consultation with the individual patient.

Just recently, an update was given on the patients from Germany described in the above mentioned study in whom an attempt to end TLM treatment was made. The sample consisted of 20 PCSOs in whom TLM treatment was discontinued and these patients were compared to 20 PCSOs in whom TLM treatment was not yet terminated. The authors reported that during a mean follow-up of 55 months, only two PCSOs in whom TLM was discontinued came into contact with official authorities because of a new sexual offense, suggesting that for some PCSOs, ending TLM treatment could be a realistic option if performed in a structured and secure setting (Sauter et al., 2018).

Ethical and Legal Framework of Pharmacological Treatment

Depending on the applied dose of TLM medication, these agents usually lead to a more or less complete reduction in sexual functioning including non-paraphilic sexual behaviors. In PCSOs at very high risk of sexual violence the complete reduction of sexual functioning may sometimes present an intended effect; however, in PCSOs with a low to medium risk the reduction of non-paraphilic sexual functioning has to be viewed as an adverse effect restricting the patient's basic human rights (Basdekis-Jozsa et al., 2013; Briken, Basdekis-Jozsa et al., 2018; Turner & Briken, 2018a). Article 12 of the European Convention of Human Rights as well as article 16 of the Human Rights Convention of the United Nations establish the right of every human being to have their own family, including the right to freely live one's own, non-criminally relevant sexuality (Basdekis-Jozsa et al., 2013). The only way to comply with these legal rules is to perform TLM treatment on a completely voluntary basis. While this is the case in almost all countries, in some countries and in some U.S. States there is the possibility of court-ordered mandatory TLM treatment (Turner et al., 2017). In our view such an approach is not compatible with the above stated human rights conventions. However, even in the countries in which TLM can be applied on a voluntary basis only, some concerns about voluntariness remain. At least for Germany it was found that patients currently placed in a forensic psychiatric hospital and who agreed to be treated with TLM were granted home leave steps earlier than patients who were not treated with TLM (Briken et al., 2009). Thus, the question arises as to how far TLM treatment can really be seen as voluntary in light of the fact that if a patient decides not to be treated with TLM he might be released from imprisonment much later. It is conceivable that under these circumstances some patients will consent to TLM treatment despite serious concerns (Briken et al., 2009; Turner & Briken, 2018a).

To avoid or at least reduce this ethical and decisional dilemma it was suggested that the person applying and supervising the treatment should always be different from the person who decides about possible home leave or other forms of detention relaxation (Basdekis-Jozsa et al., 2013). Furthermore, every patient has to be fully informed about any adverse effects that can occur with TLM treatment and only after that should the patient be asked for his informed consent. Although associated with high personal cost it would be desirable if gathering informed consent could be performed by two independent medical healthcare providers, optimally with broad experience in forensic psychiatry as well as sexual medicine. In patients with cognitive impairments or patients younger than 16 years of age the legal guardians have to be informed about the treatment and its effects and side effects as well. In patients with a permanent romantic relationship, the partners could be included in the decision-making process (Basdekis-Jozsa et al., 2013). If these suggestions are followed, one could at least speak of an ethically proper approach despite all the criticism surrounding the pharmacological treatment of sexual deviance in PCSOs.

Conclusions

Pharmacological agents present a potent treatment option to reduce paraphilic sexual fantasies and behaviors. Due to their broad spectrum of partially severe side effects and the ethical concerns that particularly relate to voluntary treatment in forensic psychiatric patients, they should be used in carefully selected patients only and the treatment process should be monitored by a multidisciplinary team of medical healthcare providers and psychologists with experience in endocrinology, sexual medicine, and forensic psychiatry (Guay, 2009). To fulfil these requirements, considerable financial resources are needed which are usually not available in forensic psychiatric settings. However, it is the ethical duty of treatment providers to at least follow the current evidence-based treatment recommendations and guidelines.

References

Adi, Y., Ashcroft, D., Browne, K., Beech, A., Fry-Smith, A., & Hyde, C. (2002). Clinical effectiveness and cost-consequences of selective serotonin reuptake inhibitors in the treatment of sex offenders. *Health Technology Assessment*, 6(28), 1–66. PMID: 12583819

Assumpcao, A. A., Garcia, F. D., Garcia, H. D., Bradford, J. M. W., & Thibaut, F. (2014). Pharmacological treatment of paraphilias. *Psychiatric Clinics of North America*, 37(2), 173–181. https://doi.org/10.1016/j.psc.2014.03.002

Bancroft, J., Tennet, G., Loucas, K., & Cass, J. (1974). The control of deviant sexual behavior by drugs. 1. Behavioural changes following oestrogens and anti-androgens. *British Journal of Psychiatry*, 586, 310–315.

Basdekis-Jozsa, R., Turner, D., & Briken, P. (2013). Pharmacological treatment of sexual offenders and its legal and ethical aspects. In K. Harrison & B. Rainey (Eds.), *The Wiley-Blackwell handbook of legal and ethical aspects of sex offender treatment and management* (pp. 302–320). John Wiley & Sons.

Beech, A. R., & Mitchell, I. J. (2005). A neurobiological perspective on attachment problems in sexual offenders and the role of selective serotonin re-uptake inhibitors in the treatment of such problems. *Clinical Psychology Review*, 25(2), 153–182. https://doi.org/10.1016/j.cpr.2004.10.002

Bradford, J., & Pawlak, A. (1993). Double-blind placebo crossover study of cyproterone acetate in the treatment of the paraphilias. *Archives of Sexual Behavior*, 22(5), 383–402. https://doi.org/10.1007/BF01542555

Briken, P., Basdekis-Jozsa, R., & Turner, D. (2018). Pharmakotherapie von paraphilen Patienten im Maßregelvollzug und Sexualstraftätern. In M. Dudeck & F. Steger (Eds.), *Ethik in der Forensischen Psychiatrie und Psychotherapie (pp. 179–188)*. Medizinisch Wissenschaftliche Verlagsgesellschaft.

Briken, P., Hill, A., & Berner, W. (2003). Pharmacotherapy of paraphilias with long-acting agonists of luteinizing hormone-releasing hormone: A systematic review. *Journal of Clinical Psychiatry*, 64(8), 890–897. https://doi.org/10.4088/JCP.v64n0806

Briken, P., Hill, A., & Berner, W. (2011). Pharmacotherapy of sexual offenders and men who are at risk of sexual offending. In D. P. Boer, R. Eher, L. A. Craig, M. H. Miner, & F. Pfäfflin (Eds.), *International perspectives on the assessment and treatment of sexual offenders* (pp. 419–431). John Wiley & Sons. https://doi.org/10.1002/9781119990420

Briken, P., & Kafka, M. P. (2007). Pharmacological treatments for paraphilic patients and sexual offenders. *Current Opinion in Psychiatry*, 20(6), 609–613. https://doi.org/10.1097/YCO.0b013e3282f0eb0b

Briken, P., Müller, J. L., Berner, W., Bödeker, R.-H., Vollmann, J., Kasperk, C., & Koller, M. (2017). Vom Scheitern einer Studie in Maßregelvollzugskrankenhäusern Klinische Prüfung zum additiven Effekt von Triptorelin auf die Wirksamkeit von Psychotherapie. Der Nervenarzt, 88, 480–485. https://doi.org/10.1007/s00115-017-0301-7

Briken, P., Nika, E., & Berner, W. (2001). Treatment of paraphilia with luteinizing hormone-releasing hormone agonists. *Journal of Sex & Marital Therapy*, 27(1), 45–55. https://doi.org/10.1080/00926230152035840

Briken, P., Turner, D., Thibaut, F., Bradford, J., Cosyns, P., & Tozdan, S. (2018). Validation of the "change or stop testosterone lowering medication (COSTLow)-scale" using Delphi method among clinical experts. *Journal of Sex & Marital Therapy*, 45(2), 148–158. https://doi.org/10.1080/0092623X.2018.1491910

Briken, P., Welzel, K., Habermann, N., Hill, A., & Berner, W. (2009). Antiandrogene Therapie und Lockerungen bei Sexualstraftätern im Maßregelvollzug Berlin [Antiandrogenic pharmacotherapy of sexual offenders and home leave steps in the forensic psychiatric hospital Berlin]. *Psychiatrische Praxis*, 36, 232–237. https://doi.org/10.1055/s-0028-1090221

Cesnik, J. A., & Coleman, E. (1989). Use of lithium carbonate in the treatment of autoerotic asphyxia. *American Journal of Psychotherapy*, 43, 277–286. https://doi.org/10.1176/appi.psychotherapy.1989.43.2.277

Cooper, A. J. (1981). A placebo-controlled trial of the antiandrogen cyproterone acetate in deviant hypersexuality. *Comprehensive Psychiatry*, 22, 458–465. https://doi.org/10.1016/0010-440X(81)90034-1

Cooper, A. J., & Cernovovsky, Z. (1992). The effects of cyproterone acetate on sleeping and waking penile erections in pedophiles: Possible implications for treatment. *Canadian Journal of Psychiatry*, 37(1), 33–39. https://doi.org/10.1177/070674379203700108

Cooper, A. J., Cernovovsky, Z., & Magnus, R. V. (1992). The long-term use of cyproterone acetate in pedophilia: A case study. *Journal of Sex and Marital Therapy*, 18(4), 292–302. https://doi.org/10.1080/00926239208412854

Cooper, A. J., Sandhu, S., Losztyn, S., & Cernovovsky, Z. (1992). A double-blind placebo controlled trial of medroxyprogesterone acetate and cyproterone acetate with seven pedophiles. *Canadian Journal of Psychiatry*, 37(10), 687–693. https://doi.org/10.1177/070674379203701003

Corona, G., Ricca, V., Bandini, E., Mannucci, E., Lotti, F., Boddi, V., Rastrelli, G., Sforza, A., Faravelli, C., Forti, G., & Maggi, M. (2009). Selective serotonin reuptake inhibitor-induced sexual dysfunction. *Journal of Sexual Medicine*, 6, 1259–1269. https://doi.org/10.1111/j.1743-6109.2009.01248.x

Corretti, G., & Baldi, I. (2010). Oxcarbamazepine reduces exhibitionistic urges and behaviors in a paraphilic patient. *Archives of Sexual Behavior*, 39, 1025–1026. https://doi.org/10.1007/s10508-010-9626-z

Czerny, J., Briken, P., & Berner, W. (2002). Antihormonal treatment of paraphilic patients in German forensic psychiatric clinics. *European Psychiatry*, 17, 104–106. https://doi.org/10.1016/S0924-9338(02)00635-1

Eher, R., Rettenberger, M., & Turner, D. (2019). The prevalence of mental disorders in incarcerated contact sexual offenders. *Acta Psychiatrica Scandinavia*, 139(6), 572–581. https://doi.org/10.1111/acps.13024

Garcia, F. D., Delavenne, H. G., de Assumpção, A. F. A., & Thibaut, F. (2013). Pharmacologic treatment of sex offenders with paraphilic disorder. *Current Psychiatry Reports*, 15(5), 356. https://doi.org/10.1007/s11920-013-0356-5

Greenberg, D. M., Bradford, J. M. W., Curry, S., & O'Rourke, A. (1996). A comparison of treatment of paraphilias with three serotonin reuptake inhibitors: A retrospective study. *Bulletin of the American Academy of Psychiatry and the Law*, 24(4), 525–532. PMID: 9001750

Guay, D. R. P. (2009). Drug treatment of paraphilic and nonparaphilic sexual disorders. *Clinical Therapeutics*, 31(1), 1–31. https://doi.org/10.1016/S0149-2918(09)00023-X

Hill, A., Briken, P., Kraus, C., Strohm, K., & Berner, W. (2003). Differential pharmacological treatment of paraphilias and sex offenders. *International Journal of Offender Therapy and Comparative Criminology*, 47(4), 407–421. https://doi.org/10.1177/0306624X03253847

Houts, F. W., Taller, I., Tucker, D. E., & Berlin, F. S. (2011). Androgen deprivation treatment of sexual behavior. *Advances in Psychosomatic Medicine*, 31, 149–163. https://doi.org/10.1159/000330196

Hucker, S., Langevin, R., & Bain, J. (1988). A double blind trial of sex drive reducing medication in pedophiles. *Annals of Sex Research*, 1(2), 227–242. https://doi.org/10.1007/BF00852799

Kafka, M. P., & Hennen, J. (2000). Psychostimulant augmentation during treatment with selective serotonin reuptake inhibitors in males with paraphilias and paraphilia-related disorders: A case series. *Journal of Clinical Psychiatry*, 61(9), 664–670. https://doi.org/10.4088/jcp.v61n0912

Kiersch, T. A. (1990). Treatment of sex offenders with Depo-Provera. *Journal of the American Academy of Psychiatry and the Law*, 18(2), 179–187. PMID: 2142608

Koo, K. C., Ahn, J. H., Hong, S. J., Lee, J. W., & Chung, B. H. (2014). Effects of chemical castration on sex offenders in relation to the kinetics of serum testosterone recovery: Implications for dosing schedule. *The Journal of Sexual Medicine*, 11(5), 1316–1324. https://doi.org/10.1111/jsm.12492

Kraus, C., Strohm, K., Hill, A., Habermann, N., Berner, W., & Briken, P. (2006). Selektive Serotonin Wiederaufnahmehemmer in der Behandlung von Paraphilien [Selective serotonine reuptake inhibitors (SSRI) in the treatment of paraphilia]. *Fortschritte der Neurologie und Psychiatrie*, 75(6), 351–356. https://doi.org/10.1055/s-2006-944261

Kravitz, H. M., Haywood, T. W., Kelly, J., Liles, S., & Cavanaugh, J. L. (1996). Medroxyprogesterone and paraphiles: Do testosterone levels matter? *Bulletin of the American Academy of Psychiatry and the Law*, 24(1), 73–83. PMID: 8891323

Lewis, A., Grubin, D., Ross, C. C., & Das, M. (2017). Gonadotrophin-releasing hormone agonist treatment for sexual offenders: A systematic review. *Journal of Psychopharmacology*, 31(10), 1281–1293. https://doi.org/10.1177/0269881117714048

Lippi, G., & van Staden, P. J. (2017). The use of cyproterone acetate in a forensic psychiatric cohort of male sex offenders and its associations with sexual activity and sexual functioning. *South African Journal of Psychiatry*, 23(1), 1–8. https://doi.org/10.4102/sajpsychiatry.v23i0.982

Maletzky, B. M., & Field, G. (2003). The biological treatment of dangerous sexual offenders. *Aggression and Violent Behavior*, 8(4), 391–412. https://doi.org/10.1016/S1359-1789(02)00065-4

Maletzky, B. M., Tolan, A., & McFarland, B. (2006). The Oregon depo-Provera program: A five-year follow-up. *Sexual Abuse: A Journal of Research and Treatment*, 18(3), 303–316. https://doi.org/10.1007/s11194-006-9021-4

McGrath, R. J., Cumming, G. F., Burchard, B. L., Zeoli, S., & Ellerby, L. (2010). *Current practices and emerging trends in sexual abuser management: The Safer Society 2009 North American survey*. Safer Society Press.

Nelson, E., Brusman, L., Holcomb, J., Soutullo, C., Beckman, D., Weldge, J. A., Kuppili, N., & McElroy, S. L. (2001). Divalproex sodium in sex offenders with bipolar disorders and comorbid paraphilias: An open retrospective study. *Journal of Affective Disorders*, 64(2–3), 249–255. https://doi.org/10.1016/S0165-0327(00)00255-X

Nishiyama, T. (2014). Serum testosterone levels after medical or surgical androgen deprivation: A comprehensive review of the literature. *Urologic Oncology: Seminars and Original Investigations*, 32(1), 38.e17–38.e28. https://doi.org/10.1016/j.urolonc.2013.03.007

Pfaus, J. G. (2009). Pathways of sexual desire. *The Journal of Sexual Medicine*, 6(6), 1506–1533. https://doi.org/10.1111/j.1743-6109.2009.01309.x

Rösler, A., & Witztum, E. (1998). Treatment of men with paraphilia with long-acting analogue of gonadotropin-releasing hormone. *New England Journal of Medicine*, 338, 416–422. https://10.1056/NEJM199802123380702

Sauter, J., Emmerling, A., Stasch, J., Voß, T., & Klemke, K. (2018). Das Absetzen antiandrogener Medikation im ambulanten Setting. Discontinuing antiandrogenic treatment in a forensic outpatient setting. *Forensische Psychiatrie, Psychologie, Kriminologie*, 12(4), 352–359. https://doi.org/10.1007/s11757-018-0498-8

Sauter, J., Turner, D., Briken, P., & Rettenberger, M. (2020). Testosterone-lowering medication and its association with recidivism risk in individuals convicted of sexual offensesTesT. *Sexual*

Abuse: A Journal of Research and Treatment. [epub ahead of print] https://doi.org/10.1177/1079063220910723

Serretti, A., & Chiesa, A. (2009). Treatment-emergent sexual dysfunction related to antidepressants: A meta-analysis. *Journal of Clinical Psychopharmacology*, 29(3), 259–266. https://doi.org/10.1097/JCP.0b013e3181a5233f

Thibaut, F., Bradford, J. M. W., Briken, P., La Barra, F. D., Thibaut, F., Bradford, J. M. W., Häßler, F., & Cosyns, P. (2016). The World Federation of Societies of Biological Psychiatry (WFSBP) guidelines for the treatment of adolescent sexual offenders with paraphilic disorders. *The World Journal of Biological Psychiatry*, 17(1), 2–38. https://doi.org/10.3109/15622975.2015.1085598

Thibaut, F., De La Barra, F., Gordon, H., Cosyns, P., & Bradford, J. M. W. (2010). The World Federation of Societies of Biological Psychiatry (WFSBP) guidelines for the biological treatment of paraphilias. *The World Journal of Biological Psychiatry*, 11(4), 604–655. https://doi.org/10.3109/15622971003671628

Thibaut, F., Cosyns, P., Fedoroff, J. P., Briken, P., Goethals, K., & Bradford, J. M. W. (2020). The World Federation of Societies of Biological Psychiatry (WFSBP) 2020 guidelines for the pharmacological treatment of paraphilic disorders. *The World Journal of Biological Psychiatry*, 21(6), 412–490. https://doi.org/10.1080/15622975.2020.1744723

Turner, D., Gregório Hertz, P., Sauter, J., Briken, P., & Rettenberger, M. (2018). Pharmacological treatment of sexual offenders in German outpatient treatment centers. *International Clinical Psychopharmacology*, 33(6), 349–352. https://doi.org/10.1097/YIC.0000000000000222

Turner, D., Basdekis-Jozsa, R., & Briken, P. (2013a). Pharmakologie sexueller Präferenzstörungen und ihre neurobiologischen Implikationen. In A. Stirn, R. Stark, K. Tabbert, S. Wehrum-Osinsky, & S. Oddo (Eds.), *Sexualität, Körper und Neurobiologie* (pp. 263–273). W. Kohlhammer Verlag.

Turner, D., Basdekis-Jozsa, R., & Briken, P. (2013b). Prescription of testosterone-lowering medications for sex offender treatment in German forensic-psychiatric institutions. *The Journal of Sexual Medicine*, 10(2), 570–578. https://doi.org/10.1111/j.1743-6109.2012.02958.x

Turner, D., Basdekis-jozsa, R., Dekker, A., & Briken, P. (2014). Which factors influence the appropriateness of testosterone-lowering medications for sex offenders? A survey among clinicians from German forensic-psychiatric institutions. *The World Journal of Biological Psychiatry*, 15(6), 472–478. https://doi.org/10.3109/15622975.2013.839052

Turner, D., & Briken, P. (2018a). Die Behandlung paraphiler Störungen mit GnRH-Agonisten unter besonderer Berücksichtigung ethischer und rechtlicher Aspekte. *Forensische Psychiatrie, Psychologie, Kriminologie*, 12(4), 244–351. https://doi.org/10.1007/s11757-018-0503-2

Turner, D., & Briken, P. (2018b). Treatment of paraphilic disorders in sexual offenders or men with a risk of sexual offending with luteinizing hormone-releasing hormone agonists: An updated systematic review. *Journal of Sexual Medicine*, 15(1), 77–93. https://doi.org/10.1016/j.jsxm.2017.11.013

Turner, D., Petermann, J., Harrison, K., Krueger, R., & Briken, P. (2019). Pharmacological treatment of patients with paraphilic disorders and risk of sexual offending: An international perspective. *World Journal of Biological Psychiatry*, 20(8), 616–625. https://doi.org/10.1080/15622975.2017.1395069

Voß, T., Klemke, K., Schneider-Njepel, V., & Kröber, H. L. (2016). Wenn ja, wie lange? – Dauer antiandrogener Behandlung von Sexualstraftätern mit paraphilen Störungen: Klinische Erfahrungen aus Auslassversuchen in der forensischen Nachsorgepraxis. *Forensische Psychiatrie, Psychologie, Kriminologie*, 10(1), 21–31. https://doi.org/10.1007/s11757-015-0346-z

Wainberg, M. L., Muench, F., Morgenstern, J., Hollander, E., Irwin, T. W., Parsons, J. T., Allen, A., & O'Leary, A. (2006). A double-blind study of citalopram versus placebo in the treatment of compulsive sexual behaviors in gay and bisexual men. *Journal of Clinical Psychiatry*, 67(12), 1968–1973. https://doi.org/10.4088/jcp.v67n1218

Wincze, J. P., Bansal, S., & Malamud, M. (1986). Effects of medroxyprogesterone acetate on subjective arousal, arousal to erotic stimulation, and nocturnal penile tumescence in male sex offenders. *Archives of Sexual Behavior*, 15(4), 293–305. https://doi.org/10.1007/BF01550364

Winder, B., Lievesley, R., Elliot, H., Hocken, K., Faulkner, J., Norman, C., & Kaul, A. (2018). Evaluation of the use of pharmacological treatment with prisoners experiencing high levels of hypersexual disorder. *Journal of Forensich Psychiatry & Psychology*, 29(1), 53–71. https://doi.org/10.1080/14789949.2017.1337801

Wong, J. S., & Gravel, J. (2018). Do sex offenders have higher levels of testosterone? Results from a meta-analysis. *Sexual Abuse: A Journal of Research and Treatment*, 30(2), 147–168. https://doi.org/10.1177/1079063216637857

19

Rehabilitating Paraphilic Disorder in Prisons

Interventions Sensitive to Shame and Trauma and the Importance of Safe Prisons

Jamie S. Walton

Midlands Psychology Services, Psychology Services Group, Her Majesty's Prison and Probation Service

Introduction

People convicted of sexual offenses comprise a substantial percentage of the prison population in many jurisdictions. In the United Kingdom (UK), recent prison statistics indicate that rates stabilized at about 18% in 2019, and decreased by 8% in 2020 (Ministry of Justice, 2019, 2020); however, this group remains one of the largest of those sentenced to prison. Although prison sentences are reserved for the most serious sexual crimes, in every prison population, invariably there are differences in people's offending histories, levels of risk, sentence lengths, and intervention requirements. People convicted of sexual offending present with different challenges, and prisons must attend to these in responsive ways. Atypical sexual interests, referred to clinically as "*paraphilias*," represent a particularly difficult challenge for prison management, forensic assessment and intervention. This chapter focuses on some of the key issues, and is divided into three sections. First, the classification and assessment of paraphilias is discussed with relevance to challenges for practitioners working in prisons. The effectiveness of prison-based interventions for paraphilias is then reviewed, after which some directions for the future are discussed. These include, firstly, the need for initiatives that foster safe prisons; and secondly, the need for therapeutic interventions that are much more sensitive to the stressors that are prevalent among prisoners with paraphilia, namely, stigmatization, and the effects of childhood adversity. The final section describes an example of such intervention delivered in HM Prison and Probation Service (HMPPS) in England and Wales.

Paraphilia and Paraphilic Disorder: Issues and Challenges for Forensic Practitioners in Prisons

The term "paraphilia" can be defined as any intense and persistent sexual interest other than a sexual interest in genital stimulation or preparatory fondling with phenotypically normal, physically mature, consenting human partners (American Psychiatric Association, 2013). "Phenotypically normal" in this case refers to the normal characteristics of adults. At first glance, the definition appears to label anything outside of a narrow range of sexual behaviors as paraphilic. Set that aside, and a paraphilia refers to a period of six months or more during which arousal to atypical stimuli must be manifest. However, this does not in

Sexual Deviance: Understanding and Managing Deviant Sexual Interests and Paraphilic Disorders,
First Edition. Edited by Leam A. Craig and Ross M. Bartels.
© 2021 John Wiley & Sons, Ltd. Published 2021 by John Wiley & Sons, Ltd.

itself imply that a person has a disorder of sexual interest. Only where a paraphilia causes distress, impairment, or acts of harm is the diagnosis of a disorder appropriate (APA, 2013). For this, the APA (2013) reserves the term "Paraphilic Disorder." This term has also been proposed by the Working Group on the Classification of Sexual Disorders and Sexual Health (WGSDSH; Krueger et al., 2017) for inclusion in the updated International Classifications of Diseases and Related Health Problems (ICD), published by the World Health Organization. This distinction between paraphilia and mental disorder is important, because many people who exhibit paraphilia resist illegally harming others (Cantor & McPhail, 2016), and many others do not experience distress or impairment (Wismeijer & van Assen, 2013). In short, it is "Paraphilic Disorder" that distinguishes the dysfunctional manifestation of a paraphilia.

Paraphilic Disorders can be divided into two types—criminal and non-criminal (Moser, 2019). Criminal Paraphilic Disorders include: recurrent and intense arousal to exposing one's genitals to an unsuspecting person(s) (Exhibitionistic Disorder); rubbing up against non-consenting individuals (Frotteuristic Disorder); sexual activity with a prepubescent child (Pedophilic Disorder); and spying on an unsuspecting individual(s) naked or undressing (Voyeuristic Disorder). Acting out any of these sexual urges necessarily entails a non-consenting person and will constitute a crime. Non-criminal Paraphilic Disorders include recurrent and intense arousal to non-living objects or non-genital body parts (Fetishistic Disorder); receiving or issuing pain, humiliation, or suffering (Sexual Masochism and Sexual Sadism Disorder respectively); and thoughts of being the opposite gender and cross-dressing (Transvestic Disorders). Fetishistic, transvestic, and sadomasochistic interests often involve consenting partners. An example would be two consenting adults engaging in sadism and masochism role-play together, with both of them experiencing pleasure. This is called 'BDSM' (Bondage and Discipline, Domination, Submission, Sadism and Masochism). These paraphilia have been proposed to be removed from the forthcoming ICD (Krueger et al., 2017). In terms of forensic implications, Pedophilic Disorder, Sexual Sadistic Disorder, and multiple paraphilia are associated with sexual recidivism (Mann et al., 2010). There are two important issues for practitioners to navigate that are especially relevant to the rehabilitation for Paraphilic Disorders in prisons. The first issue is about inferring paraphilia from offending behavior. The second is about the remission of a Paraphilic Disorder once the symptoms are manifest.

Inferring Paraphilia from Offending Behavior

Criminal paraphilias—voyeurism, exhibitionism, and frotteurism—are only specified in a sexual crime if the individual has eroticized, and is aroused to, the non-consenting aspects of the act. An individual who engages in such act, but is not actively aroused to the non-consenting aspects of it, is engaging in criminal behavior, but they are not necessarily exhibiting evidence of a Criminal Paraphilic Disorder. This is because behavior, including sexually abusive behavior, is only one possible manifestation of paraphilic arousal, and it is intense and recurrent arousal, not behavior that constitutes paraphilia. The exemption is pedophilia. This is because the APA (2013) diagnostic template for pedophilia includes "behaviors" as well as "arousing fantasies" and "sexual urges" in the definition of the sexual interest itself (rather than possible manifestations). In doing so, it permits practitioners to establish the presence of pedophilia on the basis of child sexual offending alone. However, experts suggest pedophilia should not be considered any differently from other paraphilia on this issue (e.g., First, 2014). In all cases, it is important that forensic practitioners corroborate offending behavior with evidence of an atypical arousal pattern (First, 2014; Krueger et al., 2017; Seto, 2018). This can be challenging in prisons, however, because a person's disclosure of a paraphilia could delay their sentence progression. Therefore, they may be expected to lie about their arousal patterns. To overcome this, ideally, assessments would be hard to fake, and they would assess multiple aspects of sexual response (Thornton et al., 2018). The most validated assessment for this purpose is phallometry (McPhail et al., 2019). Phallometry measures changes in penile circumference or volume while stimuli depicting different ages, sexes, and sexual activities are presented. However, whilst phallometry is the preferred assessment, there is a lack of standardization across procedures, as well as several ethical objections to presenting certain visual stimuli, and the assessment itself is intrusive, rendering it highly unappealing (see Laws, 2009). Phallometry is no longer used in HMPPS, and its use in other jurisdictions is often limited.

The APA (2013) does offer a solution to the issue of non-disclosure by clarifying that a history of *recurring* sexual offenses (for example, separate frotteuristic behavior against three or more victims) can establish satisfactory support for a paraphilia when an individual denies arousal. This is contrary to the case made above to establish an arousal pattern for paraphilias rather than infer them from behavior. The APAs advocacy of this practice is practical, but further evidence is needed to determine what level of accuracy in identifying paraphilias can be obtained from different sexual offenses and their characteristics (Beech et al., 2016; First, 2014). Rating scales such as the Screening Scale for Pedophilic Interests Revised (SSPI-2; Seto et al., 2017) and the Severe Sexual Sadism Scale (SeSaS; Nitschke et al., 2009) are of the type required. The SSPI-2 consists of behavioral indicators of child sexual offending (e.g., "any boy victim under 15 years"; "use of child sexual exploitation material") that are empirically related to phallometrically assessed arousal to children. Recent analysis of SSPI-2 data (Stephens et al., 2019) indicates that these indicators screen for a sexual interest in both prepubescent and pubescent children ("*pedohebephilia*"; see Blanchard et al., 2009). The SeSaS combines items to do with crime scene behavior, offending planning and prior sadistic behavior, and is considered to be a suitable diagnostic aid (Nitschke et al., 2013). Even with rating scales, though, practitioners should endeavor to find support for their behavioral inferences, the most obvious being to eliminate other reasons for sexual offending such as emotional dyscontrol, intoxication, and general antisociality.

Paraphilic Disorders and Their Remission (or Not)

A close read of current APA criteria suggests that a short period of significant distress could be sufficient to convert a paraphilia to a Paraphilic Disorder (Moser, 2019). Upon resolving the distress, a period of five years symptom-free in a non-controlled environment is required before an individual may be classified as having a Paraphilic Disorder in full remission, never reverting back to a paraphilia per se. In prisons, however, this specifier is irrelevant because it does not apply, since prisons are controlled. Instead, the specifier "in a controlled environment" must be used (APA, 2013). Importantly, in either case "in remission" indicates the absence of distress, impairment or harm—*not* the absence of paraphilia. Even more importantly, remission criteria of any kind are entirely absent for Pedophilic Disorder. This is a particularly contentious issue (Briken et al., 2014; Cantor, 2018; Cantor & Fedoroff 2018; Fedoroff, 2018), and to avoid misinterpretation it is important that practitioners in prisons are clear about what features of Pedophilic Disorder can remit, and what others will likely remain.

The general consensus amongst researchers is that paraphilias persist over time (Cantor, 2018; Miletski, 2017; Seto, 2012, 2017). Evidence confirming (or disconfirming) this for most of the paraphilias is in fact meagre, except for pedophilia, for which survey data appear supportive (Bailey et al., 2016; Grundmann et al., 2016). Where change in pedophilic arousal has been reported using phallometry (Müller et al., 2014), it has been robustly criticized (Bailey, 2015; Cantor, 2015; Lalumière, 2015; see Federoff et al., 2015 for a response). Despite this, some clinicians refute the view that pedophilia is non-changeable. Fedoroff (2016), in particular, suggests that clinicians should advise their participants that all available evidence suggests paraphilia can be modified. Advice of this kind is discouraged by others (e.g., Bailey, 2015; Cantor, 2018), although this dissuasion should not be conflated with the idea that individuals cannot, or *do not* change. This is where the lack of remission specifiers for Pedophilic Disorder could be confusing, because the criteria include features—distress, impairment, and harmful behavior—that can and do fluctuate. Ameliorating them, for example working with stress and shame and improving functional coping, are actually important goals of intervention for people in prison who would likely meet criteria for Pedophilic Disorder, just as they are for people with other Paraphilic Disorders (e.g., Walton, in press). In all cases, the agenda should be about expanding repertoires of strength and skill for the thriving of a whole person toward a more constructive crime-free life. When it comes to paraphilia and their dysfunction, it is these repertoires of strength and skill that are important for practitioners in prisons to assess and test. When strengths and skills are lacking, structured program interventions are often recommended.

Interventions for Paraphilic Disorders Delivered in Prisons

As explained above, sexual offending behavior is one manifestation of a paraphilia, and is not synonymous with it. This means many people in prison convicted of sexual offenses will not have a paraphilia. For example, across samples of people convicted of sexual offending, the prevalence of pedophilia is about 50% (see Seto, 2018). However, these samples include adults and adolescents assessed differently in prisons, hospitals, and clinics, and rates vary accordingly. Despite this, beginning in the late 1960s, interventions in secure settings focused solely on individuals assessed as such. Early approaches were based on behavior learning principles and extended no further than attempting to extinguish paraphilias by administering aversive stimuli directly to arousal. Techniques included active shaming (Serber, 1970), and the administration of foul odors and shocks (Colson, 1972; Evans, 1968). Astonishingly, the use of shame as an aversive stimulus was still being used in a technique called "aversive behavioral rehearsal" as recently as 2009 in 14% of institutional interventions for adults surveyed in North America (McGrath et al., 2010). Even more astonishing is that it was being used in 17.3% of institutional interventions for adolescents (McGrath et al., 2010). Intervention should aim to alleviate shame, not use it as a therapy goal.

In the decades that followed, two things occurred. Firstly, the rise of cognitive therapy produced a new treatment goal for disorders right across the mental health spectrum. For people convicted of sexual offending with (and without) Paraphilic Disorders, the new goal was to detect, challenge and change distorted (offense supportive) cognition. Secondly, Paraphilic Disorders and sexual offending seemed associated with other characteristics such as poor victim empathy, and limited social skills. Interventions expanded to address these characteristics, and then up-scaled in the early 1990s into structured group-based programs operating across prisons (e.g., Grubin & Thornton, 1994). From this point on, group-based sexual offending programs were what people in prison with paraphilia regularly accessed. A primary focus was relapse-prevention (RP), along with instilling victim empathy and eliminating offense denial often outright and usually with confrontation (Salter, 1988).

State of the art though these programs were, some of the characteristics they targeted were not associated with recidivism, as was found out years later. Cognition was also not well defined, and without the clarification that awaited them (e.g., Maruna & Mann, 2006) practitioners often conflated thoughts that support offending with functionally different cognitive processes such as minimization and denial (see Walton, 2019). During the early 2000s, experts recommended shifts toward enhancing individuals' wellbeing, using motivational interviewing, focusing on their values, and enhancing strengths for leading prosperous and safe good lives—a "Good Lives Model" (GLM; Ward & Stewart, 2003). This signified a new frontier, one that was future-focused and strength-based. However, in many programs, not necessarily confined to prison settings, GLM-integration resulted merely in the addition of a good lives module rather than a paradigm shift (see Willis et al., 2014).

The Effectiveness of Programs Delivered in Prisons

Establishing if interventions reflecting any of the major shifts in practice have reduced sexual recidivism is contentious. A key dispute has to do with what researchers are prepared to accept as the minimum standards of scientific rigor necessary to achieve accurate causal inference. Randomized controlled trials (RCTs) are the most internally valid design. However, there are organizational barriers to implementing RCTs in prisons. Most researchers have instead used observational designs that compare individuals who received an intervention with an incidental group who, for reasons to do with time, opportunity, or refusal, did not. These designs are much more vulnerable to confounding and systematic bias which render the groups non-equivalent and diminish confidence that any differences in reconviction rates are due to an intervention, rather than other factors (see Walton, 2018 for a discussion on methods).

Researchers who limit inclusion to the few RCTs available report no effect of intervention on sexual recidivism (e.g., Dennis et al., 2012). Some researchers who employ strict inclusion criteria and only accept observational studies where there are no serious doubts as to the equivalence of the groups, report a small positive effect of Cognitive Behavioral Therapy (CBT) only (Schmucker & Lösel, 2017). Others using similar criteria, albeit including fewer and different studies focusing on sexual offending against children, report no such effect (Grønnerød et al., 2015; Långström et al., 2013). Those who use the least strict criteria report the largest effects for a variety of approaches (e.g., Hanson et al., 2009; Lösel & Schmucker, 2005). Arguably, the most authoritative recent review that balances the size of the database with relative rigor is Schmucker and Lösel (2017). Notably, this meta-analysis found no effect on sexual recidivism for programs delivered in prisons. The largest observational study illustrating this result examined the outcomes of HMPPS Core Sex Offender Treatment Programme (CSOTP) from 2000 to 2012 (Mews et al., 2017). Sexual recidivism for those who received the CSOTP compared to those who did not, increased by an absolute value of 2% over an 8.2-year follow up.

Extricating the effects for people with Paraphilic Disorders from these results is challenging. Mews et al. (2017), for example, went to extensive lengths to match their groups on 87 variables. However, there were insufficient file records to confidently match on a composite variable for sexual deviancy, defined as sexual preoccupation, pedophilia, sexual sadism and multiple paraphilia. Sexual deviancy is not only predictive of sexual recidivism (Mann et al., 2010), but was a variable that likely impacted selection onto the CSOTP. The resulting selection bias from sexual deviancy and other unobserved variables would have needed to be substantial to change the result. However, the issue illustrates the challenges faced in trying to discriminate what effects prison-based programs have for those with Paraphilic Disorders.

Another option is to extract results for therapy procedures targeting paraphilic arousal, for example behavior therapy. Amidst the mass rise of CBT group-based programs for sexual offending, it became customary to incorporate behavior therapy either as a module or ad hoc according to individual need (e.g., Marques et al., 2005). A recent meta-analysis found that behavior therapy techniques reduced paraphilic arousal ("pedohebephilia" specifically), especially for people who show high arousal levels (McPhail & Olver, 2020). As to whether these reductions in paraphilic arousal lead to reductions in sexual recidivism, the picture is less clear. Lösel and Schmucker (2005) found that interventions that incorporated behavior therapy significantly reduced recidivism. More recently, Gannon et al. (2019) have reported that interventions that incorporated behavior therapy produced larger reductions in recidivism than those that did not. However, these findings should be interpreted with caution. This is because the evaluations of interventions incorporating behavior therapy included by Lösel and Schmucker (2005) were heavily confounded. In their subsequent meta-analysis using stricter scientific rigor, Schmucker and Lösel (2017) excluded a vast proportion of these evaluations. Gannon et al. (2019) included many evaluations that fall below the standards set by Schmucker and Lösel (2017). It is, therefore, perhaps expected that they would report a similar effect to Lösel and Schmucker's original meta-analysis, and for that reason, the evidence attesting to the long-term impact of behavior therapy should be considered cautiously.

Directions for Interventions in Prisons

With the ambiguity of the evidence base in mind, what can practitioners working in prisons do to support people with Paraphilic Disorders in leading non-harmful lives? There are some directions to take. Firstly, self-regulation problems associated with sexual recidivism overlap substantially with those associated with general criminality (see Bonta & Andrews, 2017; Mann et al., 2010). Neuroimaging research is also beginning to show that individuals with pedophilia who sexually offend, as compared to those who do not, differ in their gray matter volumes and prefrontal functioning relative to reduced self-regulation abilities and higher antisociality (Kärgel et al., 2015, 2017; Schiffer et al., 2017). Therefore, amidst the ambiguity, the principles of effective rehabilitation for general criminality should form the foundation. These principles are well known as Risk-Need-Responsivity (RNR; Bonta & Andrews, 2017). Accordingly, intervention intensity (dose) should be proportionate to risk; it should strengthen pro-social competencies in areas associated with sexual recidivism; it should CBT-based, and it should be delivered in humanizing ways that are responsive to personal circumstances. Recent work by way of RNR has articulated biopsychosocial processes that influence paraphilia as well as therapy procedures that aim to strengthen capacities for pro-social change (Carter & Mann, 2016; Walton, in press).

As part of identifying the important therapy procedures, practitioners have also reported on the need to work with the effects of Adverse Childhood Experiences (ACEs) and the stigmatization of sexual offending and paraphilia (e.g., Jahnke, 2018; Levenson & Grady, 2016; Levenson et al., 2018; Walton, in press). Consider pedophilia, for example. Hate for this sexual interest is found at all levels of society including the young, educated, and liberal minded (Imhoff, 2015; Imhoff & Jahnke, 2018). The effects of stigmatization are bleak. They include marginalization, stress (of disguise), anger, fear and internalized shame, all of which are threat-based states, toxic to health and change (Jahnke & Hoyer, 2013; Jahnke et al., 2015). The same can be said for ACEs, such as childhood abuse and neglect. ACEs can set in motion a cascade of neurodevelopmental changes in a child's brain manifesting as self-regulation and attachment problems leading to chronically poor outcomes decades later (Anda et al., 2010). Many of these outcomes—for example, alcoholism, emotional dysregulation, and relationship problems—are associated with sexual recidivism (Mann et al., 2010), as they are other forms of harm and adversity. Broadly, there is mounting evidence of high (but by no means universal) levels of ACEs in people convicted of sexual offending (Jespersen et al., 2009; Seto & Lalumière, 2010). High ACEs are also associated with higher sexual deviancy scores (Levenson & Grady, 2016; Levenson et al., 2016). To be clear about the point, stigmatization and trauma are areas that need more attention in assessment and intervention (see Levenson et al., 2018).

The prison climate itself also matters, a lot. Social hostility toward sexual offending can intensify in prison. Of course, prisons should work to mitigate the detrimental effects of imprisonment, and so a relevant protective measure is to house people convicted of sexual crimes in separate accommodation with other vulnerable prisoners away from the "main" population (Nicholls & Webster, 2018). This segregation creates safety. However, it can also have counter-productive effects, such as perpetuating labeling and stigmatization (Nicholls & Webster, 2018). When people convicted of sexual offending come to prison, their "vulnerable prisoner" status indicates firmly that they are at the bottom of the prison hierarchy. Often, the behaviors of most use are related to defense and survival (Schwaebe, 2005). If a prison is experienced as unsafe, the effect of an intervention delivered within it will probably be negligible, but it could easily be canceled out entirely. In some cases, the lack of safety and staff support makes intervention an unfeasible proposition altogether (Mann et al., 2013). On the other hand, research is now showing that when people in prison experience safety, their readiness to access interventions can increase (Blagden et al., 2019; Stasch et al., 2018).

Blagden and colleagues (Blagden et al., 2017; Blagden & Wilson, 2020) recently found that prisoners felt safer after their prison had re-rolled to accommodate only people with sexual convictions. Such a population shift is a huge executive directive for prisons, and further research is needed to know if co-location on this level promotes long-term pro-social change. However, there are a number of other initiatives that are associated with improved experiences of prison, and these need to become the wider focus. Procedural justice is a case in point. Procedural justice involves four principles: voice, neutrality, trustworthiness, and respect (Tyler, 2008). There is now mounting evidence that when people in prisons feel heard, when they see rules applied consistently, and when they experience authenticity in staff behavior and receive courtesy, they are more likely to cooperate and abide by rules (see Mann et al., 2019 for a discussion). Peer-support schemes are another example. In a recent review specific to people in prison with sexual offense convictions, Perrin et al. (2018) identified a number of themes related to the way peer-support can reduce anxiety, promote redemptive identities, mitigate stigma-induced stress, and extend the context for using skills in therapy to the broader prison environment.

For some people convicted of sexual offenses, the stability of paraphilia, along with the effects of ACEs and stigmatization, will make leading a continually non-harmful life challenging. Pro-social change is unlikely to hinge on a prison program. It will be ongoing, taking place *within* professional relationships in prisons and beyond. The professional relationships in which rehabilitation is shaped must ensure prison security and prison order. However, to achieve this most effectively, these relationships need to be consistent and respectful, and most importantly, they must foster the space for people to feel safe and redeemable, such that pro-social change *can* actually occur.

The Healthy Sex Program for Men with Paraphilia Delivered in HMPPS

This final section outlines a program delivered in HMPPS for adult men with paraphilic interests and convictions for sexual offending. It is called the Healthy Sex Program (HSP). The program lasts between 12 and 30 hours. It is delivered individually, therapist-to-participant and is open to those with and without mild Learning Disability and Challenges (LDC). There have been previous iterations of the program, but it was revised in 2019 and has received full accreditation from the Correctional Service Advise and Accreditation Panel (CSAAP)—a non-statutory expert advisory body for the UK Ministry of Justice. The revised program awaits evaluation. However, it incorporates a number of design and implementation principles that have been shown to moderate positive outcomes, such as being delivered by psychologists, and integrating a range of therapy procedures that make up the general bulk of evidence-based CBT competencies (Gannon et al., 2019; Schmucker & Lösel, 2017; see Hayes & Hofmann, 2018 for a review of CBT competencies). In brief, these therapy procedures include behavior therapy and self-management, modification of beliefs, mindfulness, values clarification, compassion work, urge management and intimacy / interpersonal skills practice. At its core the HSP takes a functional analytic approach, focusing on shaping new antecedent-behavior-consequence contingencies to deal with the specific stimuli that exert strong control over paraphilic arousal. These stimuli may include aversive and so negatively reinforced states (e.g., shame, disgust, loneliness, and boredom), or positively reinforced cues such as visual or auditory triggers, and/or offending memories, and sexual thoughts. Generally, a participant will practice a range of urge management and self-regulation skills in response. This work may also include efforts to achieve the functions of paraphilic arousal in alternative ways. For example, functions such as feelings of mastery, happiness, or intimate connection, or the removal of boredom, loneliness, or tension can all be achieved in healthier ways than fantasizing about abusive sex. The use of behavior therapy is optional. As described above, the early behavior therapists were naïve in seeking to eliminate paraphilia. Behavior therapy is unlikely to permanently change arousal. This is because it relies on creating new contingencies to shape new arousal responses. If, however, those contingencies are stopped (that is, a person stops practicing the technique), the conditioned response will diminish and previous arousal patterns will likely return. Furthermore, unlike the early behavior therapists that prioritized aversion therapies, HSP uses appetitive techniques such as "directed masturbation" that reward progressively healthier fantasy with masturbatory-induced pleasure, thereby steadily shaping arousal to pro-social themes. This is important. Intervention cannot just concern itself with removing risks as if a life of restriction could ever be truly fulfilling. Intervention has to offer viable alternatives that can serve a pro-social life. Behavior therapy, functional analysis, and the other procedures listed above are described in detail by Walton (in press). The remainder of this chapter is given to HSP assessment, and procedures for working with the effects of trauma and stigmatization.

Program Assessment

The HSP is accessed via one of four pathways provided in HMPPS. High-risk men without LDC who show strong needs across attitudinal, interpersonal, and self-regulation domains first access a program called "Kaizen," whilst those with mild LDC access "Becoming New Me plus" (BNM+). Medium and high-risk individuals who have greater pro-social skills access less intensive intervention, called "Horizon," and those with LDC access a program called "New Me Strengths" (NMS). These programs have been described already (see Walton et al., 2017; Ramsay, 2020; Ramsay et al. 2020). Graduates of these programs are offered an assessment for the HSP when criminal paraphilia are indicated from self-report and behavioral records. The assessment focuses primarily on the presence of criminal paraphilia, harmful sexual scripts, and sexual preoccupation, and in addition, the presence (or absence) of skills for adult intimacy.

Assessors review prison files and conduct a clinical interview(s) to establish the presence of indicators for criminal paraphilia. Similar to APA (2013) criteria, a time of six months or more is used as a guide for the presence of paraphilia, and of particular relevance is recurring sexual offending. However, self-reported sexual interests, masturbatory habits, type of pornography use (where relevant), as well as desired or practiced sexual behaviors are also important contexts to be explored. Behavior screens prove useful as adjunct tools. Crime scene behavior items on the SeSaS can be assessed using forensic records to help establish sexual arousal in the commission of sexually violent offenses. Likewise, the SSPI-2 provides a screen for pedophilia. Assessors then turn to focus on strengths in insight and sexual self-regulation. An important consideration is the impact of the sterile prison environment on arousal in determining the strength of self-regulation. A participant is eligible for the HSP if a paraphilia related to sexual offending is assessed as present, with support required in strengthening skills for safe self-management. Participant's accessing the program acknowledge their paraphilia to varying degrees. For many, their arousal is actively manifest and they are struggling to cope. For others, their arousal may have declined, although they and/or professionals may express concern about the resurgence of arousal and associated risks in less restricted environments. When a participant is impeded by sexual preoccupation, particularly manifesting as insatiable sex drive and overwhelming urges, they can voluntarily undergo assessment for pharmacological interventions coordinated from one of the HMPPS' prison clinics.

Responsivity to the Neurodevelopmental Effects of Childhood Adversity

As mentioned earlier, beneath the long-term effects of ACEs are corrosive neurodevelopmental injuries. These can manifest in many domains including verbal, attention, and memory functions, as well as emotional dysregulation and cognitive inflexibility. The HSP therefore uses a multimodal, brain-friendly approach to broadly appeal to neurodiversity. In brief, methods for sensory learning such as visual, auditory, and kinesthetic are used as much as possible besides reading. This includes in-action "body-movement" techniques, symbolizing and signing, drawing, gesturing, and brain-breaks.

The inability to regulate threat is another harmful effect of ACEs. This may present differently subject to vulnerabilities that may manifest such as antisocial orientation, intimacy seeking with children, or emotional dysregulation. Resistance may present in antisocial individuals, whilst a fear of adults, including the therapist, could be observed in others. Much of this is understandable in the context of brains shaped by abandonment and fear with little experience of a safe haven, at least from adults. Either way, pressuring engagement in the HSP is unlikely to foster alliance and a basis for change. As such, the HSP only requests that a participant invests in *learning* skills for change—trying skills, and exploring what works. No expectation is placed on long-term change itself. A lot of what is viewed as needing to change (e.g., guardedness, sexualized coping etc.), although dysfunctional, often developed as safety or soothing strategies in conditions that fall short of what is needed for pro-social success.

To work with this the HSP therapist acts as a supportive coach and a secure base. This means that they try to affirm internal strength and evoke curiosity in pro-social change. It means they provide consistent standards of warmth. It also means they try to compassionately support coping with the suffering linked to ACEs and/or stigmatization as it surfaces as anger, dismay, anxiety, fear, or self-contempt. In short, there is a sensitivity in the HSP to the fact that, even in the simple request to learn skills for change, participants will encounter uncomfortable territory, and necessarily work with it in the service of increasing their repertoire of skills for leading a non-harmful life. This is the basis of developing a compassionate mind (Gilbert, 2010; Gilbert & Choden, 2013)—an optional therapy procedure in the program for working with participants suffering from shame linked to trauma and stigmatization.

Working with Shame Linked to Trauma and Stigmatization

For people with high levels of shame linked to trauma and stigmatization, it is helpful to recognize that distress is experienced in the body (van der Kolk, 2014). Rationalizing self-talk may not be the answer, at least not at first. Often the work must begin with the body (van der Kolk, 2014). Similar to a lot of general affect regulation work (McKay, 2018; van der Kolk, 2014), the HSP uses a breathing technique focusing on a slow rhythmic breath, deep from the diaphragm, extending the exhale to activate parasympathetic arousal associated with stillness and soothing. This initial breathing work is a foundation to a further therapy goal, namely, to build the strength of a compassionate mind. Compassion is defined as a sensitivity to suffering in self and others, with a commitment to try to prevent and alleviate it (Gilbert & Choden, 2013). This means compassion requires courage. It is not "soft." On the contrary, it is almost always the "harder thing" to do, because it requires a *turn towards* our own suffering that we routinely displace; our anger, our fear and anxiety, our disgust, and our self-contempt. Compassion is also a strengthening act because it involves stimulating emotions and practicing competencies that can support effective coping, including general empathy, self-regulation, distress tolerance, and mentalization skills. Compassion training was designed for dealing specifically with trauma-based shame, as well as other painful states (Gilbert, 2010). There is evidence of positive outcomes for compassion training across the healthcare sector (Craig et al., 2020; Kirby et al., 2017), and basic elements are adaptable for participants with LDC (e.g., Clapton et al., 2018).

Rather than convincing a participant that they should be compassionate, a general approach is to depathologize painful states such as stigma-induced stress and self-criticism as normal safety responses to intense experiences of threat (Gilbert, 2010). In the case of ACEs, for example, such as an unsafe and abusive childhood environment, it makes sense for the nervous system of a child to specialize in safety strategies, such as avoidance, distancing, and withdrawal. These could keep them safe. However, as a child grows into adulthood these same safety strategies may inhibit neurodevelopmental trajectories for affiliation and healthy sexual intimacy with adults. Nobody choses this of course. It is a biopsychosocial trajectory shaped within an arbitrarily inherited environment, and this depathologizing narrative is what begins to develop the *wisdom* of compassion. This is not about absolving an individual of responsibility for their sexually harmful behavior as an adult. It is quite the opposite. It is about helping them recognize *what* about their emotional pain is a normal human response in the context of life events, such that they can take responsibility for working directly and helpfully with it, as part of being better equipped to lead a non-harmful future.

Beginning with the breathing exercises, a participant might first practice imagining aspects of a compassionate version of themselves, like a method actor—them at their kindest, bravest, and wisest etc., before moving on to practicing self-corrective thinking and acts of compassion (see Gilbert, 2010; Gilbert & Choden, 2013). As the practice progresses, the aim is for this mind-set to become a state of feeling and viewing that the participant shifts to, building insight, tolerance and perspectives around their emotional pain. Practice in basic mindful observation is key, as a means of helping the participant become aware of their mind's habits, and opening up to discomforting internal experiences (Gilbert, 2010; Gilbert & Choden, 2013; see also van der Kolk, 2014). For some, a goal may be to work compassionately with anger or self-criticism, and this will entail (bravely) venturing to face what lies beneath, perhaps the fear of being "found out," hated, or the pain of feeling disgusting, revolting or deeply flawed. The goal, with practice, is for a compassionate mind to merge and grow as the wiser and more caring perspective in the participant, carrying with it a repertoire of skills to deal non-harmfully with distress, and/or paraphilic urges, ultimately to avoid harming others.

Conclusion

By virtue of their criminal significance, Paraphilic Disorders will be a continuing public risk that prisons must try to competently deal with and rehabilitate. The classification of Paraphilic Disorders continues to be debated; forensic assessment is complicated and the last 50 years of prison-based interventions that have tried to treat them have amounted to mixed and unconvincing effects. People with Paraphilic Disorders who sexually offend can experience profound stigmatization, and a non-trivial proportion are likely to have suffered childhood trauma and other life adversity. There is mounting consensus that practitioners should recognize the prevalence of these experiences and incorporate therapy procedures into their interventions to work with their damaging effects. But prisons themselves must be conducive to pro-social change, because the prison environment will invariably moderate the effects of such interventions. Prison has the potential to be a very threatening place for this group. Safeness in people's relationships in prison is indispensable. In a safe prison, professional relationships can not only wrap around intervention, they can function *as* intervention. This is likely to be essential in helping people move in less harmful crime-free directions.

References

American Psychiatric Association. (2013). *Diagnostic and statistical manual of mental disorders* (5th ed.). American Psychiatric Publishing.

Anda, R. F., Butchart, A., Felitti, V. J., & Brown, D. W. (2010). Building a framework for global surveillance of the public health implications of adverse childhood experiences. *American Journal of Preventive Medicine, 39*, 93–98. https://doi.org/10.1016/j.amepre.2010.03.015

Bailey, J. M. (2015). A failure to demonstrate changes in sexual interest in pedophilic men: Comment on Müller et al. (2014) [Commentary]. *Archives of Sexual Behaviour, 44*(1), 249–252. https://doi.org/10.1007/s10508-014-0338-7

Bailey, J. M., Hsu, K. J., & Bernhard, P. A. (2016). An internet study of men sexually attracted to children: Sexual attraction patterns. *Journal of Abnormal Psychology, 125*(7), 976–988. https://doi.org/10.1037/abn0000212

Beech, A. R., Miner, M. H., & Thornton, D. (2016). Paraphilias in the DSM-5. *Annual Review of Clinical Psychology, 12*(1), 383–406. https://doi.org/10.1146/annurev-clinpsy-021815-093330

Blagden, N., Jones, J., & Wilson, K. (2019). "It doesn't matter what you've done you're accepted here": A multi-site qualitative exploration of the experiences of being incarcerated in prisons for individuals with sexual convictions. In N. Blagden, B. Winder, K. Hocken, R. Lievesley, P. Banyard, & H. Elliott (Eds.), *Sexual crime and the experience of imprisonment. Sexual crime* (pp. 109–141). Palgrave Macmillan.

Blagden, N., Perrin, C., Smith, S., Gleeson, F., & Gillies, L. (2017). "A different world" exploring and understanding the climate of a recently re-rolled sexual offender prison. *Journal of Sexual Aggression, 23*(2), 151–166. https://doi.org/10.1080/13552600.2016.1264633

Blagden, N., & Wilson, K. (2020). "We're all the same here": Investigating the rehabilitative climate of a re-rolled sexual offender prison: A qualitative longitudinal study. *Sexual Abuse, 32*(6), 727–750. https://doi.org/10.1177/1079063219839496

Blanchard, R., Lykins, A. D., Wherrett, D., Kuban, M. E., Cantor, J. M., Blak, T., Dickey, R., & Klassen, P. E. (2009). Pedophilia, hebephilia, and the DSM-V. *Archives of Sexual Behavior, 38*(3), 335–350. https://doi.org/10.1007/s10508-008-9399-9

Bonta, J., & Andrews, D. A. (2017). *The psychology of criminal conduct* (6th ed.). Routledge.

Briken, P., Fedoroff, J. P., & Bradford, J. W. (2014). Why can't pedophilic disorder remit? *Archives of Sexual Behaviour, 43*(7), 1237–1239. https://doi.org/10.1007/s10508-014-0323-1

Cantor, J. M. (2015). Purported changes in pedophilia as statistical artefacts: Comment on Müller et al. (2014) [Commentary]. *Archives of Sexual Behaviour, 44*(1), 253–254. https://doi.org/10.1007/s10508-014-0343-x

Cantor, J. M. (2018). Can pedophiles change? *Current Sexual Health Reports, 10*(4), 203–206. https://doi.org/10.1007/s11930-018-0165-2

Cantor, J. M., & Fedoroff, J. P. (2018). Can pedophiles change? Response to opening arguments and conclusions. *Current Sexual Health Reports, 10*(4), 213–220. https://doi.org/10.1007/s11930-018-0167-0

Cantor, J. M., & McPhail, I. V. (2016). Non-offending pedophiles. *Current Sexual Health Reports, 8*(3), 121–128. https://doi.org/10.1007/s11930-016-0076-z

Carter, A., & Mann, R. E. (2016). Organizing principles for an integrated model of change for the treatment of sexual offending. In D. P. Boer (Ed.), *The Wiley handbook on the theories, assessment, and treatment of sexual offending* (pp. 359–382). Wiley-Blackwell.

Clapton, N. E., Williams, J., Griffiths, G. M., & Jones, R. S. (2018). "Finding the person you really are... on the inside": Compassion focused therapy for adults with intellectual disabilities. *Journal of Intellectual Disabilities, 22*(2), 135–153. https://doi.org/10.1177/1744629516688581

Colson, C. E. (1972). Olfactory aversion therapy for homosexual behavior. *Journal of Behavior Therapy and Experimental Psychiatry, 3*(3), 185–187. https://doi.org/10.1016/0005-7916(72)90071-7

Craig, C., Hiskey, S., & Spector, A. (2020). Compassion focused therapy: A systematic review of its effectiveness and acceptability in clinical populations. *Expert Review of Neurotherapeutics, 20*(4), 385–400. https://doi.org/10.1080/14737175.2020.1746184

Dennis, J. A., Khan, O., Ferriter, M., Huband, N., Powney, M. J., & Duggan, C. (2012). *Psychological interventions for adults who have sexually offended or are at risk of offending.* (CD007507; Cochrane Database of Systematic Reviews Issue 12). John Wiley & Sons.

Evans, D. R. (1968). Masturbatory fantasy and sexual deviation. *Behaviour Research and Therapy, 6*(1), 17–19. https://doi.org/10.1016/0005-7967(68)90036-3

Fedoroff, J. P. (2016). Managing versus successfully treating paraphilic disorders. In S. B. Levine & C. B. Risen (Eds.), *Handbook of clinical sexuality for mental health professionals* (pp. 345–361). Routledge.

Fedoroff, J. P. (2018). Can people with pedophilia change?: Yes they can! *Current Sexual Health Reports, 10*(11), 207–212. https://doi.org/10.1007/s11930-018-0166-1

Fedoroff, J. P., Curry, S., Müller, K., Ranger, R., Briken, P., & Bradford, J. (2015). Evidence that arousal to pedophilic stimuli can change: Response to Bailey, Cantor, and Lalumière. *Archives of Sexual Behaviour, 44*(1), 259–263. https://doi.org/10.1007/s10508-014-0441-9

First, M. B. (2014). DSM-5 and paraphilic disorders. *Journal of the American Academy of Psychiatry andtheLaw,42*(2),191–201.https://www.psychiatrictimes.com/view/dsm-5-and-paraphilias-what-psychiatrists-need-know

Gannon, T. A., Olver, M. E., Mallion, J. S., & James, M. (2019). Does specialized psychological treatment for offending reduce recidivism? A meta-analysis examining staff and program variables as predictors of treatment effectiveness. *Clinical Psychology Review*. https://doi.org/10.1016/j.cpr.2019.101752

Gilbert, P. (2010). *Compassion focused therapy: Distinctive features.* Routledge.

Gilbert, P., & Choden. (2013). *Mindful compassion.* Robinson.

Grønnerød, C., Grønnerød, J. S., & Grøndahl, P. (2015). Psychological treatment of sexual offenders against children: A meta-analytic review of treatment outcome studies. *Trauma, Violence & Abuse, 16*(3), 280–290. https://doi.org/10.1177/1524838014526043

Grubin, D., & Thornton, D. (1994). A national program for the assessment and treatment of sex offenders in the English prison system. *Criminal Justice and Behavior, 21*(1), 55–71. https://doi.org/10.1177/0093854894021001005

Grundmann, D., Krupp, J., Scherner, G., Amelung, T., & Beier, K. M. (2016). Stability of self-reported arousal to sexual fantasies involving children in a clinical sample of pedophiles and hebephiles. *Archives of Sexual Behaviour, 45*(5), 1153–1162. https://doi.org/10.1007/s10508-016-0729-z

Hanson, R. K., Bourgon, G., Helmus, L., & Shannon, H. (2009). The principles of effective correctional treatment also apply to sexual offenders: A meta-analysis. *Journal of Criminal Justice and Behaviour, 36*(9), 865–891. https://doi.org/10.1177/0093854809338545

Hayes, S. C., & Hofmann, S. G. (2018). *Process-based CBT: The science and core clinical competencies of cognitive behavioural therapy.* New Harbinger.

Imhoff, R. (2015). Punitive attitudes against pedophiles or persons with sexual interest in children: Does the label matter? *Archives of Sexual Behaviour, 44*(1), 35–44. https://doi.org/10.1007/s10508-014-0439-3

Imhoff, R., & Jahnke, S. (2018). Determinants of punitive attitudes towards people with pedophilia: Dissecting effects of the label and intentionality ascriptions. *Archives of Sexual Behaviour, 47*(1), 353–361. https://doi.org/10.1007/s10508-017-1048-8

Jahnke, S. (2018). The stigma of pedophilia clinical and forensic implications. *European Psychologist, 23*(2), 144–153. https://doi.org/10.1027/1016-9040/a000325

Jahnke, S., & Hoyer, J. (2013). Stigmatization of people with pedophilia: A blind spot in stigma research. *International Journal of Sexual Health, 25*(3), 169–184. https://doi.org/10.1080/19317611.2013.795921

Jahnke, S., Schmidt, A. F., Geradt, M., & Hoyer, J. (2015). Stigma related stress and its correlates among men with pedophilic sexual interests. *Archives of Sexual Behaviour, 44*(8), 2173–2187. https://doi.org/10.1007/s10508-015-0503-7

Jespersen, A. F., Lalumière, M. L., & Seto, M. C. (2009). Sexual abuse history among adult sex offenders and non-sex offenders: A meta-analysis. *Child Abuse Neglect, 33*(3), 179–192. https://doi.org/10.1016/j.chiabu.2008.07.004

Kärgel, C., Massau, C., Weiß, S., Walter, M., Borchardt, V., Krueger, T. H., & Schiffer, B. (2017). Evidence for superior neurobiological and behavioral inhibitory control abilities in non-offending as compared to offending pedophiles. *Human Brain Mapping, 38*(2), 1092–1104. https://doi.org/10.1002/hbm.23443

Kärgel, C., Massau, C., Weiß, S., Walter, M., Kruger, T. H. C., & Schiffer, B. (2015). Diminished functional connectivity on the road to child sexual abuse in pedophilia. *The Journal of Sexual Medicine, 12*(3), 783–795. https://doi.org/10.1111/jsm.12819

Kirby, J. N., Tellegen, C. L., & Steindl, S. R. (2017). A meta-analysis of compassion-based interventions: Current state of knowledge and future directions. *Behaviour Therapy, 48*(6), 778–792. https://doi.org/10.1016/j.beth.2017.06.003

Krueger, R. B., Reed, G. M., First, M. B., Marais, A., Kismodi, E., & Briken, P. (2017). Proposals for paraphilic disorders in the International Classification of Diseases and Related Health Problems, eleventh revision (ICD11). *Archives of Sexual Behavior, 46*(5), 1529–1545. https://doi.org/10.1007/s10508-017-0944-2

Lalumière, M. L. (2015). The lability of pedophilic interests as measured by phallometry [Commentary]. *Archives of Sexual Behaviour, 44*(1), 255–258. https://doi.org/10.1007/s10508-014-0340-0

Långström, N., Enebrink, P., Laurén, E. M., Lindblom, J., Werkö, S., & Hanson, R. K. (2013). Preventing sexual abusers of children from recidivism : Systematic review of medical and psychological interventions. *British Medical Journal (Clinical Research Ed.), 347*, f4630. https://doi.org/10.1136/bmj.f4630

Laws, D. R. (2009). Penile plethysmography: Strengths, limitations, innovations. In D. Thornton & D. R. Laws (Eds.), *Cognitive approaches to the assessment of sexual interest in sexual offenders* (pp. 7–29). Wiley-Blackwell.

Levenson, J. S., & Grady, M. D. (2016). The influence of childhood trauma on sexual violence and sexual deviance in adulthood. *Traumatology, 22*(2), 94–103. https://doi.org/10.1037/trm0000067

Levenson, J. S., Willis, G. M., & Prescott, D. (2016). Adverse childhood experiences in the lives of male sex offenders: Implications for trauma-informed care. *Sexual Abuse: A Journal of Research and Treatment, 28*(4), 340–359. https://doi.org/10.1177/1079063214535819

Levenson, J. S., Willis, G. M., & Prescott, D. (2018). Incorporating principles of trauma-informed care into evidence-based sex offending treatment. In E. L. Jeglic & C. Calkins (Eds.), *New frontiers in offender treatment* (pp. 171–188). Springer.

Lösel, F. & Schmucker, M. (2005). The effectiveness of treatment for sexual offenders: a comprehensive meta-analysis. *Journal of Experimental Criminology, 1*(1), 117–146. https://doi.org/10.1007/s11292-004-6466-7

Mann, R., Barnett, G., Box, G., Howard, F. F., O'Mara, O., Travers, R., & Wakeling, H. C. (2019). Rehabilitative culture in prisons for people convicted of sexual offending. In N. Blagden, B. Winder, K. Hocken, R. Lievesley, P. Banyard, & H. Elliott (Eds.), *Sexual crime and the experience of imprisonment* (pp. 1–33). Palgrave Macmillan.

Mann, R. E., Hanson, R. K., & Thornton, D. (2010). Assessing risk for sexual recidivism: Some proposals on the nature of psychologically meaningful risk factors. *exual Abuse: A Journal of Research and Treatment, 22*(2), 191–217. https://doi.org/10.1177/1079063210366039

Mann, R. E., Webster, S. D., Wakeling, H. C., & Keylock, H. (2013). Why do sex offenders refuse treatment? *Journal of Sexual Aggression, 19*(2), 191–206. https://doi.org/10.1080/13552600.2012.703701

Marques, J. K., Wiederanders, M., Day, D. M., Nelson, C., & Van Ommeren, A. (2005). Effects of a relapse prevention program on sexual recidivism: Final results from California's sex offender treatment and evaluation project (SOTEP). *Sexual Abuse: A Journal of Research and Treatment, 17*(1), 79–107. https://doi.org/10.1177/107906320501700108

Maruna, S., & Mann, R. E. (2006). A fundamental attribution error? Rethinking cognitive distortions. *Legal and Criminological Psychology, 11*(2), 155–177. https://doi.org/10.1348/135532506X114608

McGrath, R. J., Cumming, G. F., Burchard, B. L., Zeoli, S., & Ellerby, L. (2010). *Emerging trends in sexual abuser management: The safer society 2009 North American survey*. The Safer Society Press.

McKay, M. (2018). Arousal reduction. In S. C. Hayes & S. G. Hofmann (Eds.), *Process-based CBT: The science and core clinical competencies of cognitive behavioural therapy* (pp. 245–260). New Harbinger.

McPhail, I. V., Hermann, C. A., Fernane, S., Fernandez, Y. M., Nunes, K. L., & Cantor, J. M. (2019). Validity in phallometric testing for sexual interests in children: A meta-analytic review. *Assessment, 26*(3), 535–551. https://doi.org/10.1177/1073191117706139

McPhail, I. V. & Olver, M. E. (2020). Interventions for pedohebephilic arousal in men convicted for sexual offenses against children: A meta-analytic review. *Criminal Justice and Behavior, 47*(10), 1319–1339. https://doi.org/10.1177/0093854820916774

Mews, A., Bella, L., & Purver, M. (2017). Impact evaluation of the prison-based core sex offender treatment programme. Ministry of Justice Analytical Series, London.

Miletski, H. (2017). Zoophilia: Another sexual orientation? *Archives of Sexual Behaviour, 46*(1), 39–42. https://doi.org/10.1007/s10508-016-0891-3

Ministry of Justice. (2019). *Offender management statistics bulletin, England and Wales: Quarterly April to June 2019*. Nation Crime Statistics.

Ministry of Justice. (2020). *Offender management statistics bulletin, England and Wales: Quarterly April to June 2020*. Nation Crime Statistics.

Moser, C. (2019) DSM-5, Paraphilias, and the paraphilic disorders: Confusion reigns. *Archives of Sexual Behavior, 48*(3), 681–689. https://doi.org/10.1007/s10508-018-1356-7

Müller, K., Curry, S., Ranger, R., Briken, P., Bradford, J., & Fedoroff, J. P. (2014). Changes in sexual arousal as measured by penile plethysmography in men with pedophilic sexual interest. *Journal of Sexual Medicine, 11*(5), 1221–1229. https://doi.org/10.1111/jsm.12488

Nicholls, C. M., & Webster, S. (2018). The separated location of prisoners with sexual convictions: Research on the benefits and risks. Analytical Summary 2018. HM Prison and Probation Service.

Nitschke, J., Mokros, A., Osterheider, M., & Marshall, W. L. (2013). Sexual sadism: Current diagnostic vagueness and the benefit of behavioral definitions. *International Journal of Offender Therapy and Comparative Criminology, 57*(12), 1441–1453. https://doi.org/10.1177/0306624X12465923

Nitschke, J., Osterheider, M., & Mokros, A. (2009). A cumulative scale of severe sexual sadism. *Sexual Abuse: A Journal of Research and Treatment, 21*(3), 262–278. https://doi.org/10.1177/1079063209342074

Perrin, C., Frost, A., & Ware, J. B. (2018). The utility of peer-support in enhancing the treatment of incarcerated sexual offenders. *Therapeutic Communities: The International Journal of Therapeutic Communities, 39*(1), 35–49. https://doi.org/10.1108/TC-06-2017-0018

Ramsay, L. (2020). Strengths–based programmes for men with sexual convictions, who have learning disability and learning challenges. In K. Hocken, B. Winder, N. Blagden, R. Lievesley, H. Elliott, & P. Banyard (Eds.), *Sexual crime and intellectual functioning* (pp. 59–88). Palgrave Macmillan.

Ramsay, L., Carter, A. J., & Walton, J. S. (2020). Contemporary programs designed for the tertiary prevention of recidivism by people convicted of a sexual offense: A review, and the U.K. perspective. In J. Proulx, F. Cortoni, L. A. Craig, & E. J. Letourneau (Eds.), *The Wiley handbook of what works with sexual offenders: Contemporary perspectives in theory, assessment, treatment, and prevention* (pp. 185–199). John Wiley & Sons Ltd.

Salter, A. C. (1988). *Treating child sex offenders and victims*. Sage.

Schiffer, B., Amelung, T., Pohl, A., Kärgel, C., Tenbergen, G., Gerwinn, H., Mohnke, S., Massau, C., Matthias, W., Weiß, S., Marr, V., Beier, K. M., Walter, M., Ponseti, J., Krüger, T. H. C., Schiltz, K., & Walter, H. (2017). Gray matter abnormalities in pedophiles with and without a history of child sexual offending. *Translational Psychiatry, 7*(5), e1129. https://doi.org/10.1038/tp.2017.96

Schmucker, M., & Lösel, F. (2017). Sexual offender treatment for reducing recidivism among convicted sex offenders: A systematic review and meta-analysis. *Campbell systematic reviews*, No. 8.

Schwaebe, C. (2005). Learning to pass: Sex offenders' strategies for establishing a viable identity in the prison general population. *International Journal of Offender Therapy and Comparative Criminology, 49*(6), 614–625. https://doi.org/10.1177/0306624X05275829

Serber, M. (1970). Shame aversion therapy. *Journal of Behavior Therapy and Experimental Psychiatry, 1*(3), 213–215. https://doi.org/10.1016/0005-7916(70)90005-4

Seto, M. C. (2012). Is pedophilia a sexual orientation? *Archives of Sexual Behaviour, 41*(1), 231–236. https://doi.org/10.1007/s10508-011-9882-6

Seto, M. C. (2017). The puzzle of male chronophilias. *Archives of Sexual Behaviour, 46*(1), 3–22. https://doi.org/10.1007/s10508-016-0799-y
Seto, M. C. (2018). *Paedophilia and sexual offending against children: Theory, assessment and intervention* (2nd ed.). American Psychological Association.
Seto, M. C., & Lalumière, M. L. (2010). What is so special about male adolescent sexual offending? A review and test of explanations through meta-analysis. *Psychological Bulletin, 136*(4), 526–575. https://doi.org/10.1037/a0019700
Seto, M. C., Stephens, S., Lalumière, M. L., & Cantor, J. M. (2017). The revised Screening Scale for Pedophilic Interests (SSPI–2) development and criterion-related validation. *Sexual Abuse: A Journal of Research and Treatment, 29*(7), 619–635. https://doi.org/10.1177/1079063215612444
Stasch, J., Yoon, D., Sauter, J., Hausam, J., & Dahle, K.-P. (2018). Prison climate and its role in reducing dynamic risk factors during offender treatment. *International Journal of Offender Therapy and Comparative Criminology, 62*(14), 4609–4621. https://doi.org/10.1177/0306624X18778449
Stephens, S., Seto, M. C., Cantor, J. M., & Lalumière, M. L. (2019). The Revised Screening Scale for Pedophilic Interests (SSPI-2) may be a measure of pedohebephilia. *Journal of Sexual Medicine, 16*(10), 1655–1663. https://doi.org/10.1016/j.jsxm.2019.07.015
Thornton, D., Ambroziak, G., Kahn, R. E., & Mundt, J. (2018). Advances in the assessment of sexual deviance. *Current Psychiatry Reports, 20*(8), 20–55. https://doi.org/10.1007/s11920-018-0918-7
Tyler, T. R. (2008). Procedural justice and the courts. *Court Review, Journal of the American Judges Association, 44*(1/2), 26–31.
van der Kolk, B. (2014). *The body keeps the score: Brain, mind and body in the healing of trauma*. Viking.
Walton, J. S. (2019). The evolutionary basis of belonging: its relevance to denial of offending and labelling those who offend. *Journal of Forensic Practice, 21*(4), 202–211. https://doi.org/10.1108/JFP-04-2019-0014
Walton, J. S. (2018). Random assignment in sexual offending programme evaluation: The missing method. *Journal of Forensic Practice, 20*(1), 1–9. https://doi.org/10.1108/JFP-08-2017-0032
Walton, J. S. (in press). A healthy sex programme for individuals with paraphilia convicted of sexual offending: Biopsychosocial influences and therapy procedures. In B. Winder, N. Blagden, & L. Hamilton (Eds.), *Forensic interventions for therapy and rehabilitation: Case studies and analysis*. Taylor and Francis.
Walton, J. S., Ramsay, L., Cunningham, C., & Henfrey, S. (2017). New directions: Integrating a biopsychosocial approach in the design and delivery of programs for high risk services users in Her Majesty's Prison and Probation Service. *Advancing Corrections: Journal of the International Corrections and Prison Association, 3*(1), 21–47. https://icpa.org/advancing-corrections-journal-edition-3-en
Ward, T., & Stewart, C. A. (2003). The treatment of sex offenders: Risk management and good lives. *Professional Psychology, Research and Practice, 34*(4), 353–360. https://doi.org/10.1037/0735-7028.34.4.353
Willis, G. M., Ward, T., & Levenson, J. S. (2014). The Good Lives Model (GLM): An evaluation of GLM operationalization in North American treatment programs. *Sexual Abuse: A Journal of Research and Treatment, 26*(1), 58–81. https://doi.org/10.1177/1079063213478202
Wismeijer, A. A., & van Assen, M. A. (2013). Psychological characteristics of BDSM practitioners. *Journal of Sexual Medicine, 10*(8), 1943–1952. https://doi.org/10.1111/jsm.12192

20

Behavioral Control Models in Managing Sexual Deviance

Jayson Ware[1], Lauren McIvor[2], and Yolanda M. Fernandez[3]

[1] *Corrective Services New South Wales, Australia*
[2,3] *Correctional Service of Canada, Canada*

Introduction

The explicit attempt to control deviant sexual arousal has long been a key component of sex offender treatment. Initial treatment approaches were focused almost exclusively on the notion that sexually abusive behavior occurred as a result of classic or operant conditioning processes where sexual interest in specific deviant acts was a learned behavior (McGuire et al., 1965). Contemporary sex offender treatment includes behavioral methods targeting deviant sexual arousal but these are now used in a more limited capacity and as part of a broader treatment method. We note also that, whilst these methods are labeled "behavioral," strictly speaking, they often involve cognitive methods, particularly when used in combination with expansive therapeutic strategies within a comprehensive program.

In this chapter we describe behavioral control procedures used by individuals to modify their deviant arousal. Whilst we refer to their use with sex offenders throughout this chapter, we note that these procedures have been used with individuals presenting for sexual behavior problems without charges or convictions. We commence by briefly establishing the theoretical foundations for behavioral control models and procedures. There are a number of contextual issues, which we then outline, that we believe are important considerations for treatment providers. Having established our theoretical and contextual underpinnings, we then describe the most frequently used behavioral control procedures whilst critiquing the evidence for their use. Bringing the previous sections together, and with the goal of assisting treatment providers, we provide suggestions for when each procedure could be used and for whom. At this point, we outline practice issues for these procedures in general and seek to provide some clarity or suggestions. We conclude by summarizing the various behavioral control models in managing sexual deviance, the evidence for and against their use, and offering suggestions for both treatment providers and researchers.

Theoretical Foundations

It is important that treatment providers understand the behavioral and sexuality theories underpinning each behavioral control procedure. McGuire et al.'s (1965) "sexual deviation hypothesis" and Laws and Marshall's (1990) "conditioning theory" are two theoretical models that provide rationales for the procedures we outline in the following sections.

McGuire et al. hypothesized that deviant sexual interests were acquired as a result of a single, initial, significant sexual experience that was subsequently used for masturbation. They argued

Sexual Deviance: Understanding and Managing Deviant Sexual Interests and Paraphilic Disorders, First Edition. Edited by Leam A. Craig and Ross M. Bartels.
© 2021 John Wiley & Sons, Ltd. Published 2021 by John Wiley & Sons, Ltd.

that memory of the initial experience was a preferable sexual fantasy stimulus to other options (e.g., images). As the individual repeatedly masturbated to the memory, the memory was hypothesized to gain value as a source of reinforcement. Repeated pairing of masturbation and this fantasy were said to result in the development of a deviant sexual interest though classical conditioning processes.

Laws and Marshall (1990) developed the conditioning theory of deviant sexual interests explaining the involvement of both classical and operant conditioning processes. This theory hypothesized that deviant sexual interests are learned via the same means as other non-deviant sexual interests and behaviors. Namely, a combination of conditioning processes and social learning were said to be responsible for the development and maintenance of these interests. They expanded on McGuire et al.'s classical conditioning assumption, stating that any neutral stimulus accompanying sexual arousal could eventually produce sexual arousal itself. They also emphasized that deviant interests could formulate from other sexual experiences, and not just the individual's first experience. Laws and Marshall (1990) asserted that the classically conditioned relationship between the stimulus and sexual arousal could be maintained through operant conditioning (e.g., reinforcement via repeated masturbation).

Application to Behavioral Control Strategies

Masters and Johnson's (1966) model of the human sexual response is relevant to the application of behavioral control strategies for deviant sexual interests. The human sexual response cycle is comprised of four stages: excitement, plateau, orgasm, and resolution. Kaplan (1979) also added a desire stage, prior to the excitement stage. During the desire stage, motivation to initiate sexual behaviors is established. Arousal increases during the excitement phase and then intensifies for a sustained period during the plateau phase. The orgasm phase is typically characterized by ejaculation in men, and then returns to a non-aroused state in the resolution phase. This response cycle is generally pleasurable and reinforcing for the individual.

Considering the two conditioning theories within the context of the human sexual response cycle, behavioral procedures for countering sexual deviance involve pairing sexually deviant stimuli or fantasies with punishing or unrewarding consequences and/or pairing non-deviant sexual stimuli or fantasies with reinforcement or rewarding consequences. Different conditioning strategies are relevant to different phases of the sexual response cycle. For example, masturbatory techniques are applied during the plateau and orgasm stages while satiation therapies are applicable during the resolution stage.

Contextual Issues

In considering the use of behavioral procedures the most important initial question is whether they are necessary for the individual. Marshall and Fernandez (2003) demonstrated that not all men convicted of sexual offenses display deviant sexual interests at assessment. Careful consideration of the relative merits of using these behavioral procedures with each individual is therefore warranted. The following contextual issues should be considered prior to deciding upon the use of behavioral procedures.

Use with Different Sex Offending Populations

Behavioral procedures appear to be a common option for individuals with various offense histories. They appear to be used, with small adjustments, interchangeably with those have committed sexual assaulted adults, sexually abused children, and engaged in non-contact sexual offenses. Marshall et al. (2017) noted, however, that these procedures should primarily target individuals who have sexually abused children as individuals whose offenses are limited to sexual assaults against adults, including exhibitionism and voyeurism, are less likely to demonstrate deviant sexual arousal patterns at phallometric testing (see Marshall & Fernandez, 2003).

Behavioral procedures have been used with male, female, and adolescent populations. McGrath et al. (2010), in their most recent survey of North American and Canadian sex offender programs, found that the majority of community and residential programs treating adult male sex offenders reported using one or more behavioral procedures (68% and 59%, respectively) to address deviant sexual interests. Over half of the adolescent programs also reported using at least one of these procedures and, interestingly, a significant proportion of female programs also reported using behavioral control procedures (59% and 37%, respectively).

Although aging may decrease risk of reoffending for many sex offenders (Helmus et al., 2012), behavioral procedures may still be relevant, particularly if the offending has occurred recently. Leonard and Donathy (2017) reminded practitioners of the importance of considering the impact of age on sexual functioning. Specifically, they noted the misconception that significantly decreased sexual thoughts and behaviors occur in all older individuals. While age-related declines in sexual interest and activity occur in some individuals, others' sexual functioning may remain at high levels. An understanding of the individual's recent sexual functioning including age-related issues such as their physical health and mobility and any medication side effects, is an important contextual consideration.

The use of behavioral procedures for online or internet sex offenders may be particularly important. De Almeida Neto et al. (2013), for example, argued that online sex offenders have typically paired sexual arousal with internet access/use so often that simply sitting in front of a computer can elicit sexual arousal. Behavioral control procedures can be adapted to relevant stimuli such as sitting in front of the computer, touching the keyboard, clicking through programs, and using the (controlled) internet. Once the behaviors associated with the use of the computer or internet are no longer paired with sex or heightened arousal, computer stimuli may be less likely to trigger sexual thoughts and arousal.

Behavioral procedures have long been used for individuals with intellectual or development disabilities who have sexually offended (Plaud et al., 2000). Whilst their initial use involved aversive conditioning procedures that are unlikely to be used today (e.g., electric shocks), process or procedures have remained the same. Lindsay (2009), for example, described the importance of operant and classical conditioning approaches with a sex offending cohort of developmentally delayed individuals, and outlined successful examples using aversion and directed masturbation techniques.

Use When Deviant Sexual Interests Are Present

Whilst many sex offender treatment programs routinely use behavioral procedures for all participants, we do not advocate this approach. Rather, we argue that these procedures are best used with those individuals who would most benefit from them and where there is some evidence for their use. Marshall et al. (2006) outline a helpful set of criteria to indicate which offenders might most benefit from these procedures. They noted that a history of persistent deviant behaviors over time, phallometric examinations suggesting significant deviant arousal, or self-reported persistent sexual fantasies, all indicate the suitability of behavioral control procedures. Similarly, with respect to institutional behaviors, Marshall et al. (2006) suggest using behavioral procedures with offenders who persistently display sexualized behavior toward other inmates or staff or are found to be hoarding pornography or sexualized pictures, both of which could reflect the dynamic risk factor of sexual preoccupation (Hanson & Morton-Bourgon, 2005; Marshall & O'Brien, 2009).

Use Within the Broader Context of Treatment

Any effort to modify deviant sexual interest should occur within the broader context of treatment. We agree with Marshall et al. (2009) who argued that behavioral efforts to modify deviant sexual interests should be embedded within the context of all other relevant issues addressed in the sex offender treatment program. This said, as noted by Ware and Mann (2012), initial treatment targets should focus on engaging the individual and addressing factors that may feel more comfortable or less threatening addressing during the early stages of treatment. Appropriate early treatment topics might include self-esteem, relationships, or coping with emotions. It is also important that education about appropriate and healthy sexual behaviors has been delivered, preferably before or concurrently with the section on deviant sexual interests. This ensures that the basis for the use of behavioral procedures is clear and that treatment options for issues such as sexual dysfunction are considered alongside deviant issues. Our strong recommendation is that behavioral control procedures should be introduced later, although not last, in treatment.

Behavioral Procedures

This section describes several behavioral control procedures used with individuals who have committed sexual offenses. There are two broad types of behavioral control procedures: (1) the pairing of deviant sexual images with an aversive or punishing stimuli such as a noxious odor (aversive conditioning); and (2) the pairing of appropriate sexual images with positive or reinforcing stimuli such as masturbation and orgasm (masturbatory or orgasmic reconditioning). Both approaches aim to assist the client to control, reduce, or eliminate deviant sexual interests as well as to help with the development, strengthening, and maintenance of appropriate sexual arousal and interests. It is hoped that these changes in sexual interests will impact subsequent behavioral choices. In this section, we will describe five behavioral control procedures common to sex offender treatment, their theoretical foundations, and the evidence, or lack thereof, for their use.

Aversion Procedures

Aversive behavioral rehearsal. Aversive behavioral rehearsal, originally called shame aversion (Serber, 1970), involves the individual role-playing deviant sexual behaviors in the presence of others (therapist or treatment group members) or whilst being video recorded. The theoretical underpinning of this technique is the pairing of intense shame, guilt, or anxiety with deviant sexual thoughts or behavior. It is hypothesized that the subsequent negative emotions associated with the deviant behaviors will extinguish the behavior. The shame felt by the offender is reportedly the punishing stimulus. In practice, the offender is effectively compelled to see what he looks like and sounds like whilst abusing someone (McGrath et al., 2010). Although described as a behavioral control procedure, aversive behavioral rehearsal, or variations of the original procedure, is often incorporated as part of victim empathy sessions as opposed to sexual health sessions (Webster et al., 2005). There is a lack of empirical evidence as to its effectiveness, with only older case studies available to guide its use (such as Wickramaserka, 1976).

Whilst McGrath et al. (2010) reported that 14% of residential and 22% of community-based sex offender treatment programs for adults in the USA and Canada were using this procedure, we advocate against its use. Marshall et al. (2009) have expressed significant concern over such shame-based aversion procedures, labeling them as "ethically dubious." More generally, there is a consensus amongst clinicians that shame-inducing treatment procedures result in poorer overall treatment outcomes (Proeve & Howells, 2002).

Olfactory and ammonia aversion. Olfactory and ammonia aversion involve the repeated pairing of deviant thoughts or images with the presentation of either a noxious odor or smelling salts (salts of ammonia). Whilst administered in the same manner (inhaled nasally), the two procedures differ in terms of the body's physiological response. Maletzky (1991, 1997) argued that olfactory aversion, which has involved odors produced by valeric acid, mercapto-ethanol, or rancid meat, is effective due to the nausea-inducing aspect of the smell. Laws (2001) offered a simpler explanation, suggesting that the noxious stimulus paired with the deviant thoughts or behavior has an effect due to physiological discomfort. In support of his argument, Laws noted the similarities in outcomes, from case studies, between noxious odors and the effects of ammonia aversion which is mediated by the pain system (rather than the olfactory system). Marshall et al. (2009) reported that there can be a rapid adaptation to smells which means they can lose their punishing properties quickly. They recommend using multiple different foul odors during repeated conditioning trials.

Both olfactory and ammonia aversion appear to have been used mainly with those who engage in exhibitionism but have also been used with those individuals whose deviant thoughts are frequent and triggered by multiple and varied stimuli or where the offender reports high levels of sexual preoccupation (Marshall et al., 2006). Olfactory and ammonia aversion remain popular, being used by almost 30% of community programs in the USA and Canada (McGrath et al., 2010).

Empirical support of the effectiveness of this approach remains unclear. Few empirical studies exist and all were completed over 10 years ago. The available evidence has, for the most part, come from single-case designs, mainly with individuals who have engaged in exhibitionism (Abel & Rouleau, 1990; Maletzky, 1980; Maletzky & McGovern, 1991) but also with clients who have sexually abused children (Earls & Castonguay, 1989; Marshall, 2006), an individual diagnosed with sadism (Laws et al., 1978), and an individual convicted of possession and distribution of child pornography (e.g., Campbell-Fuller & Craig, 2009). We note that there have also been inconsistencies in the case studies which necessarily limits their generalizability, such as difference in the number of trials, duration of treatment, and the introduction of new odors.

Covert sensitization. Covert sensitization was first described by Cautela (1967) as an aversion-based procedure to reduce unwanted thoughts or behaviors through their repeated imagined association with an unpleasant consequence. Initially adapted for use with sex offender treatment by Cautela and Wisocki (1971), this procedure subsequently gained popularity, perhaps due to the fact that it can be applied without the need for the therapist to facilitate the unwanted behavior (deviant sexual arousal) or the unpleasant consequences. It appears to be the most commonly used as a behavioral procedure in sex offender treatment programs with close to half of surveyed U.S. and Canadian treatment programs using a variation of covert sensitization (McGrath et al., 2010).

The basic principle of covert sensitization is that individuals are first assisted to construct offense sequences that replicate the chain of circumstances, thoughts, emotions, and behaviors that preceded their prior sexual offense behavior or, alternatively, they are instructed to detail a deviant sexual fantasy. They are then required to generate a list of several relevant and realistic negative consequences that should evoke strong negative emotions or autonomic responses when imagined. Anecdotally, offenders often need assistance with this aspect of the task as the examples they generate can often reflect what they believe the treatment provider needs to hear rather than genuinely aversive consequences (see Waldram, 2007, for a discussion of this issue). The offender is then tasked with rehearsing the offense sequences or fantasies while concurrently introducing the aversive consequences immediately prior to engaging in the deviant sexual behavior in the offense sequence or the sexual fantasy. These offense sequences and imagined aversive consequences can be written on cue cards (Marshall, 2007), recorded as audio tapes (McGrath, 2001), or completed *in vivo* in the treatment provider's office (Maletzky, 1991).

In theory, covert sensitization discourages subsequent engagement in deviant sexual behaviors by creating an association between those behaviors and the unpleasant consequence. Maletzky (1980) argued, however, that the aversiveness of covert or imagined consequences, even after repeated pairing, is unlikely to be strong enough. Similarly, Marshall and colleagues (2006, 2009, 2011) reported that the aversiveness of the imagined consequences decreases quickly. Maletzky (1980) suggested the addition of an actual stimulus effectively combining covert sensitization with olfactory aversion and calling this procedure "assisted covert sensitization."

Marshall (2007) reported the use of a modified version of covert association for which he argued that the important element of the procedure is likely to be repeated association or pairing of a stimulus and a negative emotion rather than the aversiveness of the consequence. He suggested that the individual should gradually move the aversive consequences earlier and earlier in the sequence or fantasy, so by the time the offender has gained mastery over the procedure, they are interrupting the offense sequence or fantasy at the point when they are contemplating the sequence or fantasy. Gray (1995) reported on the use of a similar approach (minimal arousal conditioning), initially developed by Jensen and Laws (1994), in which the aversive stimulus (imagined or using four odors or ammonia) is introduced when the offender first starts to experience sexual arousal. This practice appears to be increasing in popularity with a significant increase in U.S. and Canadian community-based programs adopting its use between 2002 and 2009 (from 18% to 27%).

Despite its popularity, studies examining the use of covert sensitization have declined significantly since the 1990s. There is some evidence for assisted covert sensitization in treating individuals who have sexually abused children or engaged in exhibitionism (Maletzky, 1980, 1991). However, when Rea et al. (2003) attempted to generalize the results of assisted covert sensitization procedures from a laboratory to a community setting with a client who had sexually abused a child, it was unsuccessful. Weinrott et al. (1997) have conducted the largest study involving a variation of a covert sensitization procedure in which they delivered a large number of audiotaped individualized offending sequences and subsequent videotaped representations of aversive consequences to participants over 25 treatment sessions. This study demonstrated significant decreases in phallometrically assessed and self-reported deviant arousal.

Stava et al. (1993) tried to resolve some questions about the mechanism of covert sensitization's supposed effectiveness in reducing arousal to deviant imagery. They tested whether adding aversive imagery was more effective than simply distracting the participant with neutral stimuli for reducing arousal to deviant stimuli. They also tested whether or not habituation to deviant stimuli, simply by repeated exposures, would reduce sexual arousal. They found that introducing aversive stimuli was more effective than distraction and that habituation to deviant stimuli did not reliably occur.

Masturbatory reconditioning. Masturbatory or orgasmic reconditioning uses masturbation to increase sexual responsiveness to appropriate stimuli while simultaneously decreasing sexual responsivity to deviant stimuli. Maletzky (1997) noted that three variations of orgasmic reconditioning have been used: directed masturbation, masturbatory fantasy change, and masturbatory satiation.

Directed masturbation and masturbatory fantasy change. Directed masturbation (Maletzky, 1991) simply involves directing the client to masturbate to "appropriate" sexual fantasies or masturbate whilst watching appropriate sex images or videos. This overt, positive conditioning procedure involves the pairing of appropriate sexual fantasies or stimuli with masturbation and orgasm, both perceived to be positively reinforcing behaviors. McGrath (2001) notes that appropriate fantasies should include sexual and non-sexual aspects, such as involving consenting adults, non-sexual activity and conversation, foreplay, mutual enjoyment, and after play such as hugging. Marshall and colleagues (2006, 2011) advise against the use of pornography or fantasies that are ultimately unrealistic (e.g., that involve celebrities or unlikely scenarios).

An adaptation to this procedure involves the offender masturbating to deviant fantasies until the point of orgasm inevitability, at which time he is directed to switch to an appropriate fantasy until orgasm (Marquis, 1970). If the client experiences a loss of arousal they are to revert back to the deviant fantasy until re-aroused. They then switch back to fantasizing about an appropriate partner and behavior. The individual is encouraged to introduce the appropriate fantasy earlier and earlier with subsequent masturbation events. Laws and Marshall (1991) suggested switching fantasies when the individual is aroused to above 30% of a full erection. They named this procedure "thematic shift."

Fernandez et al. (2006) noted that behavioral procedures involving the use of masturbation, which is a naturally occurring and common phenomenon, should be expected to assist in the development of pro-social sexual behaviors. Despite this, these procedures are still uncommon in sex offender treatment programs (McGrath et al., 2010), perhaps due to a lack of evidence as to their effectiveness, or to the practice issues involved in their use.

In their review of the limited available evidence, Laws and Marshall (1991) did not find any of the masturbatory procedures to be significantly better than the others and noted the lack of evidence of their effectiveness. There are case studies reporting on the effectiveness of directed masturbation for individuals who have engaged in voyeurism (Jackson, 1969) and who have sexually abused children (Kremsdorf et al., 1980; Thorpe et al., 1963), as well as those who engage in unconventional, but not deviant, fetish-related behaviors (Marshall, 1974). The thematic shift approach has been used somewhat successfully in conjunction with aversion therapies with sadistic (Davison, 1968) and fetishistic behavior (Lande, 1980). A combination of directed masturbation and ammonia aversion was also used more recently with an individual diagnosed as a pedophile in a case study by Campbell-Fuller and Craig (2009). They found significant self-reported decreases in the participant's frequency and duration of deviant fantasies and masturbation, from baseline to intervention. Increases in frequency and duration of non-deviant fantasies were also observed, but not at levels of statistical significance.

Verbal and masturbatory satiation. The underlying principle of satiation procedures is that the repeated evocation of a sexual fantasy in the absence of a rewarding consequence will lead to extinction of the behavior through a loss of valence or boredom. Specifically, this procedure is used when an individual is in a resolution or refractory state of the sexual response cycle. This period occurs almost immediately after orgasm and involves a state where the man is unresponsive to sexual stimuli which would otherwise be arousing (Masters & Johnson, 1966).

Two types of satiation therapy have been used in sex offender treatment. Masturbatory satiation was first described by Marshall and Lippens (1977). The procedure starts with masturbation to an appropriate fantasy. Post-orgasm the individual switches to a deviant sexual fantasy and continues masturbating beyond orgasm, for a significant period of time, whilst rehearsing, preferably verbally, his deviant sexual fantasies. The theory is that continued masturbation during the refractory period is uncomfortable and therefore the deviant fantasy is paired with an aversive stimulus. An important issue for this process is to ensure the individual does not continue masturbating post-orgasm to the deviant fantasy to a point where arousal returns. Verbal satiation is carried out in the same manner as masturbatory satiation except that the client does not continue masturbating post-orgasm while verbalizing his abusive sexual fantasies (Laws, 1995). In this case the deviant fantasy is paired with a general state of non-arousal, rather than the discomfort of masturbating post-orgasm. As noted by Marshall et al. (2009), satiation therapy involves two methods of action, repetition of deviant fantasies and the association of this repetition with non-reward or discomfort. Despite Marshall et al. (2017) suggesting that masturbatory satiation is problematic for offenders due to the issues with physically masturbating for lengthy periods and the risk of becoming re-aroused while verbalizing the deviant fantasy, we note that, within North American and Canadian programs, it is used more often than verbal satiation (McGrath et al., 2010).

Once again, evidence for this approach is limited, although positive. Masturbatory satiation has been demonstrated to depress deviant sexual interests in an individual who sexually abused children (Marshall, 1979) and an individual who sexually assaulted an adult (Marshall & Lippens, 1977). These case studies also included directed masturbation procedures. Similarly, Johnston et al. (1992) found that a combination of satiation therapy and directed masturbation resulted in marked reductions in arousal to deviant imagery from pre- to post-treatment. Verbal satiation has also been used successfully, in combination with directed masturbation (Alford et al., 1987; Hunter & Goodwin, 1992; Hunter & Santos, 1990). We consider satiation procedures to have the most substantial evidence base of all behavioral control procedures.

Practice Issues

A number of practical issues remain, at least to us, unclear at this point. There is a lack of clarity as to when to use behavioral control approaches and, specifically, the context in which these procedures are likely to be effective and for whom. There remains a lack of empirical evidence pointing to ideal practice conditions (i.e., how many sequences are required and how often these should be rehearsed). We have articulated what could be gleaned from the little empirical evidence that exists and from case studies.

Use of procedures combined together. Whilst the behavioral control procedures are usually described as discretely separate methods, Marshall and his colleagues have (Marshall et al., 2006, 2009, 2011) advocated for the combination of directed masturbation to enhance appropriate sexual arousal followed by satiation during the refractory period. They argued that treatment should focus on the enhancement of appropriate arousal as well as the reduction or extinction of deviancy. As noted above, many of the case studies or empirical studies have examined combinations of procedures.

Frequency of procedures/homework. The frequency and the length of time any procedure should be used remains unclear and appears largely determined by the self-reported responses of each offender, use of phallometric assessments to gauge success in terms of objective arousal responses to appropriate and deviant stimuli, or through the arbitrary time suggested by treatment manuals.

Guidance is, to a large degree, only available through case studies. Typically, each of the procedures outlined above has been used for two to four months, although there is some variation to this. Laws (2001), for example, described the successful use of olfactory aversion with an offender three times a week for eight weeks and, in a separate case, successfully used ammonia aversion four times a week for 14 weeks. Ball and Seghorn (1999) described the use of covert sensitization daily over 20 weeks of treatment, whereas McGrath (2001) suggested using this same procedure a minimum of two times per week over five weeks. Marshall et al. (2006, 2011) recommended the use of combining masturbatory reconditioning and satiation on every occasion the individual masturbates over the course of treatment, and rehearsing their covert association procedure on a daily basis.

Difficulties using imagery or fantasy. McGrath (2001) notes that clients may struggle with the use of imagery. He advocates for the use of relaxation techniques at the beginning of each procedure and using other techniques that enhance imagery, such as imagining real people or past personal events within fantasies. Clients may require assistance generating appropriate sexual fantasies due to either their lack of salience or through negative emotions associated with masturbating. Marshall (1975) specifically developed a procedure to assist with reducing feelings of guilt and other such negative emotions associated with masturbating. Treatment providers have also described using other collateral professional supports when offenders refuse to masturbate, for example, on religious grounds (Laws & Marshall, 1991; Marshall et al., 2006; McGrath, 2001).

Advantages of masturbatory procedures. Whilst masturbatory procedures appear to be less commonly favored, they do have significant advantages. In contrast to other procedures, masturbation is a normative and natural process and, as anecdotally reported by clients, does not feel artificial or contrived as more intrusive options such as olfactory stimuli do. Fernandez et al. (2006) also noted that masturbatory procedures include both reinforcing (i.e., directed masturbation) and depressing methods (i.e., satiation), promoting the understanding that healthy sexuality, versus abstinence, is the ultimate goal.

Using the procedures in an engaging and positive manner. The characteristics of the therapist, therapeutic relationship or alliance, and group climate positively influence sex offender treatment engagement and pre- to post-treatment changes (Kozar & Day, 2012). We believe a number of these characteristics are particularly important to modifying sexual interests. It is our experience that therapists who approach sexual deviance discussions in a manner perceived as confrontational, judgmental, or rigid have fewer effective outcomes. In these instances, clients typically respond by withholding information relating to sexual deviance, fabricating answers to appease the therapist, or are even openly hostile. Conversely, therapists who are confident in discussing sexual issues, demonstrate genuineness, empathy, directed discussions, and who explore issues through open ended questions generally experience greater engagement and compliance with the behavioral procedures (see also McGrath, 2001).

Conclusions

Unfortunately, there remain many unanswered questions regarding the clinical utility of behavioral control procedures with individuals who have engaged in sexual offending. Well controlled studies are needed to inform and implement better evidence-based practices. In particular, more research is required to determine which procedures are effective in increasing healthy sexual interests and decreasing arousal to deviant fantasies or behaviors, which clients are more likely to benefit from behavioral control procedures, and what dosage or frequency of intervention is best. Even more importantly, there is currently no information that indicates whether any demonstrated improvements in arousal last, whether they are generalizable outside the treatment context, or whether such changes are related to reductions in recidivism.

Sexual interests remain an important treatment target in sex offender treatment programs. Deviant sexual interests and sexual self-regulation (i.e., sexual preoccupation, sex as coping) are empirically supported dynamic risk factors, which should form the basis of intervention strategies. As such, based on the limited evidence available, we suggest that practitioners consider incorporating a combination of masturbatory procedures into treatment for individuals who demonstrate deviant sexual interests during phallometric testing, who self-report deviant sexual interests or whose behavior suggests difficulty controlling their sexual arousal. Treatment strategies should target both increasing sexual arousal (e.g., directed masturbation) and decreasing deviant sexual arousal (e.g., masturbatory or verbal satiation). Targeting sexual interests should be delayed in the treatment process until therapeutic rapport has been firmly established and should be presented in a supportive, non-judgmental, and sex positive manner. Other professionals should be included as needed in order to address any barriers to healthy sexuality (e.g., religious or spiritual guidance). Dosage considerations should be based on the level and entrenchment of deviant sexual interests and follow-up assessments should be incorporated to gauge persistence of any changes and generalization to non-treatment contexts. It is imperative that additional research is done to assess the impact of behavioral control procedures and improve precision in sex offender treatment.

References

Abel, G. G., & Rouleau, J. L. (1990). The nature and extent of sexual assault. In W. L. Marshall, D. R. Laws, & H. E. Barbaree (Eds.), *Handbook of sexual assault* (pp. 9–21). Springer.

Alford, G. S., Morin, C., Atkins, M., & Schoen, L. (1987). Masturbatory extinction of deviant sexual arousal: A case study. *Behavior Therapy, 18*(3), 265–271. https://doi.org/10.1016/S0005-7894(87)80020-5

Ball, C. J., & Seghorn, T. K. (1999). Diagnosis and treatment of exhibitionism and other sexual compulsive disorders. In B. K. Schwartz (Ed.), *The sex offender: Theoretical advances, treating special populations and legal developments* (Vol. 3, pp. 1–28.16). Kingston, NJ: Civic Research Institute.

Campbell-Fuller, N., & Craig, L. A. (2009). The use of olfactory aversion and directed masturbation in modifying deviant sexual interest: A case study. *Journal of Sexual Aggression, 15*(2), 179–191. https://doi.org/10.1080/13552600902759556

Cautela, J. R. (1967). Covert sensitization. *Psychological Record, 20*, 459–468. https://doi.org/10.1016/B978-0-08-023346-8.50007-2

Cautela, J. R., & Wisocki, L. A. (1971). Covert sensitization for the treatment of the sexual deviations. *The Psychological Record, 21*, 37–48. https://doi.org/10.1016/B978-0-08-020373-7.50029-2

Davison, G. C. (1968). Elimination of a sadistic fantasy by a client-controlled counterconditioning technique: A case study. *Journal of Abnormal Psychology, 73*(1), 84–90. https://doi.org/10.1016/B978-0-08-020374-4.50066-9

de Almeida Neto, A. C., Eyland, S., Ware, J., Galouzis, J., & Kevin, M. (2013). Brief interventions: Solving the "internet sex offender paradox". *Psychiatry, Psychology, and Law, 20*, 182–188.

Earls, C. M., & Castonguay, L. G. (1989). The evaluation of olfactory aversion for a bisexual pedophile with a single-case multiple baseline design. *Behavior Therapy, 20*(1), 137–146. https://doi.org/10.1016/S0005-7894(89)80125-X

Fernandez, Y. M., Shingler, J., & Marshall, W. L. (2006). Putting "behavior" back into the cognitive-behavioral treatment of sexual offenders. In W. L. Marshall, Y. M. Fernandez, L. E. Marshall, & G. A. Serran (Eds.), *Sexual offender treatment: Controversial issues* (pp. 211–224). Wiley.

Gray, S. R. (1995). A comparison of verbal satiation and minimal arousal conditioning to reduce deviant arousal in the laboratory. *Sexual Abuse: A Journal of Research and Treatment, 7*, 143–153.

Hanson, R. K., & Morton-Bourgon, K. E. (2005). The characteristics of persistent sexual offenders: A meta-analysis of recidivism studies. *Journal of Consulting and Clinical Psychology, 73,* 1154–1163.

Helmus, L., Thornton, D., Hanson, R. K., & Babchishin, K. M. (2012). Improving the predictive accuracy of Static-99 and Static-2002 with older sex offenders: Revised age weights. *Sexual Abuse: A Journal of Research and Treatment, 24,* 64–101. https://doi.org/10.1177/1079063211409951

Hunter, J. A., Jr, & Goodwin, D. W. (1992). The clinical utility of satiation therapy with juvenile sexual offenders: Variations and efficacy. *Annals of Sex Research, 5,* 71–80.

Hunter, J. A., Jr, & Santos, D. R. (1990). The use of specialized cognitive-behavioral therapies in the treatment of adolescent sexual offenders. *International Journal of Offender Therapy and Comparative Criminology, 34*(3), 239–247. https://doi.org/10.1177/0306624X9003400307

Jackson, B. T. (1969). A case of voyeurism treated by counterconditioning. *Behaviour Research and Therapy, 7*(1), 133–134. https://doi.org/10.1016/B978-0-08-020374-4.50068-2

Jensen, S. H., & Laws, R. (1994). *Minimal arousal conditioning.* Unpublished manuscript.

Johnston, P., Hudson, S. M., & Marshall, W. L. (1992). The effects of masturbatory reconditioning within non-familial child molesters. *Behaviour Research and Therapy, 30*(5), 559–561.https://doi.org/10.1016/0005-7967(92)90043-G

Kaplan, H. S. (1979). *Disorders of sexual desire.* Brunner Mazel.

Kozar, C. J., & Day, A. (2012). The therapeutic alliance in offending behavior programs: A necessary and sufficient condition for change? *Aggression and Violent Behavior, 17*(5), 482–487. https://doi.org/10.1016/j.avb.2012.07.004

Kremsdorf, R. B., Holmen, M. L., & Laws, D. R. (1980). Orgasmic reconditioning without deviant imagery: A case report with a pedophile. *Behaviour Research and Therapy, 18*(3), 203–207. https://doi.org/10.1016/0005-7967(80)90037-6

Lande, S. D. (1980). A combination of orgasmic reconditioning and covert sensitization in the treatment of a fire fetish. *Journal of Behavior Therapy and Experimental Psychiatry, 11*(4), 291–296. https://doi.org/10.1016/0005-7916(80)90075-0

Laws, D. R. (1995). Verbal satiation: Notes on procedure, with speculations on its mechanism of effect. *Sexual Abuse: A Journal of Research and Treatment, 7,* 155–166.

Laws, D. R. (2001). Olfactory aversion: Notes on procedure, with speculations on its mechanism of effect. *Sexual Abuse: A Journal of Research and Treatment, 13*(4), 275–287. https://doi.org/10.1177/107906320101300405

Laws, D. R., & Marshall, W. L. (1990). A conditioning theory of the etiology and maintenance of deviant sexual preferences and behavior. In W. L. Marshall, D. R. Laws, & H. E. Barbaree (Eds.), *Handbook of sexual assault: Issues, theories, and treatment of the offender* (pp. 209–229). Plenum Press.

Laws, D. R., & Marshall, W. L. (1991). Masturbatory reconditioning with sexual deviates: An evaluative review. *Advances in Behaviour Research and Therapy, 13*(1), 13–25. https://doi.org/10.1016/0146-6402(91)90012-Y

Laws, D. R., Meyer, J., & Holmen, M. L. (1978). Reduction of sadistic sexual arousal by olfactory aversion: A case study. *Behaviour Research and Therapy, 16*(4), 281–285. https://doi.org/10.1016/0005-7967(78)90026-8

Leonard, M., & Donathy, L. L. (2017). Understanding normal sexual functioning to assess sexual deviancy. In D. T. Wilcox, M. L. Donathy, R. Gray, & C. Baim (Eds.), *Working with sex offenders: A guide for practitioners* (pp. 49–58). Routledge.

Lindsay, W. R. (2009). *The treatment of sex offenders with developmental disabilities: A practice workbook.* Wiley-Blackwell.

Maletzky, B. M. (1980). Assisted covert sensitization in the treatment of exhibitionism. In D. J. Cox, & R. J. Daitzman (Eds.), *Exhibitionism: Description, assessment, and treatment* (pp. 187–251). Garland Press.

Maletzky, B. M. (1991). *Treating the sexual offender*. Sage.
Maletzky, B. M. (1997). Exhibitionism: Assessment and treatment. In D. R. Laws, & W. O'Donohue (Eds.), *Sexual deviance: Theory, assessment, and treatment* (pp. 40–74). Guilford.
Maletzky, B. M., & McGovern, K. B. (1991). *Treating the sexual offender*. Sage Publications, Inc.
Marquis, J. (1970). Orgasmic reconditioning: Changing sexual object choice through controlling masturbation fantasies. *Journal of Behavioral Therapy and Experimental Psychiatry, 1*, 263–271. https://doi.org/10.1016/B978-0-08-020373-7.50025-5
Marshall, L. E., & O'Brien, M. D. (2009). Assessment of sexual addiction. In A. R. Beech, L. Craig, & K. D. Browne (Eds.), *Assessment and treatment of sex offenders: A handbook* (pp. 163–177). Wiley.
Marshall, W. L. (1974). A combined treatment approach to the reduction of multiple fetish-related behaviors. *Journal of Consulting and Clinical Psychology, 42*(4), 613–616. https://doi.org/10.1037/h0036727
Marshall, W. L. (1975). Reducing masturbatory guilt. *Journal of Behavior Therapy and Experimental Psychiatry, 6*, 260–261.
Marshall, W. L. (1979). Satiation therapy: A procedure for reducing deviant sexual arousal. *Journal of Applied Behavior Analysis, 12*(3), 377–389. https://doi.org/10.1901/jaba.1979.12-377
Marshall, W. L. (2006). Olfactory aversion and directed masturbation in the modification of deviant preferences: A case study of a child molester. *Clinical Case Studies, 5*(1), 3–14. https://doi.org/10.1177/1534650103259754
Marshall, W. L. (2007). Covert association: A case demonstration with a child molester. *Clinical Case Studies, 6*(3), 218–231. https://doi.org/10.1177/1534650105280329
Marshall, W. L., & Fernandez, Y. M. (2003). *Phallometric testing with sexual offenders: Theory, research, and practice*. Safer Society Press.
Marshall, W. L., Hall, K. S., & Woo, C. (2017). Sexual functioning in the treatment of sex offenders. In W. L. Marshall, & L. E. Marshall (Eds.), *Handbook on the assessment, treatment and theories of sexual offending* (Vol. 3, pp. 1369–1384). Wiley-Blackwell.
Marshall, W. L., & Lippens, K. (1977). The clinical value of boredom: A procedure for reducing inappropriate sexual interests. *Journal of Nervous and Mental Diseases, 165*(4), 283–287. https://doi.org/10.1097/00005053-197710000-00009
Marshall, W. L., Marshall, L. E., & Serran, G. A., & O'Brien. (2011). *Rehabilitating sexual offenders: A strength-based approach*. American Psychological Association.
Marshall, W. L., Marshall, L. E., Serran, G. A., & Fernandez, Y. M. (2006). *Treating sexual offenders: An integrated approach*. Routledge.
Marshall, W. L., O'Brien, M. D., & Marshall, L. E. (2009). Modifying sexual preferences. In A. Beech, L. Craig, & K. Browne (Eds.), *Assessment and treatment of sex offenders: A handbook* (pp. 311–327). John Wiley & Sons.
Masters, W., & Johnson, V. (1966). *Human sexual response*. Little Brown.
McGrath, R. J. (2001). Utilizing behavioral techniques to control sexual arousal. In M. S. Carich, & S. E. Mussack (Eds.), *Handbook for sexual abuser assessment and treatment* (pp. 105–116). Safer Society Press.
McGrath, R. J., Cumming, G., Burchard, B., Zeoli, S., & Ellerby, L. (2010). *Current practices and emerging trends in sexual abuser management: The Safer Society 2009 North American Survey*. Safer Society Press.
McGuire, R. J., Carlisle, J. M., & Young, B. G. (1965). Sexual deviations as a conditioned behaviour: A hypothesis. *Behaviour Research and Therapy, 2*(2–4), 185–190. https://doi.org/10.1016/0005-7967(64)90014-2
Plaud, J. J., Plaud, D. M., Kolstoe, P. D., & Orvedal, L. (2000). Behavioral treatment of sexually offending behavior. *Mental Health Aspects of Developmental Disabilities, 3*(2), 54–61.

Proeve, M., & Howells, K. (2002). Shame and guilt in child sexual offenders. *International Journal of Offender Therapy and Comparative Criminology, 46*(6), 657–667. https://doi.org/10.1177/0306624X02238160

Rea, J. A., Williams, D., Saunders, K. J., Dixon, M., Wright, K., & Spradlin, J. E. (2003). Covert sensitization: A generalization analysis in the laboratory and natural environment through the use of a portable-penile plethysmograph. *The Behavior Analyst Today, 4*(2), 192–201. https://doi.org/10.1037/h0100119

Serber, M. (1970). Shame aversion therapy. *Journal of Behavior Therapy and Experimental Psychiatry, 1*(3), 213–215. https://doi.org/10.1016/0005-7916(70)90005-4

Stava, L., Levin, S. M., & Schwanz, C. (1993). The role of aversion in covert sensitization treatment of pedophilia: A case report. *Journal of Child Sexual Abuse, 2*, 1–14. https://doi.org/10.1300/J070v02n03_01

Thorpe, J. G., Schmidt, E., & Castell, D. (1963). A comparison of positive and negative (aversive) conditioning in the treatment of homosexuality. *Behaviour Research and Therapy, 1*(2–4), 357–362. https://doi.org/10.1016/0005-7967(63)90051-2

Waldram, J. B. (2007). Narrative and the construction of "truth" in a prison-based treatment program for sexual offenders. *Ethnography, 8*(2), 145–169. https://doi.org/10.1177/1466138107078631

Ware, J., & Mann, R. E. (2012). How should "acceptance of responsibility" be addressed in sexual offending treatment programs? *Aggression and Violent Behavior, 17*(4), 279–288. https://doi.org/10.1016/j.avb.2012.02.009

Webster, S. D., Bowers, L. E., Mann, R. E., & Marshall, W. L. (2005). Developing empathy in sexual offenders: The value of offence re-enactments. *Sexual Abuse: A Journal of Research and Treatment, 17*(1), 63–77. https://doi.org/10.1177/107906320501700107

Weinrott, M. R., Riggan, M., & Frothingham, S. (1997). Reducing deviant arousal in juvenile sex offenders using vicarious sensitization. *Journal of Interpersonal Violence, 12*(5), 704–728. https://doi.org/10.1177/088626097012005007

Wickramaserka, I. (1976). Aversive behavior rehearsal for sexual recidivism. *Behavior Therapy, 7*(2), 167–176. https://doi.org/10.1016/S0005-7894(76)80272-9

Author Index

Note: page numbers in *italics* refer to figures; page numbers in **bold** refer to tables.

Sexual Deviance: Understanding and Managing Deviant Sexual Interests and Paraphilic Disorders, First Edition. Edited by Leam A. Craig and Ross M. Bartels.
© 2021 John Wiley & Sons, Ltd. Published 2021 by John Wiley & Sons, Ltd.

C

d

g

i

j

n

O

P

x

y

z

Subject Index

Note: page numbers in *italics* refer to figures; page numbers in **bold** refer to tables.

Sexual Deviance: Understanding and Managing Deviant Sexual Interests and Paraphilic Disorders, First Edition. Edited by Leam A. Craig and Ross M. Bartels.
© 2021 John Wiley & Sons, Ltd. Published 2021 by John Wiley & Sons, Ltd.

i

n

p

t